Friend
and Hap

Friendship and Happiness

And the Connection Between the Two

TIM DELANEY *and* TIM MADIGAN

McFarland & Company, Inc., Publishers
Jefferson, North Carolina

LIBRARY OF CONGRESS CATALOGUING-IN-PUBLICATION DATA

Names: Delaney, Tim, author.
Title: Friendship and happiness : and the connection between the two /
    Tim Delaney and Tim Madigan.
Description: Jefferson, North Carolina : McFarland & Company, Inc.,
    Publishers, 2017. | Includes bibliographical references and index.
Identifiers: LCCN 2017032604 | ISBN 9781476668963 (softcover : acid
    free paper) ∞
Subjects: LCSH: Happiness. | Friendship. | Aristotle.
Classification: LCC BJ1481 .D44 2017 | DDC 177/.62—dc23
LC record available at https://lccn.loc.gov/2017032604

BRITISH LIBRARY CATALOGUING DATA ARE AVAILABLE

ISBN) 978-1-4766-6896-3 (print
ISBN 978-1-4766-2990-2 (ebook)

Front cover images © 2017 iStock

Printed in the United States of America

McFarland & Company, Inc., Publishers
    Box 611, Jefferson, North Carolina 28640
    www.mcfarlandpub.com

Acknowledgments

The authors would like to acknowledge all of our friends, especially our close and best friends, and all those who make us happy!

Tim Delaney thanks one of his former students at SUNY Oswego, Steven Belles, who helped with researching various articles used in this book; he also offers special thanks to Christina.

Tim Madigan thanks Glenn and Mindy Odden, as well as the many students at St. John Fisher College who have taught him at least as much about the meaning of friendship as he has taught them.

Table of Contents

Preface

The original conception of this book was to focus solely on friendship. The idea came to the authors when they realized that their students have found this to be a particularly interesting topic for discussion.

Tim Madigan, a professor of philosophy, often teaches about the three primary types of friendship described by Aristotle in his writings on ethics, and their relevance to the present-day.

Tim Delaney, a professor of sociology, has long taught about the role of socialization and friendship. He has also focused on the wide variety of forms of friendship *since* the time of the Ancient Greeks, especially the relatively recent emergence of electronic and virtual variations of friendships.

During the early stages of the development of this book, however, it became abundantly clear that the topic of happiness should also be addressed, as the two concepts of *friendship* and *happiness* are clearly linked together. Since the topics of friendship and happiness are worthy subjects in their own right, we will examine them in two separate sections, but throughout this book we will focus on the connection between friendship and happiness.

We will also include survey data collected on college students and their views of friendship and happiness. In addition, whether the reader is a college student or not, there are plenty of insightful revelations about friendship and happiness described throughout this book that should be of interest.

It is also worth noting that while the concept and categorization of friendship types has expanded a great deal since the time of Aristotle's writings, it is clear that there is still great relevance to Aristotle's conception of friendship in the modern world.

Our discussion on happiness includes a chapter on unhappiness. Inspired in part by philosopher Bertrand Russell's classic 1930 book *The Conquest of Happiness*, we propose that it is unhappiness that must be conquered if one hopes to achieve happiness. We then look at happiness itself from a philosophical and sociological perspective while incorporating ideas from other academic disciplines as well.

In addition, we have included "Popular Culture Scenarios" throughout the book, to help demonstrate how films, television series, music and short stories have all contributed to our understanding of friendship and happiness.

PART I

Friendship

Friendship involves an association of at least two people who share a sense of intimacy, feelings of affection, dispositions, and commonality. A friendship consists of people who refer to themselves as friends and as such are linked, or bonded, by expressions of harmony, accord, understanding and rapport. Friends come in a variety of types and categories but are generally viewed as those who are attached to one another by feelings of affection or personal regard, those who provide assistance and support to one another, are on good terms with one another and who may share certain attributes such as religious and cultural affiliations or those who share a common interest such as music or a favorite sports team.

In this part of the book, we will examine friendships from the time of Aristotle and his discussion of three specific categories of friends (utility, pleasure, and the good) through the wide variety of types and categories of friendships in the contemporary era—an era that has increasingly become dominated by virtual and electronic friendships. We will also explore the manner in which friendships are formed.

1

Aristotle on Friendship

"The desire for friendship comes quickly. Friendship does not."
—Aristotle

While he lived long ago, the ethical writings of the Ancient Greek philosopher Aristotle (384–322 BCE) still have relevance to the present day, particularly when we try to understand the meaning of "friendship." In Book VIII of his work known as the *Nichomachean Ethics,* Aristotle categorizes three different types of friendship: friendships of utility, friendships of pleasure, and friendships of the good. Briefly, friendships of utility are those where people are on cordial terms primarily because each person benefits from the other in some specific way. Business partnerships, relationships among co-workers, and classmate connections are examples. Friendships of pleasure are those where individuals seek out each other's company because of the joy it brings them. Passionate love affairs, people associating with each other due to belonging to the same cultural or social organization, and fishing buddies fall into this category. Most important of all are friendships of the good. These are friendships based upon mutual respect, admiration for each other's virtues, and a strong desire to aid and assist the other person because one recognizes an essential goodness in that person.

The first two types of friendship are relatively fragile. When the purpose for which the relationship is formed somehow changes, then the friendships tend to end. For instance, if the business partnership is dissolved, or one takes another job, or one graduates from school, it is more than likely that no ties will be maintained with the former friend of utility. Likewise, once the love affair cools, or one takes up a new hobby, or gives up fishing, the friends of pleasure will go their own ways.

Friendships of the good (which are usually referred to as *best friends*) are those which are the most important. They tend to be lifelong, are often formed in childhood or adolescence, and will exist so long as the friends continue to remain virtuous in each other's eyes. To have more than a handful

4

of such friends of the good, Aristotle states, is indeed a fortunate thing. Such friendships of the good require time and intimacy—to truly know people's finest qualities you must have deep experiences with them, and close connections. In this first chapter, we will examine in detail Aristotle's three concepts of friendship.

Friends of Utility

Sam and Bill were co-workers in the same company, doing essentially the same tasks. They enjoyed talking to each other during breaks about issues of mutual interest—sports, dating, politics, and other topics, and often engaged in joshing debates on subjects they slightly differed about. More importantly, they shared with each other information about their future aspirations and were often helpful to each other in job-related issues. When one of them fell behind on certain tasks, he could always rely on the other to come to his assistance. Since they lived near each other, they would often give each other rides to work when one of them was having car trouble.

A few months after their first meeting at work Sam and Bill started getting together for dinner once a week on Fridays. They would take turns picking up the check, and mentally kept a scrupulous account to make sure each was ordering roughly the same amount so that neither would ever "get stuck" paying more than his fair share. During these dinners, over a few beers they'd poke fun at their overbearing bosses, gossip about other co-workers with whom they were not on such good terms, and speculate about their futures with the company. Both of them agreed that these dinners were therapeutic, and each of them looked forward to this end-of-the-week get-together. They would sometimes talk about going to a ball game or a movie, too, but never quite got around to doing so, given their busy weekend schedules.

Sam and Bill had both started working at their jobs around the same time, and both advanced together at the same pace, earning the same salary. They were well aware of other co-workers who had advanced more rapidly and/or earned more money than they did, which was a constant source of their off-work discussions. While they were cordial to other co-workers it was clear to everyone at the company that theirs was a special "work buddy" relationship. Although they each liked their jobs, both were quick to agree that should another job open up somewhere else that paid more and/or had more advancement opportunities it would be ridiculous not to take it. Each applied to other companies at a regular basis.

Five years after starting with the company he and Sam worked at, Bill was fortunate to be hired at a better-paying, more prestigious place. Sam wished him well, and they agreed that there was no reason for them not to keep meeting once a week on Fridays as they had done for so many years, especially since Bill's new job was geographically close to his old company, and they could thus meet at their regular restaurant without any problem.

After a few months, though, it became clear that the two men didn't have much to talk about now that Bill was working somewhere else. Sam noticed that Bill was less and less interested in hearing tales of his old co-workers, and Bill noticed that Sam was not interested at all in hearing tales about Bill's new co-workers, none of whom he knew. More to the point, it was clear to Sam that Bill's new job gave him much more financial status—the car he was now driving was considerably more expensive than the one he had owned while still working at Sam's office, and the clothes he now wore were obviously of a higher quality than those that Sam could afford. Sam got the impression that Bill no longer found their favorite restaurant to be to his liking. And topics that once seemed to bring them together—sports, romance, and politics—now became more and more bones of contention. The minor differences they had on these issues started to seem much more serious to them both, and they stopped bringing them up at all. Eventually, all they could talk about were "the old times," but these stories grew less and less fresh with each telling.

The two men then agreed it made more sense, given their busy schedules, to meet once a month rather than every week, and soon that morphed into just every now and then. Whenever they did get together they scrupulously kept to their old pattern of alternating who picked up the check, but given how infrequently they met it became harder to remember whose turn it was. One evening when the waitress brought their bill to them each was sure that *he* had picked up the check previously. There was an awkward pause as the check sat there on the table, untouched. Finally, Bill broke the tension by saying "Why don't we just split it?" Sam agreed, but secretly was upset since he felt it was unjust for him to pay half when he had previously paid the whole bill. Bill too was secretly upset since he thought the same thing. That was the last time the two ever got together for dinner. Every so often after that they would run into each other by chance at the airport, the shopping mall, or the movie theater in town, and would exchange pleasantries, with Bill asking how things were at the old office, and Sam inquiring how Bill was enjoying his job. Bill eventually was transferred to another city, and from that point on the two men ceased all interactions with each other, although at times they'd remember the good old days when they were co-workers and friends and half-heartedly think about renewing their acquaintanceship.

While some might read the above scenario as a tragedy of sorts, the philosopher Aristotle would instead say it was a perfectly natural relationship. It fits quite nicely what he would call a "friendship of utility." Bill and Sam, while co-workers, had been useful to each other, and had formed a relation-ship based upon this mutual satisfaction. They were of help to each other during times of crisis on the job, and even at times off the job (they agreed, for instance, to pick up each other's mail at home when the other was trav-eling). But the main point was, they each kept meticulous note of how much time and money they committed to each other, and expected the same in return. Their friendship was very much based on a sense of equality, but of the crudest sort, a kind of "you scratch my back/I'll scratch yours" reciprocity. After Bill got another job, their relationship became "unbalanced" and the sense of commitment no longer seemed equal. It also became more backwards-oriented than future-oriented, focusing on what had happened in the past rather than what they would do together subsequently, since their goals were no longer essentially equivalent. As they each became more con-scious of such differences as the basis of their relationship changed. Their desire to help the other person had lessened to the point where they no longer had any real ongoing connection.

For Aristotle, this would be an example of a friendship of utility—when the two men ceased to be of use to each other, the friendship came to an end. This is a completely natural situation, in his view, and in fact one that could be expected for most of our friendships. As our hopes and aspirations change, so too quite often do our friendships. Indeed, it would be odd if we somehow retained the same relationships with all people throughout our lives. The vast majority of these are specific to given social situations, such as school, work or recreational places, all of which are likely to change as our life interests evolve.

Sam and Bill had what Aristotle would call "an imperfect" friendship, but it was still a beneficial aspect of their lives. While it lasted, it made their life situations better, and it gave each of them a foundation they could rely upon, knowing that at least one person in their work situation could be relied upon for support. More to the point, as with any sort of friendship, it was a *voluntary* relationship. Each of them chose to give his time, commitment and assistance to the other. They trusted one another, and knew that each had the other's back whenever support was needed. They were useful to each other, and there is nothing wrong with that. Aristotle felt that we all have need of such friendships to help us in our own developments as human beings. As he writes in his famous work the *Nichomachean Ethics*: "No one would choose to live without friends, even if he had all other goods" (Aristotle 1962: 214). But just *why* is this so, and more to the point why are there different types of friendship? These questions are central to Aristotle's overall concep-tion of what constitutes a good life.

It is significant that Aristotle spends so much time examining the nature of friendship, since this is a central aspect of his overall discussion of "happiness," or *eudaimonia*. In this book, we will explore in greater detail the meaning of happiness, especially in the modern world, and see how Aristotle's concept of eudaimonia still has relevance today. But before looking in more detail at why this is so, it will be helpful to briefly talk about Aristotle himself.

Aristotle

Aristotle remains one of the most influential persons who ever lived. In fact, the United Nations Educational, Scientific and Cultural Organization (UNESCO) declared 2016, the 2400th anniversary of his birth in 384 BCE, to be a year to celebrate his memory. On their website, UNESCO (2016) states that "Aristotle was one of the most emblematic and influential philosophers of humanity. He helped shape the intellectual life of Europe and laid the theoretical foundations for the idea of Democracy and the establishment of the Constitutions in Europe and in the United States; he continues to be present in the intellectual evolution of Western civilization, as an essential part of its cultural heritage. He is a figure of unquestionable universal significance with the anniversary of which UNESCO should be associated."

While he lived long ago and in a far different culture than our own, it is no exaggeration to say that Aristotle is still "alive and well" when it comes to his influence, especially in regards to his writings on ethics (of which the discussion of friendship plays a large role). His writings on various topics, such as art, astronomy, biology, logic, physics, and theology are still taught in countless institutions of higher learning, even though much of the information found within has proven to be incorrect or at least contentious. It is not so much the facts presented that remain important, but rather the methods he developed for how to search for knowledge that still are pertinent. Like all great philosophers, Aristotle was a seeker of truth, and remains inspirational as a model for how one attempts to arrive at reliable knowledge.

The contemporary Irish philosopher Fran O'Rourke, author of the 2016 book *Aristotelian Interpretations,* goes so far as to call Aristotle "the greatest thinker of all time." In an interview with *Irish Times* columnist Joe Humphreys, on why UNESCO had declared 2016 "The Year of Aristotle," O'Rourke focuses specifically on Aristotle's conception of what it means to be a human being. "We are not a species of solitary beings. We need each other and cannot live in isolation—not only for the basic needs of survival, but for the fulfillment of our highest capacities such as thought and language" (Humphreys 2016). This is a central aspect to Aristotle's overall discussion of eudaimonia. O'Rourke goes on to say that "According to Aristotle, our social nature finds its highest expression in friendship" (Humphreys 2016). We will shortly look in more detail as to why this is so.

Brief Biography of Aristotle

Born in the city-state of Stagira in the northeast part of Greece in 384 BCE, Aristotle was the son of Nicomachus, a medical doctor who became the court physician to the King of Macedon. At the age of seventeen Aristotle was sent to Athens to study at Plato's Academy, considered to be the first institution of higher learning. Plato was himself the student of Socrates, who is generally considered the greatest philosopher of all time. In 399 BCE Socrates was executed by his fellow Athenians for the crimes of "impiety" and "corrupting the youth" by teaching them to disrespect the law of Athens. Socrates vigorously defended himself, arguing that he had in fact been encouraging *all* people, not just the young, to think critically and to "know themselves" by examining their beliefs and trying to see if these correspond to what is true rather than merely expedient. Plato eventually wrote down his memories of Socrates' teachings in a series of works that came to be called *dialogues* and he founded the Academy as a way of training students in the methods of Socrates, especially Socrates' focus on the importance of the human *psyche* or soul.

The main purpose of the Academy was to train future leaders of the Greek world, and admission was highly selective. It was Plato's belief, inspired by Socrates, that societies needed to be ruled by just individuals, rather than by those who craved power for power's sake. The role of good rulers was to guide their people like good shepherds guard their sheep, and it was important for such rulers to have virtuous advisors as well. Clearly the King of Macedon was expecting great things from Aristotle when he sent him to study at the Academy. So impressed was Plato by the acumen of his student that he asked him to stay on after his graduation to become an instructor at the Academy, where he excelled. This was a high honor indeed, a sign of how much Plato admired him. Aristotle was at the Academy for twenty years as student and instructor, and it was generally assumed by those who knew him that he would inherit it after Plato's death, since one of the most vital issues stressed at the Academy was the importance of justice, especially in regards to power. Those who achieved power should merit it by their abilities, rather than receive it simply because they were related to others by birth. Surely it was a sign of Aristotle's great abilities that Plato had wanted him to remain involved with the institution for so long.

Ironically, when Plato finally died it was discovered that, rather than leave the Academy to his best student and instructor, namely Aristotle, he had instead left it to his own nephew, Speusippus, a clear case of nepotism. While Aristotle admired Plato and always wrote about him in respectful terms, his views regarding Speusippus were quite dissimilar, as he had nowhere near such a high reputation as his uncle. While willing to be second to Plato, Aristotle had no desire to serve under Speusippus. At this point, Aristotle left the Academy and returned to Macedon to become the tutor to King Philip's young son, a boy of thirteen named Alexander. He remained in this position until Alexander no longer had need of a tutor, when he became king at the death of his father. History would, of course, remember him as Alexander the Great.

Shortly thereafter Aristotle returned to the city of Athens, where he had thrived for so long. Being a man in need of a job, Aristotle decided that rather than ask for his old position back at the Academy he would instead start a rival school, which he named "The Lyceum." This relates to another concept very important to the Greeks, namely the *agon* or contest. One comes to know one's own worth through competition with others. Aristotle would now offer competition to the Academy. He ran the Lyceum for twelve years and much of the writings attributed to him which have survived, including the *Nichomachean Ethics,* are thought to be lecture notes written by his students. The students at the Lyceum were called *peripatetics,* meaning those who walk around, perhaps in part to contrast them to the students at the Academy, who merely sat and thought. Aristotle stressed *active* knowledge. He continued to do original work himself in a myriad number of topics, including art, astronomy, biology, chemistry, logic, physics, and religion.

At the same time that he was running his school, Aristotle followed with interest the career of his former pupil Alexander, who was becoming more and more powerful, uniting the independent city-states of Greece under his rule and creating an empire. Alexander took the concept of the *agon* to its highest glory, becoming the most powerful man on earth. But there was another concept important to the Greeks, namely *hubris,* which literally means to go too far or to get out of line, but which is also often interpreted as "playing God." This relates back to the charge filed against Socrates, that of impiety, where it is said that he no longer worshiped the Gods or, even worse, created new Gods of his own imagining. Socrates had denied this, but when Alexander, after conquering the Persian empire, had himself declared a living God, it was hard not to think of this as an example of hubris in the extreme.

Aristotle continued to run the Lyceum until shortly after the death of Alexander in 323 BCE. When news of Alexander's death reached the citizens of Athens they rebelled against those he had put in power over them, and many—rightly or wrongly—blamed Aristotle for this. They felt that he was guilty of corrupting the young people by teaching them to disrespect the laws of Athens, especially its political system of democracy, which Alexander had overthrown. And as mentioned above there was the view that Aristotle had encouraged Alexander's hubris, which led to the impiety of his declaring himself to be a God. These two charges, corrupting the young and impiety, had of course also been levelled against Plato's old teacher Socrates in 399 BCE, and he had been sentenced to death and executed because of this. Aristotle is famously said to have uttered the immortal phrase "I will not allow Athens to sin twice against philosophy," and he fled from Athens before he could be put on trial. Along with his family he moved to the city-state of Chalcis, the birthplace of his mother, and died there in November of 322 BCE at the age of sixty-two.

Nichomachean Ethics

While fascinated by all things, Aristotle had a special regard for trying to understand what philosophers would call "the meaning of life." He meant this quite literally—what does it mean to be a living thing? What differentiates living things, such as flowers, birds, and humans, from nonliving things such as rocks, dirt, and sand? For Aristotle, the key difference was *psyche*, or soul. All living things possess something that nonliving things lack, namely an animating principle, by which he meant something that gives a thing internal motion. (When Aristotle's writings on the soul were translated centuries later into Latin, the word *psyche* was translated into the Latin *anima,* from which the English word "animal" derives.) If a rock moves it is because something else has moved it. Should it suddenly move on its own we would be startled, to say the least. Thus, living things have animation, or motion, while nonliving things do not.

But living things have different *types* of motion. And this relates to their *telos,* or goals. What are they trying to achieve with their movements? Most living things, Aristotle argued, have very simple goals and therefore very simple needs. Their goal is primarily to survive, and to perpetuate their own species. Thus, they need nutrients of some sort, and some sort of reproductive system. Such beings possess what he called a *vegetative* soul. Using a modern day popular culture reference, if such beings had a theme song it would be the Bee Gee's "Staying Alive" since that's mostly what their goal is.

In the hierarchy of living things there is a smaller category which, while also possessing a vegetative soul, has higher goals as well, such as the ability to be perceptive to sensations, to have more advanced types of movement (not merely being rooted to the ground like vegetables, for instance, but able to run, burrow or fly), and more complex lives. In short, they are animated creatures, and thus have a *sensitive* soul. Members of the animal kingdom fall within this category.

But of all living things, there is one which possesses not only a vegetative and sensitive soul, but also an even higher goal. It seeks not only to survive and to experience sensations—it seeks *knowledge*. This creature has a special type of movement unique to it, which other living things lack, namely mental movement. Even when stationary it is still involved in an activity—the activity of thought. This highest of all creatures is, of course, the human being, which Aristotle argued possesses a *rational* soul. That is why he famously defined humans as "rational animals."

This definition is key to all of Aristotle's writings, and is perhaps best expressed in the famous opening lines of his work the *Metaphysics,* where he declares "All humans by nature seek knowledge." But he develops this idea in more detail in his work called the *Nichomachean Ethics,* which adds a further definition: humans are by nature *social* creatures. Unlike many other living things, which seem to live solitary existences without the need of companions, humans literally cannot survive without the constant assistance of other human beings.

This then leads to his extended exploration of the importance of ethics, which essentially means "how one should act." Aristotle's approach to philosophy is known as "Natural Law" or "Virtue Ethics." By "natural law" he means that in order to understand something, including human beings, you have to examine their essential nature. How do they develop properly, what talents do they possess, and what is their ultimate goal? By "virtue" he means what sort of habits will allow one to develop one's talents in the most beneficial ways (the opposite of virtue is "vice," meaning a bad habit which impedes one's proper development.) For instance, given the fact that humans possess the desire for knowledge, it is a virtue to cultivate this desire through education. When one is engaged in the pursuit of knowledge one is acting virtuously. When one seeks to avoid this search, especially if one chooses to be lazy or chooses to cheat in order to get the correct answers without really understanding them, then that would be vicious behavior.

Another key point Aristotle stresses is that not all people have the exact same abilities or talents. So, if the good life involves developing one's talents through the cultivation of good habits, one must first get a sense of what one's talents are. Some people are naturally inclined to athletic prowess; others to musical abilities; others to academic pursuits. What would be right for one might not be for another.

To quote Martin Oswald, who translated the *Nichomachean Ethics* into English: "It is here that we find the most striking difference between Aristotle and his master Plato. For while Plato's work is characterized by a passionate conviction of the unity and interdependence of all branches of human knowledge, Aristotle with his sharp analytic mind is more concerned with finding what differentiates one branch of learning from the other and what is peculiar to each" (Aristotle 1962: xiii).

Nowhere is this more the case than in Aristotle's discussion of the importance of friendship. In his seminal work the *Nichomachean Ethics* (named in honor of his father and his son Nicomachus, both of whom shared this name), he famously delineates his theory of the three types of friendship, which we will be looking at in this chapter. It is important to note that books VIII and IX of the ten book *Nichomachean Ethics* are part of the larger discussion of the nature of *eudaimonia*, a term which is often translated as "happiness" but which literally means "good soul." In this book as well as in other works Aristotle asked the fundamental question: what does it mean to be a human being, and what are the various goals we have that bring out our best?

While usually translated from the ancient Greek as "happiness," a better translation of eudaimonia would be "self-fulfillment through personal excellence." For Aristotle, the good life consisted of developing one's natural abilities through the use of reason. A virtuous life is one where proper habits are formed that allow one to reach one's full potential. Some goals, such as the desire for wealth or the desire for public recognition, can propel us to action, but these are not what Aristotle considered our ultimate goal. Rather, they are a means to an end. The ultimate end or goal (*telos*) is *eudaimonia* or happiness. This is a happiness based upon self-fulfillment. "For the final and perfect good seems to be self-sufficiency," he writes. "However, we define something as self-sufficient not by reference to the 'self' alone. We do not mean a man who lives his life in isolation, but a man who also lives with parents, children, a wife, and friends and fellow citizens generally, since man is by nature a social and political being" (Aristotle 1962: 15).

Human Beings Are Social Creatures

In the larger context of the *Nichomachean Ethics* Aristotle addresses what makes us human. We are, as the famous quote above points out, social beings. We cannot exist independently. Our very development as humans is contingent on the proper—or natural—support given to us by other human beings. Briefly we will look at such natural sources mentioned in this quote (parents, children, wife, fellow citizens) and see how these differ from the role played in our development by friends.

Family

It is obvious that human beings come into the world completely helpless. A newborn baby cannot feed itself, get around from place to place on its own, or comprehend what is happening around it. Clearly, much time and effort needs to be devoted to the proper upbringing of infants if they are to survive at all, let alone thrive. And for Aristotle the proper setting for this is a family structure. Parents are morally responsible for raising those children that they bring into the world, and children are morally responsible to honor their parents. This is why he makes the important observation that your parents, and your siblings as well, cannot be your friends. This is often misinterpreted by those who think that he means you cannot have strong emotional bonds with your family members. In fact, he means just the opposite. Such strong bonds are innate rather than assumed. This is one reason, by the way, why Aristotle differed with his own teacher Plato, who argued in his book the *Republic* that children should be taken away from their parents at birth and all raised in common, to prevent emotional bonds forming between them. If that would happen then favoritism towards family members would not occur, and all people in society would love each other equally—all children would look upon all adults as their parents. Aristotle rightly saw that this was an absurd, and indeed frightening, scenario (and one which George Orwell would return to in his nightmarish dystopian novel *1984* with its chilling refrain that "Big Brother is Watching You"). It is significant that Aristotle, unlike Plato, was a married man with children. And, ironically, for all his concern over destroying favoritism based on family connections, it was Plato who left his Academy not to Aristotle, who clearly merited it, but rather to his own less talented nephew—a blatant case of nepotism. One could define nepotism as an unjust form of familial favoritism, but in Aristotle's terms that doesn't negate familial favoritism itself. Surely, we all have more concern and love for our own children than we do for the children of strangers.

The key point here, as we examine the nature of friendship, is that we do not choose the families that we belong to. We are born into them. And in Aristotle's thinking, there is also an inequality in such a relationship. Our parents are not our friends because they are not our equals. They know all about us from our earliest days, but we do not know much if anything about their lives before our birth. Our existence came about because of them, but theirs did not come about because of us. More to the point, they are role models for us, and we must honor them by always showing proper deference.

As an example of this, one of the authors of this text has a friend who is a noted and respected judge. The judge is a large man, over six feet tall, and a well-known figure in society. He is a man whom others often defer to because of his power and reputation. But the author many times saw the judge with his own mother, who was a tiny woman, less than five feet tall, and with no power or reputation in the broader society. Yet she spoke to her son in terms no one else would dare to, telling him to put his coat on or lower his voice, even when he was well into his 80s (she lived to the age of 104!). The love between the two was obvious to all, and right up until her death he showed her the respect that Aristotle felt a parent is owed by a child. While there was definitely mutual respect, there was not what Aristotle would call "friendship" since for Aristotle friendship is a relationship based upon equality. When the judge and her mother were together it was clear to everyone who was number one in the relationship.

Such inequality is also the case when it comes to siblings and other family members. These people should be, in natural terms, our strongest supporters and the people we rely most upon, but again for Aristotle there is always a hierarchical structure when it comes to our family members which precludes friendship, as well as the fact that these relationships are not chosen but rather imposed upon us. As the old saying goes, "you can pick your friends but not your relatives."

Perhaps most disturbing to modern sensibilities is Aristotle's claim that husbands and wives cannot be friends, either. In part this is due to the fact that marriages in his time—and indeed in many other times and even in many contemporary cultures—were arranged rather than chosen, which in many cases made it more challenging for spouses to be friends. But the main reason is that, to put it bluntly, Aristotle was a sexist. He did not believe that men and women were equals, and he felt that the wife should always defer to her husband. Thus, given the inequities of their relationship, there could not be a friendship relationship between husbands and wives. He writes: "There is a division of labor from the very beginning and different functions for man and wife. Thus, they satisfy each other's needs by contributing each his own to the common store" (Aristotle 1962: 239).

Later in the book we will examine more contemporary views of friendship, which call into question some of these claims regarding the distinctions between family and friends. But for now, we hope that this brief examination will make clear Aristotle's views on the subject, and why he felt that friendship outside of the family is so necessary to our proper development as human beings.

Strangers

If the only people we knew were our family members, then our roles in life would be quite limited, as would our opportunities for development. But remember Aristotle's more complete definition that we are by nature social and political beings. *Polis* is the Greek term for "body of citizens" and relates to the fact that most of us live not just within a family structure but rather within a larger political system. The basic point here is that most of the people in such a system are strangers to each other. If they were all related then it would be clearer what roles they are to play (for instance, when a monarch has children usually the firstborn is deemed to be the next in line to rule), but in most political systems there is more flexibility, and more opportunity for people to develop their talents in different ways. If in fact all people in a given society were friends, Aristotle points out, then there would be no need for laws, since we would naturally work out all of our differences. "When people are friends," he writes, "they have no need of justice, but when they are just, they need friendship in addition" (Aristotle 1962: 215). Some utopian thinkers, such as the followers of the later Greek philosopher Epicurus, took this to mean that we should attempt to always live *only* among friends. But Aristotle is quite clear that this is not possible, for the basic reason that friendship requires commitment of time and a trusting relationship, and there are natural limits to how many such connections we can make.

An interesting example of this is the so-called "familiar strangers" experiment of the psychologist Stanley Milgram (1933–1984). Milgram is best known for his rather infamous "Obedience to Authority" experiments in the early 1960s, in which participants thought they were administering electric shocks to learners who didn't give correct answers to multiple choice questions—the purpose instead was to see how far these participants would go in administering pain (which unbeknownst to them was being simulated by those getting "shocked") merely because they were told to do so by an authority figure, who they supposedly felt was really responsible. These are indeed troubling experiments for a host of ethical reasons (a good depiction of Milgram and the Obedience to Authority experiments can be found in the 2015 film *Experimenter* starring Peter Sarsgaard as Milgram and Winona Ryder as his wife).

But Milgram was a complex figure who came up with several other fascinating "thought experiments" which he then attempted to test. For instance, he and his students at the City University of New York tried to show how close two random people might be by determining the number of connections that they had with each other. This so-called "Small World" experiment was the basis of the famous "Six Degrees of Separation," which claims that, at most, there are six people separating one from another (in popular culture this is best expressed by the "Six Degrees of Kevin Bacon" game, wherein one takes any actor from any time in history and shows how he/she is separated from appearing in a film with Kevin Bacon by, at most, six other actors).

But where Milgram most relates to Aristotle is through his so-called "Familiar Strangers" experiment. Milgram asked his students to perform a very simple experiment, so simple that at first many of them thought he was joking. Go up to someone you've seen many times but have never spoken to (such as someone you see walking the halls of the school all the time, or someone you see waiting every day for the same subway you take) and introduce yourself to that person. Then report your experience. Simple enough. But, as Milgram's biographer Thomas Blass points out, it turned out not to be simple at all—in fact, for many of the students it was emotionally overpowering. For once you've spoken to a such a "familiar stranger" you've formed a connection. They are no longer a stranger to you. You have each acknowledged each other's existence. And the next time you see them you can't just politely ignore them, as you have in the past. You have to continue to make conversation, even if it's just a banal "nice weather we're having" comment. Blass comments that "Milgram felt that the tendency not to interact with familiar strangers was a form of adaptation to the stimulus overload one experienced in the urban environment. These individuals are depersonalized and treated as part of the scenery, rather than as people with whom to engage" (Blass 2004: 180). But, while these people remain strangers for the moment, there is always the chance that that situation can change. What made the experiment so uncomfortable is that it was a forced situation, rather than a chosen one. Milgram himself makes a fascinating comment about the familiar stranger situation in the narration to his film *The City and the Self,* which Blass quotes from in his book: "As the years go by, familiar strangers become harder to talk to. The barrier hardens. And we know—if we were to meet one of these strangers far from the station, say, when we were abroad, we would stop, shake hands, and acknowledge for the first time that we know each other" (Blass 2004: 181). This nicely sums up the fact that most of us, even while being "friendly," are still shielding much about ourselves from others, even such basic information as our names, our family relations, where we work, and where we went to school. By sharing this information with others, we open ourselves up to their doing the same, at which point a relationship begins. That is also why it is easier to share such information, as well as much more personal information such as our political beliefs, our financial situations, and our sexual adventures, with perfect strangers we meet only once on a plane, train or boat. Since we aren't likely to ever see them again, we are more willing to be open, knowing that no relationship is going to form from this. But as Milgram shows in his "Small World" experiment, it pays to be cautious—how can you be sure that stranger you are talking to about how much you hate your boss or how you are cheating on your spouse isn't somehow connected, by just a degree or two of separation, from your boss or spouse?

Friendlessness

As should be clear by now, Aristotle is stressing throughout his *Nichomachean Ethics* that as social beings we need to form bonds with others, but that such bonding has natural limits. We cannot be friends to all people, and should in fact be cautious about who outside of our family structure we choose to interact with.

One possible answer would be, who needs friends at all? Why not try to be completely self-sufficient? As the 1965 Simon and Garfunkel song puts it: "I have no need of friendship/Friendship causes pain/Its laughter and its loving I disdain." The song of course is not condoning this, but rather showing to us a stilted, unhappy life. While the narrator proudly asserts his independence from all social commitments, and boldly compares himself to a rock—something hard and seemingly unchanging—it is good to reflect back on Aristotle's central point about life itself. A rock is a non-living thing, without a soul. Why in the world would a living thing, especially a highly complex social being, want to compare himself with it? Surely Paul Simon, who wrote the song "I Am a Rock," was commenting ironically upon the theologian and poet John Donne's famous 1624 sermon which begins "No man is an island entire of itself; every man is a piece of the continent, a part of the main," and memorably ends with the lines, "And therefore never send to know for whom the bell tolls; it tolls for thee." It is true that friendship may cause pain, but as Aristotle shows, such pain is a part of our development as human beings. Rocks feel no pain, and islands never cry, but they also never experience happiness either.

One of the authors of this book remembers getting a phone call from a colleague he barely knew, telling him that she had just received a grant to go to do research in Africa. He congratulated her, but couldn't help but ask, since they barely knew each other (and were not even friends of utility), why she had called to tell him this news. "Because I don't have anyone else to share it with," she said. This was a heartbreaking admission, since she was essentially saying that she had no friends of any sort. What good are any achievements when you have no one to share your happiness with you?

Philia

This then leads us to the category of social relations that Aristotle calls *philia*, or friends. The best way of defining philia is "those who hold in common what they have." Essentially this is a personal bond you have with another being, which is freely chosen, reciprocated and mutually beneficial. It breaks beyond the barrier of "familiar stranger" and thus involves a type of risk-taking. You cannot be sure, for instance, that your warm feelings for the other are actually reciprocated (see Popular Culture Scenario 1.1 for a humorous example of this from the pen of Woody Allen), and the more connected you become with this person, the more risks there are, since you are making yourself vulnerable by revealing highly private information—often information that you would not wish divulged to others, even one's own family members. One *could* choose therefore to take the "Rock/Island" strategy of the Simon and Garfunkel song, but that would in fact be detrimental, since it would impede rather than advance one's development as a human being.

Popular Culture Scenario 1.1:
Woody Allen's "The Shallowest Man"

One of the most difficult questions that arises in regards to friendship of any sort is, how do I really know what the other person thinks of me? As we have seen in this chapter, when it comes to friends of utility, the basis of the relationship is usually a job or a procedure of some sort that the two people have in common. When that changes, the friendship often ends, which is why Aristotle calls it an imperfect friendship. Such a relationship is shallow at best. But in real life it is not always clear when a friendship does come to an end or just what its exact nature really is.

This dilemma is exemplified nicely in a humorous short story by the comedian Woody Allen, entitled "The Shallowest Man," published originally in 1980 in *The Kenyon Review* and then reprinted later that same year in a book entitled *Side Effects*. It is about a group of friends who get together once a week for a card game. The people involved notice that one of them, Meyer Iskowitz, is starting to look unwell. When he suddenly stops attending the game, they learn that he has been hospitalized for cancer.

Here is an interesting case study of how one can judge the nature of one's friendship—would you choose to visit someone in the hospital? As we will discuss later in this chapter, a friend of the good (or best friend) would not hesitate to be there for a friend in need. But in cases of a friend of utility or a friend of pleasure, this becomes a more difficult question. While it may be useful to visit someone in the hospital in the sense that should you be in a similar situation, you'd want a visitor, too, this is rather problematic from a strictly cost/benefit analysis. Is it really worth my time to go through the hassle of making such a visit? And would I necessarily want someone I don't really know all that well coming to see me when I am vulnerable? In regards to friends of pleasure, surely one of the least pleasurable experiences is to enter a hospital setting when one is perfectly well, and see the suffering inside. These "shallower" types of friends often make, at best, a perfunctory visit or two, and then stop. They've done their duty, as it were.

The card players in Woody Allen's story do visit Meyer Iskowitz every now and then, but not with any frequency, which given the nature of their relationship to him is to be expected. But much to Iskowitz's surprise, and growing joy, one of them, Lenny Mendel, starts to visit him every day. He brings flowers, candy, and books, and even when Meyer, due to the medication he is taking, is unable to communicate he knows that Lenny will be there when he awakes.

The members of the card game are amazed by this deep show of concern, as they never thought the two men had been particularly close. "Word of Mendel's indulgence of Iskowitz got around and at the weekly card game he was much beloved by the players. 'What you're doing is wonderful,' Phil Birnbaum said to Mendel over poker. 'Meyer tells me no one comes as regularly as you do and he says he thinks you even dress up for the occasion'" (Allen 1980). Iskowitz finally dies. "Before expiring he told Mendel once again that he loved him and that Mendel's concern for him in these last months was the most touching and deepest experience he ever had with another human being" (Allen 1980).

A moving story indeed. However, we the readers know something that Iskowitz does not. Mendel hadn't wanted to visit at all, primarily because he is a hypochondriac who was afraid of catching something deadly in the hospital, and only does so initially after being shamed by the other card players, who've all already gone to see Iskowitz. So Mendel checks the visiting hours and sees that they end at 8 p.m. He makes sure to arrive at 7:50 p.m., and is getting ready to dash out when he notices Iskowitz's nurse. She's drop-dead gorgeous. Mendel begins to visit every evening during her shift (and gets upset when every now and then she's not on duty). Whenever he talks to Iskowitz it's to learn more about Nurse Hill. He brings the candy, the flowers and the books to impress *her,* and she is indeed moved by this show of concern that Mendel has for his friend. So much so that she breaks up with her boyfriend, and starts dating Mendel shortly after Iskowitz's death. But learning his true nature, they break up in less than a year.

The card players all agree that Mendel was "the shallowest man" who ever lived. But one of them, Abe Trochman, points out that nonetheless great good came out of Mendel's visits. When another player, Lupowitz, objects that the two weren't really friends at all, and Mendel only went out of self-interest, Trochman replies: "What's the difference? Iskowitz experienced a closeness. He died comforted. That it was motivated by Mendel's lust for the nurse—so?" (Allen 1980).

While the visit of Lenny Mendel to Meyer Iskowitz may indeed have brought about some comfort to the dying man's last days, clearly this is not a case of friendship. One person is using the other as a means to an end. At least in a genuine friendship of utility—the shallowest type of all—both parties are aware of this fact that they are, in a sense, using each other, but with each other's consent. There is no deception involved, something that Lenny Meyer cannot honestly claim.

Alexander Nehamas, Carpenter Professor of Humanities at Princeton University, writes of Aristotle that his "ideas about *philia,* which is universally taken to be equivalent to friendship, are still crucial.... *Philia* was for Aristotle a great and pure good: it is something, he explains, that no one would want to live without, no matter what else one already possesses in this life, and the tradition that follows him, with very few exceptions, has also taken friendship to be one of life's greatest possessions" (Nehamas 2016: 5). Let's look at how, in Aristotle's view, friendships begin and how they develop in three likely paths.

Utility Revisited

Remember once more Aristotle's three types of friendship, utility, pleasure and the good. What do they all have in common? For Aristotle, *philia* involves three basic attributes:

1. Men must feel goodwill (benevolence) for each other
2. Men must be aware of each other's goodwill
3. The cause of their goodwill must be loveable qualities

In other words, we experience something in the other person that resonates with us. They have a certain trait or traits that we find admirable (loveable qualities) and by associating with them we ourselves become more socially connected. By "loveable" Aristotle means traits that we find useful, pleasant or good. It would be best if all three conditions were met, but this happens rarely. For instance, we may find a hammer to be a useful tool to use in nailing a board to a wall, but it isn't necessarily something that gives us pleasure. And the hammer is not able to reciprocate by finding us useful to it. As Aristotle points out, "While there are three causes of affection or friendship, we do not speak of 'friendship' to describe the affection we feel for inanimate objects, since inanimate objects do not reciprocate affection and we do not wish for their good. It would surely be ridiculous to wish for the good of wine: if one wishes it at all, it is that the wine may keep, so that we can have it ourselves" (Aristotle 1962: 217). By the way, this is something to keep in mind in the present-day when more and more of us interact with computer-generated voices. The 2013 film *Her,* for instance, deals with a young man, played by Joaquin Phoenix, who falls in love with a computer operating system. Since the system is voiced by Scarlett Johansson, it's hard to criticize him for this, but presumably that system is not getting anything back in return.

For Aristotle, in any sort of friendship, be it one of utility, pleasure, or the good, we wish the best for the other person on a reciprocal basis, and this is known by him/her. For instance, I may wish another person, say a political figure I support, goodwill in the sense that I hope he/she gets elected to office, but if that person isn't aware of this, then you cannot say there is a friendship involved. If he/she is aware of this, and wishes me well, then at best we would have a friendship of utility. We are useful to each other—the person needs my vote, and I desire that person's wellbeing as a representative of my political views. But should I move from that politician's district, or should my political views change, then the basis of our connection has also changed. We are no longer useful allies. There is no continual and reciprocal goodwill. Such friends are not loved for their own sake, but only for the benefits that accrue from them. Or, as Aristotle puts it, "usefulness is not something permanent, but differs at different times" (Aristotle 1962: 219).

Friendships of utility, therefore, are similar to trading relationships. We are both aware at all times of what we are getting out of it, and as long as there seems to be a balance of trade, all is well. It is like frequenting a restaurant and being friendly with the waiter. If the food and service are to our liking, then there is a good ongoing relationship. But if another restaurant opens with lower prices but just as tasty food and just as acceptable service, we will likely stop going to the original restaurant and our friendly relationship with the waiter will end as well.

In chapters 2–4 we will examine modern examples of changing social relationships, in cases where, for example, friends from high school or college who once shared activities, interactions, sentiment and norms come to drop such friendships when life circumstances (such as finding a job or getting married and raising a family) change. As in the opening case study of Sam and Bill, when they were working together as office mates they shared common interests, and were very useful to each other. But when their life situation changed, the basis of their friendship did as well. They were no longer useful to each other and the friendship came to an end at that point.

An Imperfect Form of Friendship

Because of the fragile nature of such relationships, Aristotle calls friends of utility "imperfect." They are vulnerable to changing life situations, and are relatively shallow in nature. They are often based upon specific social needs, and are easily dissolved. The pain of ending such relationships is usually not very great, and soon forgotten. For those of us of a certain age, it can be quite difficult to even remember the names of former friends of utility we went to school with or worked with decades earlier. And it can be shocking to meet them years later, when their physical conditions have often altered considerably. One of the authors of this book recently attended the funeral of a person he had worked for twenty years early. Several people came up to greet him by name, and he was flustered to realize, having not seen them for so long, that he had no memory at all of who they were, let alone their names.

Aristotle comes close at times to saying that friends of utility are not a real type of friendship at all, but it is better to use his terminology and say that they are "imperfect," given their ephemeral nature. One thing that immediately differentiates such friendships from the other two types is the fact that there is a very limited pleasure involved in seeing the other person. That is to say, with friends of utility we are always focused upon what it is that unites us—our taking a class together, our working together, our being engaged in a common project—rather than our desire to be with that person for his/her own sake. This, by the way, is why office Christmas/holiday parties are often so awkward. A party is usually something that you wish to attend, but when it comes to office parties there is often a requirement (stated or unstated) that one must attend. And mingling with people—even office friends of utility—you don't normally associate with outside of a given context can be off-putting. One can quickly run out of conversation points and the danger of drinking heavily because of this can cause unpleasant repercussions.

In the next section of this chapter we will examine a higher level, but still imperfect, form of friendship, namely friends of pleasure. But perhaps the most important point to make here in regards to friends of utility is that the time we spend with them and the emotional commitment we make towards them is usually quite limited.

Friends of Pleasure

Emily and Jane attended the same high school. At first, they barely acknowledged each other's existence as they passed one another in the hall. But when they became teammates in lacrosse they started to appreciate each other's athletic abilities. They relied upon each other and, like friends of utility, helped each other in playing the game. Also like friends of utility they started taking the same classes and studied for exams together. They knew that if one missed a class she could always get notes from the other.

But as they continued to play on the same team and take the same classes it became clear to Emily and Jane that they genuinely *liked* being together. They appreciated each other's company. Emily was more outgoing, Jane was more self-contained, but in many ways they complemented each other. When Emily broke her leg and had to drop off the lacrosse team their friendship still continued. And when they graduated from high school and each went to a different college in their home town they still stayed close, and continued to study together. More to the point, they freely chose to pal around, going to movies, the beach, even traveling together on cross-country trips, and eventually went out on double-dates. They remained friends for their entire lives, even after moving to different cities, and whenever one called—or eventually Skyped—the other, it brought a smile to each of their faces just to know they'd once again be in contact.

The friendship of Emily and Jane was different in nature than that of Sam and Bill described earlier. Whereas Sam and Bill's friendship ended when their job situations changed, Emily and Jane continued long after what initially drew them together—their mutual participation in a sporting activity—came to an end. Why was this the case? Because they had what Aristotle would call a friendship of pleasure. Like Sam and Bill's original friendship it involved reciprocity, in the sense that each got roughly the same thing back from the other. But in Emily and Jane's case, what they were getting back was not something as crude as a ride to work, a meal at a restaurant, or help in studying for an exam. What they got back was the pleasure of each other's existence.

Aristotle on Friends of Pleasure

Strictly speaking, the above scenario doesn't really fit Aristotle's concept of a friendship of pleasure, because it involves two women rather than two men. As mentioned earlier, Aristotle's writings on friendship were geared specifically towards men, primarily because he thought only men were truly capable of experiencing reciprocal relationships. As Alexander Nehamas points out, "Aristotle thought that in a relationship between a man and a woman, the woman is necessarily inferior to the man (*Nichomachean Ethics*, VIII, 7, 1158b11–14), and he doesn't discuss friendship between women at all" (Nehamas 2016: 231). Nonetheless, there are still some pertinent questions about friendship raised by Aristotle which bear exploration, such as: *Is* there such a thing as a friendship of pleasure, and if so how does it differ from a mere friendship of utility?

Surely the key point here is the importance of the emotions. Emily and Jane have an emotional commitment to each other, much more so than Sam and Bill had. When Sam and Bill began to drift apart and then ceased to connect at all it really didn't bother either of them to any great extent. Truth to tell, they didn't actually like each other all that much as persons. It was what each got from the other—support at work, a ride, a meal, a chance to gossip about common acquaintances, etc.—that connected them, and they were always conscious of situations where one seemed to be getting a bit more than the other. Once it no longer seemed possible, because of their growing economic disparity, for Sam and Bill to reciprocate on the same level they ceased to be friends.

Emily and Jane, on the other hand, even after their life situations began to dramatically change (Emily married, became a housewife and had a large family; Jane remained single, had many love relationships and a vibrant career) continued to stay in touch because each enjoyed the other's personality. In many ways, it was the differences between them that in fact kept them united. It was their *affection* for each other that continued to be reciprocated. The goodwill that that bore for one another was of a higher level than that of Sam and Bill. As Aristotle puts it, "Now, when the motive of the affection is usefulness, the partners do not feel affection for one another *per se* but in terms of the good accruing to each from the other" (Aristotle 1962: 218). That would seem to typify the relationship of Sam and Bill—it was one purely of utility.

However, Aristotle would likely say that Emily and Jane are also not truly interested in one another *per se* (meaning "as is"), but rather because of the pleasure each one experiences in the other's company. "The same is also true of those whose friendship is based on pleasure," he writes. "We love witty people not for what they are, but for the pleasure they give us" (Aristotle 1962: 218). In other words, should Emily and Jane no longer continue to amuse or please each other, their friendship too would begin to fray, and eventually come to an end. Emily, for instance, might become depressed by what she perceives as the hollowness of her existence. When Jane calls her up, instead of getting the cheerful person she has been friendly with, she may be disconcerted by the sadness she experiences in Emily's voice. Her calls may start to be less frequent, and as was the case with Sam and Bill, the friendship itself may end when Jane no longer feels that she is receiving back from Emily what she is providing.

This is why Aristotle says that friendships of pleasure, while of a higher nature than friendships of utility, are nonetheless still "imperfect." They are vulnerable for a similar reason—the reciprocal condition may cease to be met.

In Aristotle's words: "Friendships are most durable when each one receives what he gives to the other, for example, pleasure, and not only that: he must also receive it from the same source, as happens, for example, in friendships between witty people" (Aristotle 1962: 221). And here he makes another interesting observation, namely that friendships of pleasure are more likely to occur among young people rather than older people, for the simple reason that the young are more likely to be guided by their emotions. Young people, he felt, enter into such relationships because they are more willing to try new experiences and meet new people. Friendships of pleasure, thus, are less calculated than friendships of utility. In the latter, it is quite clear to each what exactly they are getting out of the friendship, and as long as that experience continues—such as sharing a ride, helping someone at work, or relying on each other as teammates—then the friendship will continue. Pleasure per se is not the motivating factor. But obviously with friendships of pleasure that *is* the motivating factor. Thus, when one or both no longer experiences that sense of joy, then the basis for the friendship ceases. "That is why," he writes of young people, "they form a friendship and give it up again so quickly that the change often takes place within the same day. But they do wish to be together all day and to live together, because it is in this way that they get what they want out of their friendship" (Aristotle 1962: 219).

One senses here the notion of *intensity*. The very thing that draws the friends together, namely the desire to be together because of the pleasure they take in each other's company, can also be the thing that eventually draws them apart. In some cases, this can be because of mistaken identity—each person may identify with a factor that they think the other one has, such as wittiness, that turns out to be incorrect (they may not be witty but rather just boorish, for example). In other cases, it can be because that thing that drew them together, such as wittiness, may no longer bring pleasure. After a while, for instance, one may tire of being around someone who jokes around all the time.

Imagine friendships of pleasure formed early in life when one is relatively carefree. The experiences mutually engaged in, such as drinking to excess, racing fast cars, or playing vigorous sporting activities, may all be great fun. But as one's life situations change these experiences may no longer draw people together. Once you start working full time, raising a family and/or taking on household responsibilities, these activities may cease to be feasible. The hangover one experiences after a night of carousing, the fear of getting a speeding ticket for driving too fast, or the likelihood of getting a serious injury playing a pickup football game, may all preclude one from engaging in such shared activities. When that becomes the case, these friendships of pleasure are likely to end.

Friendship of Bad People

Let us return to Aristotle's "Virtue Theory," briefly examined earlier in this chapter. It is important to note that Aristotle's discussion of friendship is not simply about why such relationships are important. It is also about the larger question of how one develops one's character in the best way possible. At this point in Chapter VIII of his *Nichomachean Ethics* Aristotle makes a further distinction about the nature of the different types of friendships. Vicious people (meaning those who deliberately engage in bad activities or vices) as well as virtuous people (meaning those who purposefully engage in good habits) can experience friendships of utility and pleasure. "To be friends with one another on the basis of pleasure and usefulness," he writes, "is, accordingly, also possible for bad people, just as it is for good men with bad, and for one who is neither good nor bad with any kind of person at all" (Aristotle 1962: 222).

Think for a moment about people who you enjoy being around, but whose character you find somehow less than stellar. The antics of such people may bring you pleasure, much like celebrities who "you love to hate" often make you smile when you read about their outrageous behavior. But there is an inequality at the basis of such a relationship. Unless one wishes to somehow emulate these bad habits, and thereby lower one's own character, then one is encouraging behavior in the other which one recognizes to be morally unacceptable. As we will explore in more detail later in this chapter, Aristotle argues that friends of the good, the highest type of friendship, would discourage such behavior in each other. In friendships of the good, friends have an obligation to always try to achieve a higher sort of connection with each other than friends of pleasure achieve. The basis of the latter is the emotions; the basis of the former is reason.

The Tripartite Soul

To understand what Aristotle is getting at here, it will be helpful to return to his model of the human soul. Aristotle was highly influenced by Plato (who in turn had been influenced by Socrates) in focusing upon the importance of the *psyche,* or soul. Remember his view that all living things contain a vegetative soul, that aspect of us that desires to live. It is the most selfish part of us, since its primary concern is "how does this benefit me?" The sensitive part of the soul belongs to those creatures—namely animals—that live within societies, and need to cooperate with others in order to survive. This is the basis for emotions. Plants, for instance, have no need of emotions. They get by just fine by absorbing sunlight, spreading their roots in the ground, and releasing seeds, without any concern for other members of their species. But dogs and cats and elephants have emotional connections with members of their groups. They protect their offspring, they frolic and play, and they even seem to mourn those of their group who have died. Finally, there is the highest form of soul, the rational soul, which only humans possess. It is this part of us which allows us to contemplate reality, including such questions as "what is friendship"?

One can say that for Aristotle friendships of utility are the lowest type, and correspond to the vegetative part of our soul. Their quid pro quo nature is ultimately selfish, in that the main question always being asked is "what's in it for me?" Friendships of pleasure correspond more with the emotional part of our soul. They give us pleasant feelings akin to that provided by being a member of a family. Such deep feelings strengthen the bonds that unite us, which is why when a friendship of pleasure ends it tends to be more painful than when a friendship of utility ends.

Nonetheless, for Aristotle—and indeed for most philosophers—the emotions are a shaky foundation on which to base one's actions. Their very instability makes them suspect when it comes to forming bonds with others. Indeed, it is good, he felt, that friendships of pleasure are more related to the young than to the old, since younger people are better able to break away from such feelings. As we become more responsible agents as we mature, we should become less motivated by our emotions and more reliant upon our reasoning facilities. That, by the way, is also why Aristotle felt that arranged marriages make more sense than romantic engagements. When the romance fades, as it usually does, then the married relationship is likely to become unpleasant. If one marries because the partner is complementary in many ways, then—as the Tina Turner song would put it—what's love got to do with it?

Friendship and Hedonism

While Aristotle doesn't allude to this, one can make a clear connection between "friends of pleasure" and what today are called "friends with benefits." (Note: "friends with benefits" will be discussed in more detail in Chapter 2.) Maura Kelly, in *Marie Claire* magazine asks: "Would 'friendships with benefits' fall into this category [friendships of pleasure]—because you're both enjoying the sexual pleasure? Or into the first category [friendships of utility] because you're using each other for sex? Good question. But I think casual sex is a bit closer to #2, because the Big A. [Aristotle] says friendships of pleasure come about because we do like some—or many—aspects of the friend. We might like his wit, her compassion or his flirty manner, for instance. Friendships of utility, on the other hand, exist mainly because the person can help us out in some way" (Kelly 2010).

The English philosopher Mark Vernon, in his 2010 book *The Meaning of Friendship,* takes this exploration a bit further: "There's a place for 'friendly lovers' too' in Aristotle" he writes. "They belong in his second category of friendship, the kind that form because of some mutual shared pleasure, in this case that being sex. A sexual friendship will thrive insofar as the pleasure it brings to both parties appeals and remains vigorous. However, if the erotic attraction dips or falls away, then the friendship is at risk: it hasn't got much more else to go on" (Vernon 2010: 61).

While one can certainly draw such an implication, it's important to note that Aristotle himself would be skeptical about this. For him, the sex drive should never be an end in itself, but rather should be the means by which new life enters the world. The sex drive would therefore relate to both the vegetative and sensitive parts of our souls, in that it perpetuates life and gives pleasure, but not to the rational part of the soul, which understands that making pleasure one's aim is to lower one's status as human. *Hedonism,* or the pursuit of pleasure, may be acceptable for those who follow a different philosophical perspective, but it would not be the case for Aristotle. It should be noted that this is one of the reasons why the Catholic Church, influenced by the Natural Law tradition through Aristotle's Christian interpreter St. Thomas Aquinas, is still to this day officially opposed to any use of artificial birth control devices, since preventing the possibility of reproduction is deemed by the Church to be unnatural, and therefore sinful. As mentioned earlier, Aristotle would likely say that those who are friends because of the sexual pleasure it gives them are not truly moral beings, and have perverted or unnatural natures. The Catholic writer Conor Gallagher nicely captures Aristotle's critique here when he writes that "Pleasure is perhaps the weakest of all glues that hold people together. It came as no surprise to Aristotle, nor should it to you, that fornication leads to loneliness and misery. In a very real sense, fornication and other sexual vices are contrary to our nature precisely because they prevent people from developing true friendships" (Gallagher 2012: 81–82). In Chapter 2 we will return to this issue by looking at contemporary views on "friends with benefits" and how this often differs from Aristotle's strictures.

Fragility of Friends of Pleasure

As with friendships of utility, friendships of pleasure are fragile and easily shattered. Because emotion is their basis, if they do come to an end it is likely that there will be pain involved, but it is usually fleeting. This type of friendship is more intimate than that of a friendship of utility, and the friends expose much more of themselves to each other. But ultimately, in Aristotle's view, the relationship remains on a rather superficial level and the friends do not truly enter into one another's deepest thoughts and aspirations. Thus, this too is an imperfect type of friendship. In the next section of this chapter we will look in detail at what he considers to be the perfect form—namely friendships of the good.

Popular Culture Scenario 1.2:
Seinfeld: Keith Hernandez's Furniture

In later chapters, we will be exploring the nature of friendship in the modern age, especially as expressed through popular culture. And no television show has better dealt with friendship in all its aspects than *Seinfeld.* Not only does it address the ongoing relationships between four harried urbanites in 1990s New York, it also has a myriad of other characters who come into the four protagonists' lives in varied and hilarious ways.

One of the most memorable of these was the two-part episode called "The Boy Friend." In it, Jerry gets to meet his idol, New York Mets baseball player Keith Hernandez (who good-naturedly plays himself). Jerry is delighted when Keith wants to form a friendship. For Jerry, it is very much a friendship of pleasure, since just being around his idol gives him joy.

However, Jerry's neighbor and friend Kramer is *not* at all happy about this state of affairs, since he is convinced that Hernandez spit on him and on Jerry's nemesis, Newman, after a Mets' game at Shea Stadium. To further complicate things (as is usual in a *Seinfeld* episode), Hernandez is attracted to Jerry's friend—and former lover—Elaine, and asks her out. Jerry becomes jealous, and begins to wonder about the nature of his relationship with his newfound friend. Things become even *more* complicated, however, when, while Elaine is visiting him in his apartment, Jerry receives a phone call from Hernandez.

ELAINE: Who was that?
JERRY: That was Keith.
ELAINE: What's going on?
JERRY: He wants me to help him move.
ELAINE: Help him move? Move what?
JERRY: You know, *furniture.*
ELAINE: So, what did you say?
JERRY: I said yes, but I don't feel right about it. I mean I hardly know the guy. That's a big step in a relationship. The biggest. That's like going all the way.
ELAINE: And you feel you're not really ready for ...
JERRY: Well we went out *one* time. Don't you think that's coming on a little too strong? [*Seinfeld* 1992].

While a very funny scene, it also expresses a genuine dilemma in any friendship relationship. The reciprocal nature of the friendship is now in question. While the basis of the friendship for Jerry was the pleasure he experienced in being in his idol's company (and the assumption that Hernandez must equally feel such pleasure in knowing Jerry), now he is beginning to feel like he is being taken advantage of. Perhaps, for Hernandez, Jerry is at best a friend of utility, one he can rely upon to do a task that no one eagerly wants to perform, moving heavy furniture. And no doubt Jerry is wondering whether or not Keith would be willing to do the same thing for him. Suddenly the pleasure aspect of the friendship is being called into question.

Being asked to help someone move heavy furniture can be a deal breaker for any friendship. One of the authors of this book well remembers getting a call from a friend who said, "I wanted to warn you not to answer your phone." It turned out a mutual friend had just called to let him know that that friend's mother had been sent to an assisted living facility, and her apartment needed to be vacated by the end of the month, which was the very next day. And that happened to be December 31st, New Year's Eve! He had rented a moving van and was calling on friends to help him. His mother, by the way, in addition to having many heavy pieces of furniture, was also a collector of books, record albums, and other items of great weight. All of these had to be put on a truck, and then unloaded into a storage unit.

But since this was a friend of the good, the author took the call—knowing full well what was going to be asked of him—and agreed to be there the next morning. As the old saying goes, "a friend in need is a friend indeed." Still, it was *not* a pleasant experience. The motivating factor here was knowing that, should the situation have been reversed, the caller—who had in fact many times previously demonstrated his goodwill and reliability—would have not hesitated to do the same.

For Jerry, though, this request from Hernandez is asking too much of him. As is his wont, Kramer comes barging in to the apartment at that very moment and asks why Jerry seems so glum.

> [Kramer enters]
> KRAMER: What's going on?
> JERRY: Keith Hernandez just asked me to help him move.
> KRAMER: *What?* Well, you hardly know the guy…. What a nerve. You
>   see, wasn't I right about this guy? Didn't I tell you? Now, you're not
>   going to do it, are you?
> JERRY: … I said yes.
> KRAMER: YOU SAID YES!? Don't you have any pride or self-respect? I
>   mean, how can you prostitute yourself like this? I mean what are
>   you going to do? You're going to start driving him to the airport?
> JERRY: I'm NOT DRIVING HIM TO THE AIRPORT! …
> KRAMER: Yeah, yeah.
> JERRY: Hey Kramer do me a favor.
> KRAMER: What?
> JERRY: Don't mention it to anybody.
> KRAMER: I wish you never mentioned it to ME. [exits] [*Seinfeld* 1992].

This episode of *Seinfeld* brilliantly captures what for New Yorkers would actually be asking something even worse than helping someone to move heavy furniture—giving them a ride to the airport! At this point, Jerry realizes his friendship with Hernandez is a sham, and breaks it off. Later in the episode, Hernandez, in a brilliant parody of Oliver Stone's film *JFK*—which starred Wayne Knight, the actor who plays Newman— proves to Kramer and Newman that he was in fact *not* the one who spit on them. They are so apologetic over their error that *they* then freely offer to help him move his furniture.

Friends of the Good

One of the most famous stories relating to what Aristotle would call a friendship of the good goes back to Ancient Greek times, and it is one he likely would have been familiar with. It is the story of Damon and Pythias, two men who have come to exemplify the importance of "true friendship."

In this tale, Damon and Pythias are followers of the mathematician and mystic Pythagoras (one of Aristotle's predecessors who is credited with coining the word "philosophy," which means "love of wisdom"). They live in Sicily in the town of Syracuse, which was dominated at the time by a tyrant named

Dionysius I. Dionysius was noted for his cruelty, violence and vindictiveness. (Interestingly enough, one of the people who tried to encourage Dionysius to temper his tyranny was Aristotle's old teacher Plato—unsuccessfully, we should add).

Pythias, appalled by the injustice he and others are experiencing, plots the king's overthrow, but is discovered and sentenced to death. He asks the king if he can return to his mother's home to settled his affairs there and say goodbye to his family. After doing so he promises to return and be executed. Dionysius laughs at this ridiculous request, sure that Pythias would never come back. However, at this point Pythias' good friend Damon offers to be held captive in Pythias' place until he returns. Dionysius, who suspects that Damon too has been plotting against him, agrees, but only under the condition that should Pythias not return, Damon will be executed in his place.

On the scheduled date of execution there is no sign of Pythias. "Dionysius, in the meanwhile, had been amusing himself by taunting Damon, constantly telling him that he was a fool to have risked his life for a friend, however dear. To anger him, he also insisted that Pythias was only too glad to escape death, and would be very careful not to return in time. Damon, who knew the goodness and affection of his friend, received these remarks with the scorn they deserved, and repeated again and again that he knew Pythias would never break his word, but would be back in time, unless hindered in some unforeseen way" (Gruber 2010).

Damon is taken out to be killed. But lo and behold, Pythias suddenly comes running up to the execution scene. He profusely apologizes for the delay, relating that pirates had captured his ship (a regular occurrence in those days) and had thrown him overboard. He had had to swim all the way back to Syracuse. "Dionysius, who had come to see the execution, was so touched by this true friendship, that for once he forgot his cruelty, and let both young men go free, saying that he would not have believed such devotion possible had he not seen it with his own eyes" (Gruber 2010). In fact, Dionysius is so amazed by this show of friendship that in some versions of the story he tries to become their friend as well but is rebuffed, since Damon and Pythias recognize that he has not truly reformed and remains at heart a vile character.

This story is a popular culture favorite and has often been retold in song, opera, television adaptations, and comic books. One particularly notable variation is the 1957 movie *The Delicate Delinquent* starring Jerry Lewis (his first film after his break with comic partner Dean Martin) and Darren McGavin. It is the story of Sidney L. Pythias (played by Lewis), a young janitor mistaken to be a juvenile delinquent (a common theme of many 1950s films) who is befriended by a cop named Mike Damon (played by Darren

McGavin—perhaps best known now for his later role as the harried father in the classic 1983 film *A Christmas Story*). Unlike others who think he is a bad seed, Officer Damon sees the good in young Pythias, and judges him on his true character. He also remembers back to when he was young and also considered a troublemaker, and had been befriended by a cop who had done much the same for him. Pythias, in typical Jerry Lewis style, causes various goof-ups and mayhem but ultimately is cleared of blame and eventually becomes a police officer himself. The two men, like Damon and Pythias of old, become role models for others.

In his *Nichomachean Ethics*, Aristotle writes that such intimate friendship is only possible with a few people: "In friendships of bosom companions not many people are included, and the friendships celebrated in stories are always between two people" (Aristotle 1962: 268). It is not surprising that many of Aristotle's translators and interpreters give a reference at this point to Damon and Pythias, as well as to Achilles and Patroclus in Homer's *Iliad*, as examples of what Aristotle means by a friendship of bosom companions.

Clearly Damon and Pythias represent the strongest of all friendships by demonstrating the willingness to die for one another if need be. Theirs is definitely a relationship that goes far beyond mere utility and pleasure. In fact, Aristotle goes so far as to argue that in such cases of friendship one can say that there is a single soul living in two bodies, a rather startling claim which will be examined in more detail below.

Whether or not they shared a single soul, what is most remarkable about this story is the willingness that each friend has to sacrifice his life for the other. Surely in cases of friendships of utility or of pleasure this would be a deal breaker. And here we can see why Aristotle calls such a relationship "a perfect friendship." It has strength akin to the strongest natural bonds we feel for our family members (since we would naturally be willing to sacrifice ourselves for our parents or our children if need be). The two men's love for each other is based not upon crude quid pro quo conditions, since sacrificing one's life is not something that can ever be returned. Nor is it based upon pleasure, since fear of death is an overpowering force that overcomes any positive feelings. Rather, it is based upon the fact that the two men honor each other's character. Damon knows for certain that Pythias will not betray him—it was only the unforeseen circumstances that delayed his return. And Pythias knows that no one else would have been willing to take the chance that Damon did on his behalf, so that he could visit his aged mother and other family members one last time. It is no wonder that the story, in all its variations, continues to move people. How many of us can honestly say we would do what Damon did on behalf of another?

"Pythias," by the way, was also the name of Aristotle's first wife, with whom he had a daughter of the same name. Tradition tells us that Pythias was, like her husband, a biologist and scientist, as was their daughter, named Pythias, which makes it all the harder to understand how Aristotle could write so disparagingly of women, especially in regards to friendship.

The Highest Form of Friendship

We have previously examined why Aristotle refers to friendships of utility and pleasure as so-called "imperfect" versions. Let us now turn to see why he calls friendships of the good the "perfect" version. First of all, the word "perfect" is perhaps not the best translation from the Greek, since in English it implies being unbreakable or flawless, which is not at all Aristotle's meaning. It would be better perhaps to refer to this as the "highest" form or the strongest type of friendship. Clearly his meaning here is that friendships of utility and pleasure, while important to one's development, still pale in comparison to friendships of the good. Just what makes this so?

Goodness

The key point here is the word "good." Returning back to the notion of the human soul, Aristotle asks what is it that makes humans unique from other living things? It is the fact that we alone possess the ability to reason. And because of this, we alone ask the question—what is "good"? Is the good merely that which is expedient? If so, then all we really would need would be friends of utility, since they could help provide us with the provisions we seek for a good life. Or is the good merely that which makes us content and brings us joy? If so, all we would need would be friends of pleasure. But while usefulness and pleasure might be sufficient for other creatures, they are not sufficient for humans. What we seek most of all is the fulfillment of our talents. We desire to be the best that we can be, to *thrive*. And it is only friendships of the good that can lead us to this highest of all goals. For in this type of friendship two people mutually recognize the excellence in the other and encourage the most virtuous of behaviors. It is the love of the good that is the basis of this type of friendship. "The perfect form of friendship," Aristotle writes, "is that between good men who are alike in excellence or virtue. For these friends wish alike for one another's good because they are good men, and they are good *per se* (that is, their goodness is something intrinsic, not incidental)" (Aristotle 1962: 219).

Two quick examples come to mind here that can show the differences between the three types of friendship. Imagine for a moment that you unexpectedly inherit a large amount of money, or win a good amount in the lottery.

How would your different friends react? Friends of utility might well feel that, in recompense for all they have done for you, they deserve part of your winnings, and should you not share it with them, they may break off the friendship in anger, sure that if they were in your shoes they would certainly give *you* a large amount. Friends of pleasure would immediately see the wonderful opportunities such newfound wealth could bring: wild parties, travels to exotic places, and sensual experiences otherwise unavailable. Should you not bestow largesse for such purposes they may call you a spoilsport, and say you're no longer any fun to be around.

What might a friend of the good do in such a situation? Most likely, rather than expecting any of the money, that friend would be concerned about *you*. Many a person has come into great wealth only to squander it (it's amazing, for instance how many winners of large lotteries end up bankrupt or ruined, primarily *because* they listen to their friends of utility and pleasure). A friend of the good might well say that this money should be invested, or that you should use it to pay off your debts so that you can have peace of mind. The key point here is that a friend of the good is concerned about your wellbeing, and will only be satisfied in knowing that you have used these resources for your own good. That is reward enough for such a friend.

Consider another scenario. You are in a car accident and have been hospitalized for several weeks. As discussed earlier, it is unlikely that friends of utility or of the good will spend much time visiting you. But you can sure that a friend of the good will be there for you, not just to visit but also to be of assistance in watering your plants, walking your dog, picking up your mail, and making sure that once you are back home you still continue to receive good care.

A friend of the good shares your joys and concerns. Your success is his success. Your pain is his pain. That is the highest form of reciprocity. It goes far beyond that of friendships of utility. It is not merely keeping tabs. True friends don't keep accounts of how much each has spent on the other—in fact they will fight over who picks up the check. This is similar to the ways in which family members treat each other (at least ideally). There is not mere reciprocity but rather *mutuality*. Nothing makes a parent happier than seeing a child succeed. Good parents don't keep track of how much time and commitment they've devoted to their children—they give their money and time out of love. And while justice would demand that children reciprocate in giving their time and commitment back, in a good relationship this is done naturally rather than through a sense of imposition. The same is true of friends of the good. "Those who wish for their friends' good for their friends' sake are friends in the truest sense, since their attitude is determined by what their friends are and not by incidental considerations" (Aristotle 1962: 228–229).

Reliability and Trustworthiness

Another important point which Aristotle stresses is the fact that friends of the good can be relied upon, in ways that friends of utility and pleasure cannot. They have your back, as it were. This is nicely demonstrated in the classic 1993 film *Tombstone,* which focuses on the real-life friendship between Doc Holliday (played by Val Kilmer) and Wyatt Earp (played by Kurt Russell) in 1880s Arizona. Earp falls afoul of the dreaded Clanton gang, who have killed one of his brothers and gravely wounded another. He sets out to bring them to justice. Doc Holliday, who is dying from tuberculosis, rises from his sickbed and join the hunt. He is asked by a fellow member of the posse why, given his dire condition, he's helping Wyatt Earp. "Because he's my friend," Holliday answers. "Hell," the other member says, "I've got lots of friends." There's a dramatic pause, and Holliday quietly responds, "I don't." Earp and Holliday have a friendship of the good. They trust each other without having to say a word— each one knows that the other will be there for him through thick and thin.

Vicious People Cannot Be Friends of the Good

Earlier we saw another differentiation between the three types of friendships. Even vicious people (like the members of the Clanton gang for instance) can have friends of utility and friends of pleasure. But Aristotle holds that only virtuous people can be friends of the good. The reason for that is because it is the mutual recognition of each other's goodness that draws them together in the first place. "Hence their friendship lasts as long as they are good, and that means it will last for a long time, since goodness or virtue is a thing that lasts" (Aristotle 1962: 220). That is why this is the strongest of all friendships. Its basis is not something fleeting or changing, like a job situation or a pleasant activity which brings people together. Rather it is the strength of each other's character that binds them.

One can see here that friendships of the good contain elements of the other two types. Each person is definitely useful to the other—Earp is in need of Holliday's help, for instance, in the sense of utility. And each also bring pleasure to each other. This is memorably demonstrated in *Tombstone* when Earp, who has just moved to town, smiles broadly when he sees Holliday, whom he didn't know had also moved there. Wyatt's brothers Morgan and Virgil, who are not so fond of the gunslinger, are rather less pleased to see him. But more importantly in this relationship there is mutual and reciprocal respect.

Is It Better to Give Than to Receive?

Aristotle writes that "friendship appears to consist in giving rather than in receiving affection…. Since, then, friendship consists in giving rather than in receiving affection, and since we praise those who love their friends, the giving of affection seems to constitute the proper virtue of friends, so that people who give affection to one another according to each other's merit are lasting friends and their friendship is a lasting friendship" (Aristotle 1962: 229). Such friends do not size each other up and constantly ask "what's in it for me?" Rather, by bestowing their affection on the other they are demonstrating their own genuine self-love. They realize that what is of the highest importance is the maintenance of their friendship, since each brings out the best in the other. Aristotle goes on to say that most such friendships begin early in life, and develop over time. The immediate affection that relates to friendships of pleasure blossoms into something much deeper—namely, an appreciation of the other's virtues. This relates more to the rational than to the sensitive part of our soul, since that is the part of us that analyzes and understands. It makes *judgements,* in this case judging the good nature of the other.

Should Friends Live Together?

Since friends of the good are so important to each other's wellbeing and proper development, Aristotle goes so far as to argue that it would be best if they live in close proximity (how fortunate for Earp and Holliday to find themselves together in Tombstone). He writes that "only by living together can the perception of a friend's existence be activated, so that it stands to reason that friends aim at living together. And whatever his existence means to each partner individually or whatever is the purpose that makes his life bearable, he wishes to pursue it together with his friends" (Aristotle 1962: 270). Of course, this is true not only for friends of the good but of the other two kinds as well. We need friends of utility around us on a constant basis, since our needs are many and most of us can't fulfill them on our own. And in social activities, we definitely prefer to be around those who give us pleasure. He continues: "That is why some friends drink together or play dice together, while others go in for sports together and hunt together, or join in the study of philosophy: whatever each group of people loves most in life, in that activity they spend their days together. For since they wish to live together with their friends, they follow and share in those pursuits which, they think, constitute their life together" (Aristotle 1962: 270). It's not surprising, given Aristotle's own chosen profession, that he would list studying philosophy together as one of the highest activities friends could engage in!

Rarity and Time

Another key point that differentiates the three types of friendship is the fact that each of us is likely to have many friends of utility and of pleasure, but not many friends of the good. "Such friendships are of course rare, since such men are few. Moreover, time and familiarity are required. For, as the proverb has it, people cannot know each other until they have eaten the specified measure of salt together" (Aristotle 1962: 220). Given our health concerns today we might not consider "sharing salt together" the best way to judge a friendship's strength, but it's clear what Aristotle means by this proverb. You've got to devote a good amount of time and commitment to make the relationship work.

Here we see a most important aspect regarding the highest sort of friendship—something that will be examined in detail later in the book when we look at modern types of relationships. For Aristotle, friendships of the good don't come easily, and they must be cultivated over time. In such relationships, we reveal our innermost thoughts and aspirations to another. The trust between such friends is unlimited, and thus should not ever be given lightly. You have to get to know the other person, and that cannot be rushed. Your judgement should be a rational one, not one made in haste due to expediency or pleasure. "One cannot extend friendship to or be a friend of another person until each partner has impressed the other that he is worthy of affection," Aristotle warns, "and until each has won the other's confidence. Those who are quick to show the signs of friendship to one another are not really friends, though they wish to be; they are not true friends unless they are worthy of affection and know this to be so. The wish to be friends can come about quickly, but friendship cannot" (Aristotle 1962: 220–221). It takes time and effort.

One of the best examples of this can be found in Antoine de Saint-Exupéry 1943 classic children's book *The Little Prince*. A visitor from another planet comes upon a fox whom he wishes to befriend. But the fox tells him that he must first be tamed. "What does *tamed* mean?" the little prince asks. "It is something that's been too often neglected," the fox replies. "It means 'to create ties'..." (Saint-Exupéry 1943/2000: 59). When the little prince replies that he doesn't have time, the fox poignantly replies, "The only things you learn are the things you tame.... People haven't time to learn anything. They buy things ready-made in stores. But since there are no stores where you can buy friends, people no longer have friends. If you want a friend, tame me!" (Saint-Exupéry 1943/2000: 59–60). As the fox understands, real friendship comes slowly, over time. If you tame me, the fox says, then I will be unique to you, and you will be unique to me. We won't just another little boy and another little fox—we will be friends. The little prince understands and a beautiful friendship is formed.

Soulmates

One of the most famous, but startling, things that Aristotle says about friends of the good is that they share a common soul. There has been much debate as to just what exactly this means. It seems on the face of it to be a reference to another famous Ancient Greek concept, that of the "soulmate," which the comic playwright Aristophanes relates in Plato's dialogue the *Symposium* (which means drinking party). The *Symposium* is an exploration of the meaning of love. Humans, Aristophanes said, were once completely happy. They each had two faces, four arms, and four legs and were self-contained and totally satisfied. The gods grew jealous, and feared that the humans no longer needed them. So Zeus sent a thunderbolt that split each human into two, and from then on each of us has sought to find his/her other half, or soulmate, in order to be complete. Love did not exist before the split; for love is the longing to return to one complete soul.

It is a beautiful story, and one that Aristotle was surely aware of. But it is important to remember that Aristophanes was a *comic* writer, and there is something absurd about this tale. Socrates, later in the dialogue, dismisses it out of hand. But something else significant happens in the dialogue. A drunken, beautiful young man named Alcibiades barges into the party. When told that there is a contest (*agon*) occurring to see who can praise love in the highest way, Alcibiades takes up the challenge. He looks at Socrates, his long-time friend and mentor, and describes in great detail how ugly he is. Rather strange praise, one might think. But then Alcibiades says that Socrates reminds him of the gargoyle statues one can find in the marketplace, which when opened reveal a hidden jewel. That is the key point—Socrates' outer form may appear ugly, but his inner self, his soul, is beautiful, and Alcibiades, as his friend, recognizes this.

This seems to be what Aristotle has in mind when he says that true friends share a common soul: each sees the real self of the other, and their friendship helps to bring about the best within both. It is not so much that they are, as Aristophanes would have it, soulmates but rather that they see the true worth of the other, and in doing so they better understand their own worth as well. Aristotle writes "In loving a friend they love their own good. For when a good man becomes a friend he becomes a good to the person whose friend he is. Thus, each partner both loves his own good and makes an equal return in the good he wishes for his partner and in the pleasure he gives him. Now friendship is said to be equality, and both those qualities inhere especially in the relationship between good men" (Aristotle 1962: 224).

Ultimately the friendship between Alcibiades and Socrates as expressed in the *Symposium* is a tragic one. While Alcibiades sees the true worth of Socrates, Socrates likewise sees the true vicious nature of Alcibiades, who while outwardly beautiful and charismatic, is becoming more and more obsessed with power for its own sake, and seeks to manipulate and use other people. He recognizes, for instance, that Alcibiades is only pretending to be drunk, in order to take advantage of those around him, and that he enjoys disrupting events as a way of showing his superiority. In an important passage of the dialogue, Alcibiades says of Socrates that he is the only person who can make him feel *ashamed*, because Socrates alone knows how much his vicious actions are betraying the goodness within himself in his quest for power.

Limited Number

Another important point that Aristotle makes is that it is not possible to have many friends of the good, because there are natural limits to the amount of time and effort we can put into cultivating such relationships. "To be friends with many people in the sense of perfect friendship is impossible," he writes, "just as it is impossible to be in love with many people at the same time" (Aristotle 1962: 225). It *is* possible to have many friends of utility and also to have pleasurable friendships. But while good, these two types of friends are not fully sufficient for people. "They should, however, look for friends who are good as well as pleasant, and not only good, but good for them; for in this way they will have everything that friends should have" (Aristotle 1962: 225).

Thus, in order to have friends of the good you must yourself be virtuous, for that is what will attract the other, much like the fox was attracted to the virtuous little prince. But you also have to be fortunate, since there is no guarantee you will ever meet such virtuous people. You must constantly be on the lookout, and be ready to open yourself slowly to such goodness. And you must remain geographically connected as well. Distance will not necessarily end a friendship of the good. "But, if the absence lasts for some time, it apparently also causes the friendship itself to be forgotten. Hence the saying: 'Out of sight, out of mind'" (Aristotle 1962: 223).

Is there a natural limit to how many friends of the good one can have? Aristotle feels that this is definitely the case. If you have a handful of such relationships in your entire life, consider yourself fortunate. What might that number be? "Perhaps," he writes, "it is the largest number with whom a man might be able to live together, for, as we noticed, living together is the surest indication of friendship; and it is quite obvious that is it impossible to live together with many people and divide oneself up among them. Furthermore, one's friends should also be the friends of one another, if they are all going to spend their days in each other's company; but it is an arduous task to have this be the case among a large number of people" (Aristotle 1962: 268).

Interestingly enough, some modern thinkers are giving independent verification to Aristotle's claims. In Chapter 4 we will examine the British psychologist Robin Dunbar's research showing that, no matter how many people we may claim to have as genuine friends, that number is necessarily finite. "'There is a limited amount of time and emotional capital we can distribute, so we only have five slots for the most intense type of relationship,' Mr. Dunbar said. 'People may say they have more than five but you can be pretty sure they are not high-quality friendships'" (Murphy 2016). Five friends of the good is probably about all you can really have.

The Perils of Friendship of the Good

As we saw earlier, to calls friends of the good "perfect" is not to imply that there are no dangers involved in forming such relationships or no possibilities that they might end.

While they are the strongest type, they are not invulnerable. For instance, there is always the danger that one may lose a friend due to death, or the friend's moving away. This occurs in *The Little Prince,* when the title character says that it is time for him to return to his home planet. "'Ah!' the fox said. 'I shall weep.' 'It's your own fault,' the little prince said. 'I never wanted to do you any harm, but you insisted that I tame you…'" (Saint-Exupéry 1943/2000: 61). But the fox replies that it has been worth it, "because of the color of the wheat" which will always remind him of the little prince's hair and the friendship they once had.

Another danger is the possibility of making a mistake, misjudging another person as worthy of your friendship when their true nature is not what one may think. But perhaps most disturbing of all: what if the friend ceases to be virtuous? Suppose he was initially a good person but, like Alcibiades (or Obi Wan Kenobi's former friend Darth Vader for that matter!), turns to the dark side?

Aristotle has some advice about this. "If we accept a person as a friend assuming that he is good, but he becomes, and we think he has become, wicked, do we still owe him affection? Surely, that is impossible, since only the good—not just anything—is the object of affection" (Aristotle 1962: 251). What should one do at this point? "Should the friendship, then, be broken off at once? Probably not in every case, but only when a friend's wickedness has become incurable. But if there is a chance of reforming him, we must come to the aid of his character more than to the aid of his property, inasmuch as character is the better thing and a more integral part of friendship" (Aristotle 1962: 251).

And here we see an important reason why, in a literal sense, friends of the good do not in fact share one common soul. "But no one would regard a person who breaks off such a friendship as acting strangely, because the man who was his friend was not the kind of man he turned out to be: his

friend has changed, and since he is unable to save him, he severs his connections with him" (Aristotle 1962: 251). You must do all you can—as Socrates
tries in the case of Alcibiades and Obi-Wan Kenobi tries in the case of Darth
Vader—to help your friend return to the good. But should that friend not
do so, you must worry about the bad effect he will have upon you if you continue to associate with him. Your highest duty, ultimately, is to save your own
soul.

Enemies

Another peril of friendships of the good is the fact that such people
know more about you than anyone else, including often your family members.
You have trusted them completely and revealed your innermost self to them.
But suppose, as in the case above of Obi-Wan Kenobi and Darth Vader, they
turn against you? Such people will then be your worst enemies.

This is nicely captured in the 2016 Amazon show *Goliath,* starring Billy
Bob Thornton and William Hurt as former law partners who despise each
other. David E. Kelley, creator of the show, as well as other classics like *Ally
McBeal* and *L.A. Law,* understands how perfect friends can become perfect
enemies. "'There's a profound contempt that these two have for each other
but the nucleus was a long-standing love,' Kelley says. Billy and Donald were
'at one time best of friends; they founded this law firm together. It's only that
deep kind of friendship that can give rise to such a malignant hatred'" (Ryan
2016).

Because they know you the best, former friends of the good can do you
the most harm. They know your innermost secrets; your real desires; and all
your weaknesses. By revealing such information, you have made your vulnerable, and—in the famous last words of Cardinal Wolsey after he fell afoul
of King Henry VIII—naked to your enemies.

Is It Worth It?

But consider the alternative. What if you keep to yourself and form no
relationships at all? In that case, Aristotle holds, you won't develop properly
as a human being. In the worst case, you will be completely alone (like the
character in Simon and Garfunkel's "I Am a Rock"), living an unnatural solitary life. But even if you only have friends of utility or of the good, your life
will still be unfulfilled and superficial. Recent studies, by the way, have shown
that having friends of the good is an actual health requirement: "According
to medical experts, playing it safe by engaging in shallow, unfulfilling or non-
reciprocal relationships has physical repercussions. Not only do the resulting
feelings of loneliness and isolation increase the risk of death as much as smok-

ing, alcoholism and obesity; you may also lose tone, or function, in the so-called smart *vagus* nerve, which brain researchers think allows us to be in intimate, supportive and reciprocal relationships in the first place" (Murphy 2016). This is the kind of experimental verification that Aristotle would have appreciated.

There are no guarantees that friendships of the good will form and blossom, but Aristotle argued you must always be at the ready for them. You must take chances—but make sure they are *reasonable* chances. Don't reveal too much too soon (good advice in the internet age). Use your reasoning powers to properly evaluate the nature of your relationship with your friends. Is it one of utility? Pleasure? Or most fortunate of all, a friendship of the good?

Criticisms of Aristotle's Friendship of the Good Concept

We'd like to point out some criticisms of Aristotle's views on friendships of the good, which will also be addressed in more detail in the following chapters. First of all, one can certainly say that his notion of friendships of the good is too elitist, especially since he limits this primarily to upper-caste males. Also, the conditions that Aristotle lays out—especially the need for equality and the necessity of living together—can be too much to ask in a hectic environment. Surely the living conditions of many humans have changed dramatically since Aristotle's times. We can stay in touch with friends who've moved to other cities and other countries (although not yet to other planets, as in the case of the little prince and the fox). Would no longer "sharing salt" together really mean the end of friendships of the good? And do we really need to drop friends of pleasure and utility, especially when social networking makes it far more convenient to stay in close contact with people from throughout our lives?

Another possible objection to Aristotle is the question, can vicious people in fact have friends? Did Hitler or Stalin, for instance, have only superficial relationships or might they really have been on close personal terms with others? More to the point, the actual Wyatt Earp and Doc Holliday were, it seems, far more vicious than portrayed in the film *Tombstone*, yet nonetheless did indeed seem to be close friends. Was it really the goodness in each other's souls that brought them together?

Perhaps most pertinently, are there really just three categories of friendship, utility, pleasure and goodness? In the following chapters, we'll explore many other options and show that in fact it can be quite complicated figuring out the exact nature of one's friendship relationships.

Can Men and Women Be Friends?

Last but not least, Aristotle's writings on friendship seem most outdated and unacceptable when it comes to his views regarding men and women. His assertion that husbands and wives cannot be friends because there is no equality seems outrageous today. And as mentioned earlier, he never discusses the possibility of friendship among women at all in his *Nichomachean Ethics,* nor the question whether men and women could ever become friends of the good.

One of the best depictions of a friendship of the good in popular culture was that of the two lawyers Alan Shore (played by James Spader) and Denny Crane (played by William Shatner) in the 2004–2008 television show *Boston Legal* (also created by the aforementioned David E. Kelley). At the end of every episode these two men would smoke cigars on a balcony, drink brandy, and ruminate on philosophical topics. Theirs was a genuine "bro" relationship, although given some of the questionable legal tactics they resorted to in the series it is arguable whether or not they constituted virtuous people.

At the end of one episode they raised a question which naturally comes to mind when reading Aristotle's exploration of friendship: namely, shouldn't married partners be the truest of best friends?

> DENNY CRANE: Well, I have nothing against marriage. I've done it five times. But here's the thing about wives. They don't let you play with your friends. I mean, I couldn't be standing outside here every night on this balcony if.... I'll take a friend over a wife every time.
>
> ALAN SHORE: Shouldn't a wife be your best friend? You know, Ralph Waldo Emerson said he reckoned a friend to be the masterpiece of nature. I'm not sure I truly understood that before I met you, Denny.
>
> DENNY CRANE: I'm not having sex with you.
>
> ALAN SHORE: Just the same [*Boston Legal* 2008].

One should note that in the final episode of the series Denny and Alan in fact get married to each other (by an actor playing Supreme Court Justice Scalia no less!) Gay marriage had just been legalized in Massachusetts in 2008, so it was a timely way to end the show. But the reasons had nothing to do with sex. Denny throughout the series was increasingly worried that he was succumbing to Alzheimer's Disease, and Alan fought to get him access to a non–FDA approved drug that could potential slow the onslaught of the disease. Alan wanted to also make sure that, when his friend Denny finally was unable to take care of himself, Alan would have full power of attorney to make decisions on his behalf, and so the two were married for protective reasons. In this episode, Alan beautifully summed up his true feelings: "Denny is my best friend. I love him with all my heart. If I could yank that horrible disease out of his body, I would fight it and I would win. I would use every ounce of my strength and I would win, if I could—but I can't" (*Boston Legal* 2008).

In the words of *Entertainment Weekly* writer Mandi Bierly, "When you're asked the trivia question, 'What was the final line spoken on *Boston Legal*?,' smile when you answer that it was Denny Crane (William Shatner) saying 'It's our wedding night' to Alan Shore (James Spader) as they slow danced on the balcony of the Chinese-acquired Chang Poole & Schmidt. I know I will. That was the most satisfying series finale I've seen in years" (Bierly 2008). Crane and Shore may not be the modern Damon and Pythias, but they sure come close.

Aristotle's Friendship in the Modern Age

It is important to note that we are not claiming by any means that everything Aristotle had to say was correct. Rather, we have been spelling out his views on friendship in part to see what they are, for they have been very influential, and also in part to set the stage for our further explorations. But we should point out that one of the best-known exponents of Aristotle's philosophy in the present-day, and someone who has made a strong case that his writings are still relevant and work exploring, is the University of Chicago Professor of Philosophy Martha Nussbaum (we will explore her work on the concept of eudaimonia in Chapter 6). She clearly exemplifies the fact that women are not inferior to men by nature, and she has persuasively argued that the best way to understand Aristotle is to expand his categories to allow more and more people to thrive. The two Pythiases—Aristotle's wife and daughter—would surely appreciate that!

Popular Culture Scenario 1.3:
When Harry Met Sally

One of the best explorations of the question of whether men and women can be friends is found in the 1989 film *When Harry Met Sally,* directed by Rob Reiner and written by Nora Ephron. It has stood the test of time as one of the best-loved romantic comedies ever made. And in fact, as *New York Times* writer Neil Genzlinger observes, it has even become a holiday classic. "What qualifies that as a holiday film? Three things:

1. It has a Christmas tree in it. Several, actually.
2. Its pivotal scene involves a New Year's Eve party.
3. It is, on one level, all about taking a leap of faith into a hopeful future, certainly appropriate for a holiday season that ends on New Year's Day" [Genzlinger 2016].

The film details the 12-year relationship between Harry Burns (Billy Crystal) and Sally Albright (Meg Ryan), who initially meet in college and have an immediate attraction for each other. But Harry warns Sally that "men and women can't be friends because the sex part always gets in the way." Indeed, he has a strict "rule" (very Aristotelian in fact) that male-female friendships are completely impossible. Throughout the movie, the two debate this topic, sometimes good-naturedly and sometimes rather heatedly, as in the following exchange:

> SALLY: We are just going to be friends, OK?
>
> HARRY: Great, friends. It's the best thing.... You realize, of course, that we can never be friends.
>
> SALLY: Why not?
>
> HARRY: What I'm saying is—and this is not a come-on in any way, shape, or form—is that men and women can't be friends, because the sex part always gets in the way.
>
> SALLY: That's not true. I have a number of men friends and there is no sex involved.
>
> HARRY: No, you don't.
>
> SALLY: Yes, I do.
>
> HARRY: No, you don't.
>
> SALLY: Yes, I do.
>
> HARRY: You only think you do.
>
> SALLY: You're saying I'm having sex with these men without my knowledge?
>
> HARRY: No, what I'm saying is they all *want* to have sex with you.
>
> SALLY: They do not.
>
> HARRY: Do too.
>
> SALLY: They do not.
>
> HARRY: Do too.
>
> SALLY: How do you know?
>
> HARRY: Because no man can be friends with a woman that he finds attractive. He always wants to have sex with her.

One of the charms of the film is the delightful banter between the main characters. Eventually Harry concedes that his "rule" is not an absolute. In the original screenplay by Nora Ephron, the two decide to just remain friends, but eventually Ephron and Reiner decided that—since it was a romantic comedy after all and people would be expecting it—Harry and Sally would in fact get married at the end. But the film nonetheless raises many fascinating questions about the nature of men and female friendship, and challenges Aristotle's assertion that husbands and wives can never be friends of the good.

Summary

In this chapter, we looked at the life and teachings of the Ancient Greek philosopher Aristotle and how his views regarding the nature of friendship continue to influence modern-day discussions of the topic. In particular, we examined his threefold categorization of friendship—utility, pleasure and the good.

We began by examining Aristotle's claim that we are by nature social beings, and that in order to develop in the best possible ways we need connections with many other humans. This begins with the family, which in Aristotle's view is an unequal relationship. Parents cannot be friends, in his view, since the relationship with them is not on equal terms, nor is it a chosen one. The same holds for siblings and other family members.

We next looked at the role that strangers play in our lives, particularly what psychologist Stanley Milgram calls "familiar strangers." Most of those we associate with fall within this category; we are not truly friends because there is no reciprocal relationship involved.

Friends of utility are those whom we choose to be involved with. We rely upon each other, and in doing so help each person to develop. But such relationships are fragile, and in Aristotle's terms "imperfect." They are likely to end when our life situations change and we are no longer of use to each other.

We then learned about Aristotle's second category of friendship, friends of pleasure. We saw that, unlike friends of utility, which are based upon a crude quid pro quo relationship, friends of pleasure are based upon human emotions, especially the joy that people feel in being in each other's company. Such friendships are thus of a higher nature, and tend to be more important to one's development.

This was then related to Aristotle's concept of the tripartite nature of the human soul—vegetative, sensitive, and rational—with friendships of pleasure relating to the sensitive part of the soul. He argued that these types of friendships are usually associated with the young, who are more prone to being led by their feelings.

We examined the concept of "friends of the good" and saw that, according to Aristotle, the basis of such friendship is a deep appreciation of the goodness or virtue of the other. This is a "perfect" form of friendship because it is the strongest as well as the longest-lasting. "Perfection" does not imply that such friendships will never end or have no flaws, but it does mean that their foundation is the most solid, since the basis for them is the concern each has for the other's continued well-being. Friends of the good encourage virtuous behavior, and are reliable and trustworthy to the highest degree.

Aristotle goes so far as to claim that such friends share a common soul, although the exact meaning of this phrase is open to interpretation. He also says that only virtuous people can experience such relationships—vicious or bad people can only have, at best, friendships of utility or pleasure.

Another key condition for Aristotle is the need for friends to live together or at least be in close proximity. Such friendships take time to develop, and because of the commitment necessary one can only have a limited number of friends of the good.

While stronger than the other two types, friendships of the good can also come to an end, due to death, leave-taking, mistaken identity, or in the worst-case scenario when one of the friends ceases to be virtuous. Our greatest enemies are often our former best friends. Still, it is important to open one's self up to such relationships, since they allow us to develop in the highest of ways, and life would be inadequate without such friendships.

We ended with a brief look at criticisms that Aristotle's views are elitist, sexist, and not in tune with changing realities, all of which will be examined in greater detail in subsequent chapters, as well as pointing out that Aristotle's threefold concept is still relevant in trying to understand the nature of friendship in the present day.

Chapter 2

Forming a Friendship

Ten-year-old Nikki sits alone in the front yard of her home. She is distraught. Her best friend, and former next door neighbor, has just moved away with her family. Her world is crumbling. How could her friend's family move away from the neighborhood? Didn't they consider the feelings and the friendships of the little girls hurt by this decision? Nikki is too young to understand that variables beyond her control can have such an adverse effect on her life. She has no idea things like this will happen the rest of her life—in fact, in just four short years, her new best friend will stop hanging out with her because she will get a boyfriend and will spend all her time with him. But, that's a problem for future Nikki; right now she yearns for a new best friend.

Before too long, Nikki's parents inform her that the vacant house her best friend once lived in has been sold and that the new owners will be moving in very soon. Nikki hopes that there is a girl near her age so that they can become best friends. Nikki hasn't paid much attention to the fact that her parents were upset when the family moved away because they were good friends with the other parents. The moving van appears the next day and lo and behold there is a young girl Nikki's age and the two hit if off immediately. Nikki and the new neighbor girl are now besties and all is good in the world. Unfortunately, Nikki's parents and the parents who bought the next-door home do not get along with each other right away and, as it turns out, they never will become close friends. The fact that the neighbor children are now close friends means that the adult parents will have to learn to tolerate one another but they are not particularly happy about it.

This story provides a glimpse into the sometimes complicated world of contemporary friendship. In this chapter, we will learn about the value of group formation, the manner in which the socialization process helps us to form friendships, significant categories of friends (including casual friends, good friends and best friends), characteristics of good friendships, and it concludes with a look at why many friendships end.

Group Formation

In the first chapter of this book we discussed Aristotle's three categories of friends: friends of utility, friends of pleasure and friends of the good. Aristotle's observations on friendships have, for the most part, stood the test of time; they do not, however, represent a complete understanding of the nature of friendship, especially in regards to the starting point of group formation and friendships. In fact, humans, like most animal species, have long formed groups. Alligators form congregations; apes and baboons group into troops; antelopes, reindeer and others in herds; bees in hives; elephants, elks and others as herds; geese fly in flocks; mosquitoes in scourge; owls in parliament; hyenas, wild dogs and wolves in packs; and zebras in zeals, cohorts or herds. As Aristotle observed, humans too are social creatures. They also form groups and have done so throughout history for the primary purposes of safety and basic survival. Never the fastest nor the strongest creatures of the animal kingdom, humans found a way to survive by sharing food, caring for infants, hunting and gathering food supplies for group members and collecting and sharing tools. The development of groups and the formation of strong social bonds improved the group's probability of survival. Even as humans continued to evolve physically and intellectually over hundreds of thousands of years the need for companionship and a strong communal bond with others would remain intact.

In contemporary society, people still value group formation for safety and basic survival but also for a variety of other reasons as well. The social interaction between group members, for example, serves an important role in an individual's life, as everyone wants to feel part of a group or community (Maslow 1954). It is important for individuals to experience a sense of unity with their fellows and by joining together in groups, individuals become a part of a greater whole. Group membership provides individuals with a sense of identity. The group provides members with an identity because of their various connections (e.g., cultural ancestry and subcultural associations). Individual personalities allow for the maintenance of self-identity.

Integrative Bonds

Peter Blau (1918–2002) describes how human beings choose between alternative potential associations or courses of actions (group formation) by evaluating the experiences, or expected experiences, of each in terms of preference ranking and then select the best alternative (Blau 1964). Blau believed that the main force that draws people together is social attraction (Farganis 2000). Attraction is defined in terms of potential rewards to be granted for participating in the social exchange. When there are inadequate rewards, the deterioration of the social ties between individuals, and groups is (more) likely to occur. Irrational as well as rational behaviors are governed by these considerations. Of particular importance is the realization that not all individuals (or groups) prefer or value the same alternatives equally (Delaney 2004). Blau also makes distinctions between intrinsically rewarding exchanges (e.g., love relationships) and associations primarily concerned with extrinsic benefits (e.g., a posse member for a famous rapper who gets paid to run errands).

As it pertains to group formation, social attraction involves the development of integrative bonds that unite individuals in a cohesive unit. Some of the integrative bonds discussed by Blau (1964) include:

1. Impressing Others—Expectations of rewards make associations attractive. Strategies to appear impressive include taking risks, performing well at difficult or valued tasks, and the ability to exhibit both strain and ease depending on the social occasion.
2. Social Approval—Humans are anxious to receive social approval for their decisions and actions, for their opinions, and suggestions. The approving agreement of others helps to confirm their judgments, to justify their conduct, and to validate their beliefs. Preoccupation with impressing others impedes both expressive involvement and instrumental endeavors. Restraints imposed by social approval are confined to circles of significant others.
3. Attractiveness—Opinions that are met with approval, and one's approval of another's opinion, increase one's level of attractiveness; whereas serious and persistent conflicts of opinions lead to personal rejections (unattractiveness). The role of first impressions is involved in perceived attractiveness, for they may be self-fulfilling as well as self-defeating. One must be cautious of first impressions for their reflections may be distorted. Bluffing is a mechanism utilized by some people in hopes of creating a positive early impression; however, the cost of having a bluff called may be too high. For example, if one is at a social gathering and does not know most of the people there, she may be tempted to impress others by claiming to be a medical doctor when she really is not, as a means of increasing her level of attractiveness. However, this bluff will backfire if a medical emergency arises and that person cannot properly execute the claimed doctor's role (her bluff is called).
4. Love—The extreme case of intrinsic attraction is love. Love appears to make human beings unselfish, since they themselves enjoy giving pleasures to those they love, but this selfless devotion generally rests on an interest in maintaining the other's love. The

exchange process is most evident in love attachments, but the dynamics are different because the specified rewards are not as clear as in many other social exchanges. Ironically, freely granting expressions of love depreciates their value. Such is the dilemma of love! It is also interesting to note that in love relationships, there is quite often one person who is "more in love" than the other. This has been referred to as "the principle of least interest." The person "in less love" has the power advantage (an edge), and may manipulate this advantage to gain more rewards.

Integrative bonds promote the development of group formation. Blau reasoned that group cohesiveness further promotes the development of consensus on normative standards and the effective enforcement of these shared norms because integrative ties of fellowship enhance the significance of the informal sanctions of the group (e.g., group disapproval and ostracism directed toward the group member who does not heed the norms of cohesiveness). For example, a couple who have expressed to one another their attraction and love for the other are expected to abide by standardized norms that they have created together, such as remaining loyal to one another. A violation of normative expectations may lead to a "break-up" (ostracism).

Social Groups

Not all congregations of people constitute a social group as there are clear distinctions between social groups, aggregates and categories of people. A social group is defined as two or more people who interact regularly and in a manner defined by some common purpose, set of norms, and a structure of statuses and roles (social positions). Two general requirements must be met for a number of people to qualify as a group: (1) they must interact with one another in an organized fashion, and (2) they must identify themselves as group members because of shared views, goals, traits, or circumstances. Core members of a street gang would qualify as a social group, for example. Gang members identify one another based on such qualities as wearing certain colors and clothing, tattoos, hand signals, language, jewelry, activity, and the use of graffiti (Delaney 2012a). As a matter of distinction, an aggregate consists of a number of people who happen to be clustered in one place at a given time—for example, a number of tourists climbing the Great Wall of China, movie patrons, travelers at an airport, train station or bus stop, and spectators at a sporting event. A category includes a number of people who share a particular attribute but who may have never met. Examples of categories include all eldest daughters, all left-handers, Democrats, Republicans, sports fans, and so on.

The Group System

A social group can be viewed as a type of social system. As with all social systems, there are key elements that help to preserve the continued existence of the social group. Sociologist George Homans (1910–1989) described four key elements of the group system: activity, interaction, sentiment, and norms. *Activity* refers to what the members of the group do as group members (e.g., a support group must meet regularly and help provide support to one another). *Interaction* involves group members getting together with one another and engaging in activities. Traditionally (including during Aristotle's era) it was implied that such interaction must be conducted on a face-to-face basis. Recall Aristotle's admonition that "as the proverb has it, people cannot know each other until they have eaten the specified measure of salt together" (Aristotle 1962: 220). But, as we will learn in chapters 3 and 4, such interactions are now often conducted electronically. The *sentiment* of the group is seen as the sum of the feelings of group members with respect to the group. The *norms* of the group refer to the code of behavior adopted consciously or unconsciously by the group.

As a means of underscoring the traditional idea of group activity predicated on face-to-face interactions, Homans (1950) defined a group as "a number of persons who communicate with one another often over a span of time, and who are few enough so that each person is able to communicate with all the others not at secondhand, through other people, but face to face" (p.1). Homans, then, viewed a social group as a plurality of people relatively small in number who interact with one another on a somewhat regular basis via face-to-face interactions. When the members of the group maintain an active involvement with one another and share activity, interaction, sentiment and norms, they have formed a social system. Homans explained that the collapse of entire civilizations can be explained by the failure of a number of small groups to properly meet these group needs. "A civilization, if it is in turn to maintain itself, must preserve at least a few of the characteristics of the group.... Civilizations have failed in failing to solve this problem" (Homans 1950:456) and are, thus, subject to collapse.

In the tradition of Vilfredo Pareto (1848–1923), Homans' group system involves the realization that both external (physical, technical and/or social) and internal (necessary elements of behavior among group members that are mutually depended) needs must be secured. Homans (1950) used the term *feedback*—borrowed from the property of electrical circuits (that he noted in his famous studies of the Bank Wiring Observation Room)—to describe the relationship between the internal and external group systems. He stated that there is always a process of "buildup" in which the internal system is subject to change as a result of fluctuations from the group members themselves. Changes in attitudes, sentiments, and norms among divisive members of the group will cause the need for an internal system's adjustment in activity.

While Homans put forth the notion that entire civilizations could collapse due to the failure of a number of key groups to meet system needs (e.g., the banking and mortgage industries), most of us have experienced the collapse of a tight-knit friendship group. As we saw in Chapter 1, friends from high school or college once shared activities, interactions, sentiment and norms only to see active involvement dissipate due to changing life circumstances (external fluctuations) such as group members finding a job or getting married and raising a family. It's one thing when a group of college friends go out every night and party until the wee hours only to repeat the same behavior the next day, but such activities cannot continue when one has responsibilities such as raising and providing for a family. (This topic will be revisited later in the chapter.)

The Group Structure

Once a group has formed it may continue indefinitely, become modified, or completely dissolve. The maintenance of the internal group system is at least partially dependent on the group structure itself. Individual decision-making, on the part of group members, whether they behave selfishly or in the best interests of the group, will affect the effectiveness of group action. The action of the group members is often dictated by one's status within the group structure as each member has a varying degree of commitment to maintain the social system. For example, if a child has little interest in playing baseball but has joined the team because of pressures from his parents, he will have little interest in maintaining a commitment to the team's goals and expectations of behavior.

In addition to the degree of commitment that group members possess is the issue of social equality. From the social exchange perspective (first articulated by George Homans), social behavior is an exchange of rewards and costs between persons. Unless all the members of a group are equal, social inequality will manifest itself in a number of ways including a differentiation in esteem and in recognized status (Homans 1961). The more valuable to other members of a group are the activities an individual emits to them, the higher is the esteem in which they hold that individual. The higher the esteem that one member holds, the lower the esteem that is available for the rest of the members of the group. The higher the rank of a person within the group, the more esteem and privilege that person enjoys compared to other members of the group. The military adage "with rank comes privilege" comes to mind as a general possesses far more privilege and esteem than a private. The higher-ranking group member also enjoys more perks which may lead to jealousy among lower ranking group members.

Regardless of individual esteem and status within the group structure, each member has certain role obligations. These role obligations are not always met, but generally they are. When these role obligations are met, the group has a better chance of survival (maintenance). Homans (1961) believed that most members of the group will meet their group needs due to the acknowledgment of mutual obligations. Within groups, individuals may occupy any of several social positions, referred to by sociologists as statuses. There are two general types of social statuses: ascribed and achieved. An *ascribed status* is any status a person receives through birth, such as one's ancestry, race/ethnicity, and gender. Because ascribed statuses are assigned to us at birth, we cannot, generally, alter them. (An exception to this would be a transgendered person.) Depending on the type of group(s) one belongs to, ascribed statues may or may not play an important role in dictating one's social position or role within the group. An *achieved status* is any status that a person attains or earns through individual effort, choice, competition, or luck. There are far more examples of achieved statuses than ascribed statuses. College graduate, full professor, professional athlete, workplace bowling champion, nurse, restaurant owner, or chicken wing eating champion are just a few examples of achieved statuses. Think of the social groups you belong to and ascertain why those with the highest statuses have attained their privileged standing.

Everyone possesses many social positions, or social statuses, and with specific social positions come corresponding expectations of behavior. Sociologists refer to such cultural expectations as roles. A social role may be defined as entailing culturally determined rights, duties, and expectations associated with specific social positions. The role of a college student involves attending class, reading assigned materials, participating in class discussions, completing assignments (e.g., tests, term papers), attending school-sponsored events (e.g., lectures by prominent guest speakers, art exhibits and sporting events), and representing the college in a positive manner within the greater community. A college student also holds many other social statuses simultaneously, such as being a son or daughter, a sibling, a parent, an employee, a friend, an athlete, and so on. The idea of multiple statuses extends to all people, not just college students as every one of us has many roles in life.

The possession of multiple statuses at any given time may lead to role conflict, a stressful situation that occurs when opposing expectations are attached to different statuses held by the same person. For example, friends may want you to join them for a night on the town to celebrate the achievement of one of the group members and yet you know you have a busy day ahead of you at work tomorrow, and you already promised your sister that you would watch her kids tonight while she works. Ultimately, this individual will have to prioritize her life. The status deemed most important will take precedence. Sociologists refer to a prioritized status as a "master status." A master status is the status that dominates one's identity. If the individual feels a strong commitment to her group of friends she is likely to join them in a night of celebration; or, if the individual chooses to help out her sister and watch her children, she has chosen her status within the family as a master status.

In addition to role conflict, individuals are likely to experience role strain. Role strain occurs when conflicting expectations are placed on an individual within one role, such as that of a college student. Most students have undoubtedly heard that the college years may be "the best years of their lives" and if that is the case, they feel compelled to experiment with a variety of behaviors typical of many students. Then again, the college student also realizes that with the rising costs of tuition, room and board, books and general life expenses, that she must find the balance between enjoying a social life while meeting academic expectations. Is it more important to hang out with friends all night partying or playing video games, or to study for a test or work on a term paper? Trying to do too much results in the cliché of "burning the candle at both ends," which eventually leads to strain within the role of the college student (Delaney 2012a).

Within the context of the group, each member has certain role obligations. When these role obligations are met, the group has a better chance of survival (maintenance). Most members of the group will meet their group needs due to the acknowledgment of mutual obligations and because they find such activities and interactions rewarding. Thus, conformity is met with approval and the group structure remains intact (Homans 1961). However, if a group member is slacking off in their commitment and obligation to the group, the other group members may exert some form of pressure (e.g., verbal teasing) in attempt to steer the member back toward the goals of the collective. For example, when one member of a group of friends who regularly get together every Wednesday night to play video games suddenly begins to offer excuses for not attending the weekly gatherings may experience pressure from the other group members to maintain his commitment. Still, if the person missing the weekly gatherings has a new girlfriend, he may choose to spend his time with her and his new developing group of friends that consists of other couples. The original gaming group of friends might have to find a new member for their group or risk complete dissolution.

The group structure is also influenced by its type of leader. Every group has a leader, whether that leadership position is formal or informal—a distinction determined by the type of social group. Years ago, Cartwright and Zander (1968) stated that groups have two types of leaders: the instrumental leader and the expressive (emotional) leader. The instrumental leader is consumed with achieving goals and attempts to keep group members focused and on target toward achieving desired ends. The effective instrumental leader possesses critical-thinking and problem-solving skills and is a skilled communicator. Instrumental leaders generally adopt an authoritarian style of leadership because they feel the need to keep everyone in line. The less formal the group, the less likely they abide by the demands of an authoritarian style leader; by contrast, formal groups may need an instrumental leader in order to achieve specified goals. The expressive leader focuses on maintaining harmony among members. Such a leader shows concern for the members' feelings and works to ensure that everyone stays satisfied and happy. In this regard, expressive leaders tend to adopt a laissez-faire style of leadership. Expressive leaders are common within informal friendship groups, especially when trying to direct the group with its plans for a Saturday evening of entertainment plans. An expressive leader is also more likely than an instrumental leader to adopt a democratic leadership style, which encourages input from group members. Instrumental leaders that possess an authoritarian leadership style, conversely, are less likely to incorporate input from others.

Group formation and the comprehension of role expectations and group obligations are a matter of individuals being properly socialized. Sociologists view the socialization process as the key to learning and understanding one's position in social groups, in particular, and for all of life, in general.

The Socialization Process

Socialization involves developmental changes brought about as a result of individuals interacting with other people (Schaffer 1984). Sociologists view socialization as a lifelong process of learning—one that spans from birth to death. Although early-childhood development is generally emphasized as the most critical time for learning, each of us will continue to learn new things throughout our lifetimes. We learn by interacting with others.

Every infant, from the time they are born until years later, is nearly completely dependent on caregivers for survival. These caregivers (e.g., parents, other family members, legal guardians, friends, and babysitters) teach the child necessary, basic rules of life designed to aid the infant's survival. At birth, infants are very narcissistic, meaning that they think only of their own needs and crave immediate gratification. If they are hungry or thirsty, they will usually cry and scream (as if dying!), regardless of the time of day or night or whether other family members are trying to sleep or are busy with chores. Infants do not behave badly on purpose; rather, it's that they have not learned (through the socialization process) how to behave properly. They have biological needs (for food, warmth, removal of discomfort, etc.), and they respond to these needs biologically by acting out in primal ways (e.g., crying, throwing a temper tantrum, and as toddlers by name-calling and other childish displays of poor behavior).

Despite the fact that children, like adults, have biological needs that must be fulfilled, they live in a social world where innate urges must be controlled. The child must learn to conform to societal expectations. The "spoiled" child continues to scream and throw temper tantrums in an attempt to get what he or she wants but this behavior is considered very annoying by most people and is seldom tolerated in society. Consider the fact that we certainly would not want people in positions of authority (e.g., teachers, administrators, professional sports managers, or political leaders) resorting to name calling and throwing temper tantrums just because things are not going their way, as such acts could be considered signs of mental illness or, at the very least, poor socialization.

The socialization process is responsible for taming narcissism (defined as an inordinate fascination with oneself, excessive self-love; and vanity). One of the goals of socialization is to teach children that they cannot have whatever they want whenever they want it. The real world seldom provides instant gratification for all individual needs, biological or social. It is hoped that, by the time they reach school age, all children will have learned this basic fact. Adults who act in a childish and narcissistic manner are seldom taken seriously. The notion that each of us are expected to "grow up" and "act our age" by leaving narcissistic tendencies behind as we near adulthood and certainly as we become adults is challenged today because of the development of technology that is designed for individuals to make themselves the center of attention (narcissism). We will discuss this phenomenon in Chapter 3.

As described thus far, social learning is an important aspect of the socialization process. Social learning is also a life-long endeavor. Consequently, we can define socialization as a process of social development and learning that occurs as individuals interact with one another and learn about society's expectations of proper behavior so that they can fully participate and properly function within cultural standards. While it is true that individuals are learning to conform to cultural expectations during socialization, they also acquire a social identity. Loy and Ingham (1981) explain that socialization is "an interactional process whereby a person acquires a social identity, learns appropriate role behavior, and in general conforms to expectations held by members of the social system to which he belongs or aspires to belong" (p. 189).

The socialization process is effective only if individuals learn to internalize the messages being sent to them. In this manner, the expectations of significant others and that of society in general are added to a "script" of response patterns of individuals; they have learned to respond to various stimuli in a routine fashion (everyday courtesy and manners, formal etiquette, knowing when to speak and when to remain quiet, etc.). In a broader sense, people who are properly socialized and have internalized the cultural expectations of the greater society are able to function properly in a variety of settings. Recall our earlier discussion of roles and statuses within varying social groups. Each of us performs a number of social roles in a society; in some settings, an individual may be in a position of power due to their specific role within the group structure (e.g., an owner of a business) but in other settings this same person may have little or no power (e.g., the business owner is now a customer at a grocery store, a spectator at a ball game, or a motorist stuck in "rush hour" traffic). Within this matrix of statuses and their contingent role demands, individuals must be capable of transforming identities. The socialization process prepares individuals to act properly and correspondingly in all social settings. After all, while your boss may be able to dictate your behavior, he or she cannot dictate my behavior; indicating that their power is limited to a particular setting.

It should be noted that the socialization process plays a vital role at the macro level too as it is critical for the survival and stability of the greater society itself, as members of a society are socialized to support and maintain the existing social structure. It is through the socialization process that members of society learn about their culture. Thus, the socialization process prepares the individual to perform appropriately in all social settings.

The socialization process, as noted, helps individuals to form their own sense of identity as they learn various values and norms while interacting with others. Other people become either attracted or repulsed by our social identities and may choose to be our friends or not to be our friends based on our individual identities.

The Neglected or Abandoned Child

We just learned a fair amount about the importance of the socialization process. Its importance cannot be overstated as we could argue that it is via the socialization process that we learn how to be human. In the ideal situation, every child would be raised in a loving and nurturing familial environment. This was certainly a central point of Aristotle's *Nichomachean Ethics*. Unfortunately, this is not always the case, as far too many children are neglected, abused or abandoned. The topic of family abuse is far too serious and extensive to be reviewed here but suffice it to say that child abuse may take many forms with the most common (and relevant variation of interest to us in this book) being child neglect. Child neglect refers to the failure of caregivers to provide adequate emotional and physical care for a child. Horrific examples of neglect involve cases of children being deprived of meaningful contact with other humans, children being tethered to a bedpost, underfed and undernourished, and children who are physically beaten.

In extreme cases of child neglect, a child may be abandoned and left to survive, or die, on his or her own. Studies of feral children (children raised in social isolation without human contact or who receive minimal human contact from a very young age) reveal just how important the socialization process is. Although documented cases of feral children are very rare, they are quite profound nonetheless. When a feral child is raised by animals, he or she may exhibit (within certain physical and mental limits) behaviors similar to those of the care-animal (Benzaquen 2006; Newton 2002; Harlan and Pillard 1976). One documented case of a feral child involves Ivan Mishukov, an abandoned Russian child who was protected by a pack of stray dogs and who came to learn to howl and bite when humans attempted to separate him from the dogs. Born in 1992 in Reutov, Russia, Mishukov left his home at age 4 so that he could avoid continued child abuse at the hands of his mother and her abusive boyfriend. For two years Ivan lived with a pack of stray dogs in Moscow. Relying on the limited language skills he had developed before he became abandoned, Mishukov would beg for food and share it with the dogs. In turn, the dogs would protect him from human and other animal threats. On several occasions police attempted to separate Ivan form his pack of dogs. But Ivan refused to come forward and the dogs would viciously guard him. The police then set up a meat-bait trap in the storage room of a restaurant where the dogs searched for leftovers. After the dogs were trapped, social workers rescued the boy, who howled and attempted to bite them. Ivan was quarantined in a children's home where he received medical and psychological treatment (Whitehouse 1998). This story highlights the fact that without human socialization from intimate caregivers, Ivan took on the features of his adopted family—a pack of dogs. Ivan was lucky to have had some human experience before isolation as such children are more easily rehabilitated after being rescued. Mishukov did successfully acclimate back to back into human society, he learned to speak intelligently, and later served in the Russian Army.

Many child-development theorists believe it is critically important for certain aspects of human development to be nurtured in infancy (Levine and Munsch 2016; Steinberg, Bornestein, Vandell and Rook 2011; Masten and Gewirtz 2006; Elkind 2001; and Farran and Haskins 1980). As Turner (2006) explains, "Human potentials that are hard-wired into our neuroanatomy must be activated within a certain timeframe; if they are not activated, it will be difficult to acquire in full human measure those capacities that make us human and allow us to participate in society" (p. 119). Socialization, then, becomes a critical, if not *the* critical, aspect of human development.

Theories and Human Development

The previous discussion of neglected and feral children highlights the nature-nurture continuum regarding how human development occurs. Biology (nature) certainly dictates a number of physical attributes (e.g., skin color, hair color, eye color, ancestry, and genetic markers that may indicate potential hereditary health disorders) and plays a role as to whether an individual is physiologically capable of learning, but does it dictate human behavior? Sociologists and other social scientists believe that socialization, past experiences, modeling and motives—in short, the environment (nurture)—most significantly influence human behavior. It is helpful to think of social forces and natural innate traits, in terms of their significance for human behavior, as two ends of a "nature-nurture continuum." Both forces play a role in human development; in philosophy there tends to be, as with Aristotle, an emphasis on nature, but in sociology the pendulum swings toward nurture.

A number of significant theories have been developed over the past few centuries in an attempt to explain how human development occurs. In the following pages we will take a quick look at a couple of theories that lean toward the nature side of the continuum and a couple of theories that lean toward the nurture side of the continuum.

Sigmund Freud and Psychoanalysis

Sigmund Freud (1856–1939), who developed a theory of psychoanalysis, proposed a theory of human development centered on how the individual personality develops. His model of personality is based on the concept of a dynamic unconscious, which gives rise to drives, instincts, and urges that are nearly uncontrollable. Freud believed that the personality is composed of three aspects: the id, the ego and the superego. The "id" (Latin for "it") is totally unconscious of, or unconnected to, a controllable consciousness and is consumed with satisfying basic human drives, or instincts. An instinct is an innate impulse, or tendency to act, that is common to a given species. Whether humans possess instincts is a matter of debate, but for Freud, among the chief instincts are the need for sexual gratification and our natural aggressive tendencies (Freud 1989). The id is what accounts for the young child being so self-centered and preoccupied with immediate gratification, even at the expense of the needs of others. As children age, their instincts become suppressed by societal expectations of proper behavior, an idea reflected by Freud's concept of the "superego" (Latin for "above or beyond the ego"). The development of the superego as a personality trait means that individuals have learned to impose self-control and conform their behavior to the rules of society. Freud's use of the concept of the "ego" (Latin for "I") reflects the manner by which individuals seek to balance the needs of the id within a superego framework.

At one time, psychoanalysis was a very popular theory in human development. Today, it is not.

Jean Piaget and Cognitive Development

In contrast to Freud's psychoanalytic theory, which emphasizes the importance of unconscious thoughts, cognitive theories highlight conscious thoughts (Santrock 2007). Cognitive-development theories are aptly named because the cognition itself involves the mental process of knowing and includes such aspects as perception, awareness, reasoning, judgment, and learning. The leading proponent of the cognitive-development perspective is Jean Piaget (1896–1980). Piaget ([1936] 1952, 1954) proposed that every child goes through four stages of development, each associated with increasingly complex cognitive abilities to learn and reason. The first stage of development is the sensorimotor (from birth to age two) wherein the child is still in the sensory phase—his or her understanding of the world is limited to direct contact, such as sucking, touching, listening, or looking. At this stage, infants do not know that their bodies are separate from the environment and they are unable to recognize cause and effect (Flavel, Miller, and Miller 2002). By age two, the child should have developed simple problem-solving skills, such as how to find a toy that is not immediately available (Gunter, Oates, and Blades 2005).

The second stage of development is called the preoperational (ages two to seven) and at this stage the child learns to understand and articulate speech and symbols, progressing from basic words and phrases to lengthy sentences, as well as gaining the abilities to read and write. The concrete operational stage (ages seven to eleven) is the third step in cognitive development according to Piaget. At this point, the child is capable of performing specific (concrete) tasks that involve basic formulas, such as mathematical calculations. The child is also replacing intuitive thought with logic and reasoning so long as they are applied to concrete examples. Children at this age are also capable of playing team games. The final stage of cognitive development is the formal operational stage (ages twelve through adolescence). During this final stage, children have learned to think abstractly and to use logical deductive skills and reasoning. The adolescent is capable of looking at a problem, thinking of courses of action, and deciding which course of action might be best.

Cognitive-development theories such as Piaget's reflect the definition parameter of socialization as a learning *process*. The word "process" is important as it implies development occurs as a result of a systematic series of actions and that the situation is on-going. In the decades since Piaget first proposed his theory, critics have pointed out that not all children follow this script of development as some children may, for example, lack the physiological or mental capacity to develop at a "normal" pace. In addition, it is not difficult to argue that some adults, let alone teenagers, lack—or at least do not make use of—the ability to think abstractly (stage 4).

Social Learning Theory

Scientists and social thinkers who believe that human behavior is not scripted based on innate, natural causes (nature) put forth the notion that human behavior is not fixed or predetermined but instead is a matter of freewill (nurture). This freewill notion does not ignore the fact that social structures and achieved and ascribed statuses may limit the choices available to each of us.

Proponents of the social learning perspective focus on the process of learning itself; that is to say, how does learning actually occur? The most common variation of social learning theory states that learning is a three-step procedure that entails critical aspects: acquisition, instigation, and maintenance. *Acquisition* refers to the initial introduction of a behavior; *instigation* occurs when the individual actually participates in some form of behavior; and *maintenance* refers to the repetitive and consistent participation in a behavior over a period of time. An individual initially learns of a behavior either through direct interaction with others, wherein such behavior is reinforced, or indirectly through observation. As a result, human development occurs because of environmental experiences.

Social learning takes place through two primary methods: conditioning and modeling. Conditioning is a learning process whereby individuals associate certain behaviors with rewards and others with punishments. Reinforcement is used as a powerful tool in human development as it attempts to influence individuals to conform to specific norms and values. Individuals also learn behavior through observation and modeling. Observing how others behave represents a learning opportunity via modeling. Many people choose friendship groups based on conditioning and/or modeling opportunities. Group behavior that is deemed rewarding is likely to be continued whereas group behavior that is deemed to be too costly (e.g., in time commitments or because of negative experiences) is likely to be suspended. An examination of your own friendship groups can be tested based on the social learning theory perspective.

Symbolic Interactionism

Symbolic interactionism is a sociological theory based on the premise that social reality is constructed in each human interaction through the use of symbols. Symbolic interactionism was created by Herbert Blumer in 1937 but made famous by George Herbert Mead (in his posthumous publication *Mind, Self and Society*) and continues to remain a top sociological theory due to the research of a slew of contemporary social thinkers. While Mead—like other social learning theorists—acknowledges the role of social forces from social institutions and organizations on individuals and the ascribed and achieved statues of individuals, he believes that humans have the capacity to think and decide on their own how they should act in a given situation and they react on the basis of their perceptions and definitions (Cockerham 1995). Mead felt that social experience is the sum total of dynamic realities observable by the individual who is a part of the ongoing societal process (Kallen 1956).

The concept of "self" and all the other related off-shoots of "self" (e.g., development of self, self-esteem, and self-concept) is very important to symbolic interactionists due to their focus on micro behaviors. Mead believed that the self, which is essentially an object to itself, is basically a social structure that arises from social experience. Borrowing from John Locke's usage of the concept *tabula rasa*, Mead insisted that a baby is born with a "blank slate" (not literally blank, of course, as a child is born with a vast number of instincts), without predispositions to develop any particular personality. The personality that develops is a product of that person's interactions with others. Mead described the self as composed of two parts: the "I" (the unsocialized self) and the "me" (the socialized self). Both aspects of the self are part of an individual's self-concept (Cockerham 1995). The "me" is the judgmental and controlling side of the self that reflects the attitudes of other members of society, while the "I" is the creative and imaginative side of the self (Pampel 2000). The combining of the "I" and the "me" leads to the creation of individual personality and the full development of self (Pfuetze 1954).

The development of self is critical for the creation of consciousness and the ability of the child to take the role of the other and to visualize her own performances from the point of view of the others. The development of self, then, represents the human development aspect of symbolic interactionism. According to Mead, there are four stages to the development of self: imitation, play, game, and generalized other.

1. Imitation Stage—Born with a "blank slate" implies that babies must learn everything, including the basics such as grasping, holding and using of simple objects such as spoons, bottles, and blankets. As their physical and mental skills further develop, they learn to play with objects by observing and imitating their parents/caregivers. For example, a parent might roll a ball to the infant and encourage the child to roll it back. The infant is capable of under-

standing simple gestures and begin to imitate the behaviors of others. While imitation is a simplistic form of behavior, it represents the earliest stage of learning and development.

2. Play Stage—At this stage of development the child learns to use language and comprehends the meanings of certain symbols. They are capable of *acting out* the roles of others and their imaginations allow them to pretend to be that person (Pampel 2000). While at play, the child will try to use the tone of voice and attitudes of whom he is "playing" (Mead 1964). The child has learned to take the role of specific others, an important step in the development of self.

3. Game Stage—At this stage, the child is now capable of putting herself in the role of several others at the same time and to understand the relationship between those roles. Mead used the game of baseball to illustrate his point. When the ball is hit, the fielder must make the play, but he must also know the role of his teammates in order to understand the game complexities as where to throw the ball if there are already runners on base, and so forth. Understanding the roles of others is just one critical aspect of the game stage. Knowing the rules of the game marks the transition from simple role taking to participation in roles of special, standardized order (Miller 1973).

4. Generalized Other—The final stage of development involves individuals being able to take on the role of the greater community or society as whole (the generalized other). There are times in life when individuals come to realize that they need to act in the best interests of others, to do the greater good for the greater number of people. At this point of development, the individual not only identifies with significant others (specific people), but also with the attitude of a society, community, or group as a whole. The ability of individuals to adopt the attitude of the generalized other is what allows for diverse and unique persons to share a sense of community.

Mead also discussed the importance of "the act." To act implies that the individual has undertaken some sort of social action. Social action is the critical element in forming friendship groups. Social learning may involve conditioning and modeling (as articulated by the social learning perspective) but individuals must still act, make a move, toward joining or forming a friendship group. Mead identified four basic and interrelated stages in the act.

1. Impulse—The impulse involves "gut" reactions or immediate responses to certain stimuli. It refers to the "need" to do some-

thing. For example, if the child is bored and sees a group of other children playing, he becomes stimulated by the activity.

2. Perception—The individual must know how to react to the impulse to act. The individual assesses the situation the best she can to ascertain whether or not taking social action is warranted, safe, or worthwhile.

3. Manipulation—Now that the impulse has been manifested and the object (e.g., a playgroup discovered) has been perceived, the individual must take some action with regard to it (Ritzer 2000). The individual walks over to the playgroup and asks to join in.

4. Consummation—At this, the final stage, the individual has taken a course of action and consummates the act by participating in group activities.

Interestingly, Mead described "the act" as involving one person while the "social act" involves two or more people. Initiating social action is the key to forming or participating in friendship group activities.

Agents of Socialization

It is the socialization process that leads to the development of friendship groups. There are a number of key agents of socialization that assist in the development of friendships. Agents of socialization include, among others, parents and other close family members, peer groups, schools, the mass media, religion, employers, and the government. For nearly everyone, parents and close family members and/or peer groups are especially important in the development of friendship groups. Many other people find closeness with members of their own religions and/or coworkers. The mass media and the government often influence the way in which we view the world and consequently impact our friendship circles. For all of us, the most important agent(s) of socialization are those that are most highly revered and trusted. They are primary groups.

The Primary Group

Socialization is most effective in primary groups. Charles Horton Cooley (1864–1929) was the first social theorist to describe primary groups (and to also contrast them with secondary groups). Cooley (1909) describes primary groups as "those characterized by intimate face-to-face association and cooperation.... The result of intimate association, psychologically, is a certain fusion of individualities in a common whole, so that one's very self, for many purposes at least, is the common life and purpose of the group" (p. 23). These associations are primary in several senses, but chiefly in that they are fundamental in forming human nature. Cooley was trying to show that even though we are born bound to our natural self, in the end our true goals are aimed to help the whole. The result of primary group association leads to a shared sense of "we-ness" among group members wherein mutual identification for which saying "we" is a natural expression. For example, this can be seen when one person is asked what he/she did over the past weekend and the other responds, "we all...."

Cooley's idea of the "primary group" was influenced by William Graham Sumner's distinction between the "in-group" and the "out-group" (an example of "we" and "them"). What draws one to a particular group involved a moral unity. Ferdinand Toennies had distinguished between *gemeinschaft* (a type of society or social setting characterized by intimacy, closeness, strong emotion, cooperation, and common values and beliefs) and *gesellschaft* (a type of society or social setting characterized by formality, emotional reserve, superficial relations between individuals, and a lack of universally agreed upon values and beliefs).

Sharing fundamental components of Aristotle's view of friendships, Cooley described *primary groups* as intimate, face-to-face groups that play a key role in linking the individual to the larger society. The primary group is relatively small, informal, involves close personal relationships and has an important role in shaping the self (similar to gemeinschaft). In contrast, secondary groups (or secondary friendships) involve a collectivity whose members relate to one another formally and impersonally (similar to gesellschaft). In our later discussion on categories of friends we can see how most "regular friendships" fall into the secondary group category while most "good" and "best" friends qualify as primary group membership.

Cooley detailed five fundamental properties of the primary group:

1. Face-to-face association (close physical proximity)
2. Unspecified nature of associations (group members do not need an excuse to get together as it is expected that they will get together to join in group activities)
3. Relative permanence (group participation and membership will continue indefinitely)
4. A small number of persons involved (it is counter-intuitive to think that there can be large numbers of people who can all remain close to one another)
5. Relative intimacy of participants (closeness breeds understanding of one another)

Similar to Aristotle, Cooley stated that the most important primary group is the family because it is the earliest and most basic grouping of social unity. The playgroups of peers in childhood become the second source of primary groups for most people. Throughout our lifetimes, if we are lucky, we will possess at least one key primary group whom we can depend on and with whom others can count on us to always be there for them. Cooley also noted that a neighborhood or community group is important for elders as they will become increasingly dependent upon one another. Nonetheless, primary groups are especially important for children as it helps them to develop a sense of self. "The self develops in a group context, and the group that Cooley called the primary group is the real seat of self-development" (Reynolds 1993:36). Secondly, they provide the initial source of socialization and interaction with the larger society. Cooley (1909) insisted that primary groups are fundamental in forming the social nature and ideals of the individual. Primary groups provide children with their first experience of interacting in the social world. Successful socialization occurs when the child learns to behave and interact "properly" in the larger society (Delaney 2004).

Primary groups include individuals with whom we form our closest relationships and, because of this, individuals learn to share their expectations with one another (Meltzer, Petras, and Reynolds 1975). These close relationships give individuals a sense of "we" or belonging; an element that is critical to their sense of self. As Cooley (1909) explained, "The group self or 'we' is simply an 'I' which includes other persons.... One identifies himself with a group and speaks of the common will, opinion, services, or the like, in terms of 'we' and 'us'" (p. 209). The group self or "we" can only be understood in relations to the larger society, just as the "I" can only be understood in relation to other individuals in the primary group. Although those relationships can change, the bond for a "common spirit" remains, which makes it difficult to sever ties with our primary groups (Cooley 1909). Interestingly, Cooley believed that in order for individuals to grow, new primary groups must be sought out. This helps to explain why high school buddies find a new primary group in college, another primary group after college, and perhaps another one or two more throughout the life cycle. Some people will be lucky enough to maintain friendship groups through all stages of human development. What is most important for one's sense of self, identity, and well-being, is to be sure to always have at least one primary group association.

We can conclude our discussion on the importance of primary group participation by restating that Cooley felt it important for individuals to form primary groups wherein the expression of "we" is natural. Humans do this despite their instinctively and initially bounded selfishness. Thus, Cooley believed that individuals are born with biological needs that must be fulfilled; yet the fulfillment of these needs can only be met through group participation. Cooley (1909) stated that the most important primary groups are the family, good and best friends (peers), and the immediate community or neighborhood. Dependence on a group leads to mutual appreciation among group members. Group membership becomes a valued commodity, and the opinions of primary, or friendship group members, understandably, are very important.

Categories of Friends

Friendships involve an association of people who share a sense of intimacy, feelings of affection, or dispositions. They consist of people who refer to themselves as friends and as such are linked, or bonded, by expressions of harmony, accord, understanding and rapport. Friends come in a variety of types and categories but are generally viewed as those who are attached to one another by feelings of affection or personal regard, those who provide assistance and support to one another, are on good terms with one another and who may share certain attributes such as religious and cultural affiliations or those who share a common interest such as music or favorite sports team.

Some friendships are likely to stay in one category indefinitely as they fit the needs of the friends involved. For example, many of us have "work friends"—those with whom we are friendly toward while at work—and we are quite content with keeping it that way as we have no desire to spend time with them outside of work. This corresponds to Aristotle's concept of "friends of utility." Some friendships, however, grow from the casual to the very close (best friends), or what Aristotle called "friends of the good." But the nature of friendship seems more complex than the trifold categorization employed by Aristotle: friends of utility, pleasure, or the good. The type of friendship one has with others depends on the people involved, their expectation level, their needs, and how much time and effort they are willing to spend on nurturing and devotion to the friendship. Other friendships may start out as good friends but over time those involved begin to drift apart. In other words, friendships are fluid and subject to change for any number of reasons.

Aristotle argued that there are only three categories of friends, those of utility, pleasure and of the good. In the contemporary era we recognize a wider variety of types of friendships. In the following pages, we will discuss some of the more common types of face-to-face friendships (we will discuss types of electronic friends in Chapter 4).

Casual Friends

There are many characteristics of a "friend" including the idea that this is a person whom you know and presumably like and trust, one who supports you in a time of need, one who cheers you on as you attempt some goal; and yet still is someone who may "bust your chops" and bring you back down to reality when you get a little too full of yourself. Friends are so important that there are well over 100 slang words used to describe them. In fact, the *Online Slang Dictionary* (2016) lists 139 slang words for "friends." Here are some examples: ace, ace buddy, bitch, bof, boo, bra, bro, brohan, brohanski, brother, brother from another mother, bruddah, bruh, bud, cat, chica, chicka, chum, cousin, crew, cuz, dawg, dog, dogg, Ese, fam, fella, flatmate, g funk, girl, habib, hobo, hoe, home boy, home girl, home skillet, homey, homie, kemo sabe, kid, man, my boy, pal, partna, partner, peaches, pimpette, pookie, posse, potna, raw dog, road dawg, road ho, rock, roll-dog, sista, sister, sister from another mister, son, sweetie, thick, thick as thieves, thug, top dog, weezy, and wingman (*Online Slang Dictionary* 2016).

All face-to-face friendships share the implied assumption that you've actually spent time together and bonded to some degree (or as Aristotle would put it, "shared salt" with one another). A casual friend would be someone with whom you do spend some face-to-face time with but yet this person is not really close to you and your encounters with one another are friendly but not very intimate. In contrast, friends of a more intimate nature tend to be placed in such categories as "close friends" or "best friends." Casual friends may come and go while closer friends may remain in your circle of acquaintances for an extended period of time, perhaps even a lifetime. Casual friends may slowly fade away and yet in other instances, such friendships may end spectacularly. Research shows that the quickest way to end a friendship is because of betrayal, where the trust necessary for a continuing relationship is shattered (Creedon 2001).

Close Friends

A step above the "casual friend" is the "close friend." Close friends may also be known as "good friends," but we will use the term "close friend" as that category of friends that falls in-between casual friend and best friends. A close friend is someone you would consider part of your inner circle. Cherie Burbach (2016), a self-described "Friendship Expert," describes close friends as those "people who know the most about your life, and have likely been through a few ups and downs with you. You may have several friends and one or two people you would consider 'good friends.' Good friends are generally those you see and talk to the most often." From this quote, we can note that Burbach seems to use close friends and good friends interchangeably. We agree with Burbach that we are more intimate with close friends than we are with casual friends and that we are likely to have shared some ups and downs with close friends. However, we disagree with her conclusion that we are likely to have just one or two people we would consider close friends. Such a quantitative limitation is reserved for the "best friend" category.

As described in the Preface, the authors conducted original research on friendship and happiness topics. The first question we asked our respondents (190 students from both a private college and a public university) was, "How many close friends do you have?" For males, the data revealed that the most common response was 4 close friends (14 respondents; 17.72 percent). However, the second most common response was a tie between 6 close friends and 11 or more close friends (15.18 percent), with one respondent claiming he had 75 close friends (see Table 2.1). For females, the most common response was 5 close friends (32 respondents; 29.09 percent), followed by 6 close friends (19 respondents; 17.11 percent). Nine female respondents reported that they had 11 or more close friends, with one female reporting 25 close friends (see Table 2.1).

Table 2.1: Number of Close Friends by Gender, Number and in Percent

Males (N=79)			Females (N=110)		
# of Friends	*Respondents*	*Percent*	*# of Friends*	*Respondents*	*Percent*
0	0	0.00	0	0	0.00
1	1	1.26	1	0	0.00
2	5	6.33	2	5	4.54
3	11	13.92	3	10	9.09
4	14	17.72	4	12	10.90
5	5	6.33	5	32	29.09
6	12	15.18	6	19	17.11
7	2	2.53	7	5	4.54
8	6	7.59	8	5	4.54
9	0	0.00	9	0	0.00
10	11	13.92	10	13	11.81
11+	12	15.18	11+	9	8.18

Good friends are people we are close with in a limited scope of life scenarios (compared to the best friend). Thus, a close friend might know a great deal about certain aspects of your life (e.g., your work life, love life, or family life) but, would not know as much about you as a best friend (who would know about all, or nearly all, the major aspects of your life).

There are many subcategories of "close friends" including the following:

- The Old Friend—An old friend is someone with whom you have developed a lifelong bond that can be revitalized whenever the two of you get together again. Just being with each other stirs fond feelings and cherished memories (Creedon 2001). The old friend may also be known as the "long-time" friend, a person you've known most of your life, or for a long portion of your life, and therefore you have quite a bit of knowledge of each other.

- The Older Friend—Someone your senior who often serves as a mentor by sharing their wit and wisdom with you. Author and columnist Mitch Albom illustrates this mentor/friendship relationship in his best-selling book *Tuesdays with Morrie*.
- The New Friend—An interesting type of close friend as they can generally do no wrong, that is, perhaps, until you have spent sufficient time with them and realize they are not as perfect as you once believed. The new friend is valued because they interact with you based on their current knowledge of you rather than your past history—a history that may include baggage you have attempted to leave behind you. Creedon (2001) explains, "New friends are more likely to enjoy your stories and show up on time. It's also easier to be who you are with a new friend, as opposed to who you *were*— which is what you end up being most of the time with your old friends."
- The Wild Friend—Many of us have that person in our life that can best be described as "The Wild Friend"—the friend whose bad behavior never ceases to entertain and yet may inspire, or lead to, trouble (e.g., barroom fights, arrests, or a bachelorette party out-of-control). The wild friend often receives a bad rap, but many people, especially those who lead boring, conventional lives, are in great need of wild friends (Creedon 2001). They add spice to one's existence.
- The Scary Friend—A friend who not only nudges you out of your comfort zone, but also engages in behaviors that really concern you. One of the authors of this book once woke up in bed with his girlfriend (during his undergraduate years) only to find his college roommate (and friend) standing over them with a samurai sword and a scary-looking smile saying, "I will protect you both!" It was never clear what we needed protection from but protection from such a roommate would be a good place to start.
- The Confidant—A friend who manages to get more information out of you than you planned on sharing. Unfortunately, many confidants are also talented gossips who may soon share your deepest secrets with someone else (Creedon 2001). This is especially the case when it comes to social media.
- The Dormant Friend—This friend is different from the "old friend" in that the dormant friend is someone you dropped from your close circle of friends and yet every now and then reappears in an attempt to spring to life a dead friendship. "The reawakened friendship speaks to the mystery of friendship in general—especially if you've forgotten why you drifted apart. But give it time; you *will* be reminded" (Creedon 2001).

It is the "close friend" category of friendship that is perhaps the most important to us and our analysis of the connection between friendship and happiness in life. According to Reach.Out.com (2016), "The better the quality relationships you have the more likely you are to be happy. Therefore it's good for your happiness to be a great friend to someone and to have a group of good friends supporting you." Close friends, then, can bring you happiness. We propose that the more close friends you have, and the better the *quality* of these friendships, the more likely they are to bring you happiness. This will be explored in more detail in our later discussion of happiness in chapters 6 and 7.

There are many qualities of a close friend including the following provided by ReachOut.com:

- Someone who shows loyalty
- Someone who will support you no matter what
- Someone you can trust and who won't judge you
- Someone who won't put you down or deliberately hurt your feelings
- Someone who is kind and has respect for you
- Someone who will love you because they choose to, not because they feel like they should
- Someone whose company you enjoy
- Someone who will stick around when things get tough
- Someone who makes you smile
- Someone who is there to listen
- Someone who will cry when you cry (ReachOut.com 2016).

In our own research, we asked college students to name some qualities of a close friend. Their responses often included the same qualities described above by ReachOut.com but were far more varied. While we separated responses from males and females there was, as expected, a clear overlap in shared views of what qualities constitute a close friend. (See Table 2.2 for our survey results.)

Table 2.2: Qualities of a Close Friend by Gender

Males	*Females*
* Hard working	* Trustworthy
* Can share anything	* Dependable
* Funny	* Funny
* Drink together	* Respectful
* Supportive	* Honest
* Hang out when bored	* Faithful
* Trustworthy	* Available
* Nice	* Nice
* Respectful	* Nonjudgmental
* Sympathetic	* Loyal
* Outgoing	* Kind
* Fun to be with	* Enjoy company

Males

* Easy going
* Similar interests
* Good listener
* Trust worthy
* Dependable/Reliable
* Loyal
* Not an asshole
* Caring
* Allows me to vent
* There in thick and thin
* Honest
* Open-minded
* Helpful
* Light-hearted
* Understanding
* Empathetic
* Enjoys good music
* Friendly
* Consistent
* Understands you
* Back-stage behavior
* Cool
* Not an idiot
* Inquisitive
* Similar interests
* Exciting
* Easy to talk to
* No hidden agendas
* Gives good advice
* Can ask anything of them and vice versa
* Help you when you are in trouble
* Doesn't make you feel bad about yourself
* Can ask anything of them and vice versa

Females

* Understanding
* Caring
* Reliable
* Relatable
* Real with me
* Kind
* Smart
* Easy-going
* Listens
* Gives advice
* Help during hard times
* Makes me laugh
* Insightful
* Responsible
* Outgoing
* Supportive
* Common interests
* Positive
* Smart
* Helpful
* Compassionate
* Well-rounded
* Fair
* Same hobbies
* Good listener
* Good morals
* Open-minded
* Intelligent
* Motivating
* Generous
* Stern and firm
* Understanding
* Optimistic
* Sweet
* Has your back
* Confident
* Kind
* Nice
* Understands my flaws
* Cares about my well-being
* Doesn't leave you hanging
* Gives you space when needed

There is a solid link between friendship and happiness. A sampling of the research on friends and happiness is provided here. The World Health Organization (WHO) (2016a) reports that the environment and our personal circumstances are determinants of health. "To a large extent, factors such as where we live, the state of our environment, genetics, our income and education level, and our relationships with friends and family all have considerable impacts on health, whereas the more commonly considered factors such as access and use of healthy care services often have less of an impact" (WHO 2016). The National Institute on Aging (NIA) (2009) reports that one person's happiness triggers a chain reaction that benefits not only their friends, but their friends' friends, and their friends' friends' friends, with the effect lasting for up to a year. In their article appearing in the U.S. National Library of Medicine National Institutes of Health, Helliwell and Huang (2013) report that "the number of real-life friends is positively correlated with subjective well-being (SWB) even after controlling for income, demographic variables and personality differences. Doubling the number of friends in real life has an equivalent effect on well-being as a 50% increase in income. Second, the size of online networks is largely uncorrelated with subjective well-being. Third, we find that real-life friends are much more important for people who are single, divorced, separated or widowed than they are for people who are married or living with a partner."

In our own research on college students, we asked participants if, overall, they were happy with the quality and quantity of their close friendships. Overwhelmingly, both males (92.4 percent) and females (91.9 percent) responded that they are happy with the quality of their friendships (see Table 2.3). Among the comments we received from males who were happy with their friendships are:

- My close friends are important to me and they are the greatest people I know
- My close friends have proven themselves [to me] over time.
- They treat me well
- Yes, quality is better than quantity

Among the comments made by female respondents who are happy with the quality of their friendships include the following:

- I love the traits of my close friends
- They are caring and there for me
- We are all different but, open-minded and respect each other's opinions
- They are a shoulder to cry on and the first people I tell when I have good news

Among the comments from males who were not happy with the quality of their friendships are:

- Some of my close friends do not always have my back
- I wish some of my friends had interests similar to mine

Among the comments from females who were not happy with the quality of their friendships are:

- Our personalities don't really match, I settled.
- Sometimes they are dishonest.
- Sometimes I wish I had a stronger group of friends.

**Table 2.3: Are You Happy with the Quality
of Your Close Friendships? by Gender, in Percent**

Males (N=79)		Females (N=111)	
Yes	92.4	Yes	91.9
No	7.6	No	8.1

We also asked participants about the quantity of their close friendships and whether they were happy with the number of friends they had (see Table 2.4). Both male and female respondents made comments centered on the idea that they only need a few close friends; that having too many friends is a burden because of the inability to spend quality time with large numbers of friends; that it is easier to communicate with friends when they are fewer in number; too many close friends makes life complicated and adds too much drama to one's own life; and that their needs are met with the number of friends they had. Perhaps summing up the sentiment of those respondents happy with the quality of friendships and sharing the belief that fewer "real" friends are better than "fake" friends is this quote, "I'd rather have 4 quarters than 100 pennies!"

The few respondents that indicated they were not happy with the quantity of their friends stated that they wish they had more friends to hang out with to do more things.

**Table 2.4: Are You Happy with the Quantity
of Your Close Friendships? by Gender and in Percent**

Males (N=78)		Females (N=109)	
Yes	93.6	Yes	91.7
No	6.4	No	8.3

With our discussion on close friends completed, we turn our attention to best friends.

Best Friends (BF)

Casual friends and close friends are important to us for a variety of reasons, but it is the select few that can claim the title and sentiment expressed by the term "best friend." The best friend is the "gold standard of friendships" (Creedon 2001) and relates to what Aristotle calls "friends of the good." Best friends possess all the qualities of "close friends" but much more. They are the friends we are very close to; they are our confidants; they are the people we can count on at all times including the good and bad, sad and happy, excited and bored, or when we just want to hang out with someone who will understand us.

In our own research, we asked college students to name some qualities of a best friend. Their responses did include many of the same qualities attributed to close friends but a number of other unique comments (see Table 2.5). While we separated responses from males and females there was, as expected, a clear overlap in shared views of what qualities constitute a close friend. See Table 2.5 to see the answers provided by respondents to the question, "What characteristics does your best friend(s) possess?"

Table 2.5: Characteristics of a Best Friend by Gender

Males	*Females*
* Very supportive	* Understanding
* Primary confidant	* Fun to be with
* Great to be around	* Passionate
* Nice person	* Has your back
* Reliable, there for me	* Caring
* Sympathetic	* Tolerant
* Trustworthy	* Trustworthy
* Honest	* Always there for you
* Easy to talk to	* Similar leisure interests
* Easy-going	* Similar world views
* Respectful	* Honest
* Similar interests	* Kind
* Fun to be around	* Reliable
* Dependable	* Adventurous
* Non-judgmental	* Outgoing
* Always has my back	* Non-judgmental
* Creative	* Considerate
* Loyal	* Realistic
* A bit reckless	* Loyalty
* Honest	* Supportive
* Smart ass	* Loving
* Long-time friend	* Positive
* Love of sports	* Smart
* Loves to play sports	* Generous
* Cynical	* Chill
* Generous	* Highly motivated
* Gives good advice	* Good listener
* Joke around with	* Resilient
* Like-minded	* Accepting
* Supportive	* Open-minded
* Political	* Sweet
* Snarky	* Will protect you
* Not superficial	* Funny

(Males)

* Inclusive
* Smart
* Talented
* Kind
* Chill
* "He's my boy!"
* Sarcastic
* A giving person
* Similar Interests
* Checks up on you
* Does favors
* Doesn't judge me
* Funny
* Goal-oriented
* Adventurous
* Honest
* Dependable/Reliable
* Set of personal values
* Outgoing
* Good sense of humor
* Crazy

(Females)

* Intelligent
* They know your secrets but friends anyway
* Sweet
* Reliable
* Candid
* Smart
* Athletic/into sports
* Candid
* Happy
* "Ride or die"
* Down to earth
* Loud
* Sarcastic
* Never get bored with them
* Accepts me as I am
* Sometimes a pain in the ass
* Willingness to help you at your worst
* No words need to be spoken
* Can laugh or cry with them
* Makes you feel appreciated
* Brutally honest when need be

According to the *Urban Dictionary* (2016a), a *best friend* is someone you can be yourself around and not give a care in the world about your actions or feelings because they will not judge you for the stupid things you may do or say. For example, you can wear your most comfortable clothes, no matter how old, torn or trashy they appear; you can eat junk food together without receiving any guilt; and you can enjoy favorite passions (e.g., watching B-movies like *Sharknado* or enjoying trashy reality TV shows). Having a best friend is also a critical element in our pursuit of happiness. (Note: See "Popular Culture Scenario 2" for a look at best friends on TV and in the movies.)

As with the term "friend" there are many slang terms used to describe a "best friend." The most commonly heard terms are "bestie" (an adoring nickname for one you hold in the highest esteem) or BFF (best friends forever). There are well over 100 slang terms for "best friend" and while the sex of the BF is not always important when categorizing these nicknames, *Hub-Pages* (2015) provides a list based on gender. Among the nicknames for guys are: amigo, bambino, big guy, braniac, bro, bub, bubba, bud, buddy, chico, chip, chipmunk, con, cowboy, doobie, freak, goob, gordo, guapo, mack daddy, moose, muggie, pickles, psycho, sherlock, slick, slim, sport, stud, superman, tank, tough guy and vito. Among the nicknames for gals: Amiga, amour, beautiful, belle, biffle, bitch, boo, buttercup, cheeky, chica, cinnamon, cookie, cupcake, cutie, darling, diamond, dimples, doll, dolly, flower, foxy lad, foxy mama, gams, juicy, lovely, pookie, princess, sassy, senorita, shorty, sugar, sunshine, toots and tootsie.

A best friend is cherished because this person is someone you can have a good time with, but is also someone who will be there for you when you are in the greatest need of comfort and companionship. You can trust a best friend with your life because, as the expression goes, they would take a bullet for you rather than see you in pain. A best friend is someone with whom you have secret "in" jokes and someone with whom you have shared stories untold to others. A best friend can make you smile without trying. You trust them and they trust you (*Urban Dictionary* 2016a).

By implication, it is nearly impossible to have more than one best friend in your life at any give time; after all, the word "best" means just that—the *best,* the most critical, the most important of all friends. While some people may go through life with one special BFF, it is more common for people to have different besties throughout their life course. The designation of someone as your best friend can be tough on other very close friends who might think of you as their best friend. Consequently, a number of people will claim to have more than one best friend. For example, a best friend from one's youth may be replaced by someone who has grown closer to you in adulthood and, yet, when these childhood best friends get together their feelings of closeness may resume and they embrace the best friend category once again. Incidentally, if you have a best friend, June 8th is the day designated as "National Best Friends Day!"

Table 2.6: Number of Best Friends (BF) by Gender, Number and in Percent

	Males (N=79)			Females (N=111)	
# of BF	Respondents	Percent	# of BF	Respondents	Percent
0	4	5.06	0	4	3.60
1	27	34.17	1	24	21.62
2	14	17.72	2	47	42.34
3	8	10.12	3	24	21.62
4	9	11.39	4	6	5.40
5	10	12.65	5	2	1.80
6+	7	8.86	6	4	3.60

In our own research, we asked participants how many best friends they had (see Table 2.6). As the data in Table 2.6 indicates, the most common response for males was one best friend (34 percent) and the second most common response was two best friends (18 percent). To the surprise of the authors, many males reported having three, four, five or six or more best friends; the highest number of best friends claimed by a male respondent was ten. For females, having two best friends was the most common (42 per-cent) and one or three tied for the second most common response (22 per-cent). A far lower percentage of female respondents (11 percent) than male respondents (33 percent) claimed to have four or more best friends; one woman did claim to have 11 best friends.

Table 2.6 reveals that four males and four females claimed to have zero best friends. In all but two cases these eight respondents reported that they were not happy with their current friendships; in the other two cases, two female respondents stated that they could not possibly choose between all their friends and designate one as the *best* friend.

Working with the premise that someone can only have one "best" friend, we asked survey participants to explain if they responded to having more than one best friend. The most common response indicated that one best friend was a relative (e.g., brother, sister, or parent) and the other(s) were non-relative friends. The second most common response involved respon-dents saying they like having a male and a female best friend so that they could better understand both males and females. As our survey was con-ducted on college students it was not surprising that a number of respondents said that they had a best friend at school and one "back home." Another fairly common explanation centered on the idea that one best friend was the person they were dating and the other best friend(s) were friends outside of dating.

If you have a best friend, and whether it's June 8th ("National Best Friends Day!") or not, you might want to get a tattoo with them. The best friend tattoo has become an increasingly popular way to express your feelings of closeness with your BFF. It would be a good idea to first assess whether or not you think the friendship is deep enough to warrant the rite and, second, you have to then find the perfect symbol to forge the bond (Wortham 2016). "Instagram and Pinterest are awash with ideas: Beavis and Butthead, two halves of an avocado, yins and yangs that nestle when two arms are pressed together" (Wortham 2016: 21). While matching tattoos are a reflection of the times in which we live, they do not ensure the longevity of a friendship and having half of matching tattoo of a former BFF might be awkward when con-sidering doing it again with a new BFF. The best friend tattoo gone bad is similar to the tattoo of a former lover that the new lover must always endure. The authors have met some people who have had a list of names of former lovers inked somewhere on their bodies. Perhaps is just a matter of time before we see the same thing again with BFFs.

Now that we have discussed "casual" friends, "close" friends and "best" friends, we can turn our attention to a few other categories of friends, many of which overlap with the three previously discussed types of friends. One of the more interesting of all other categories of friendship is "frenemies."

Frenemies

A frenemy (sometimes called a "frienemy") is a blending of the two words "friend" and "enemy" that has a dual meaning to either an enemy who pretends to be your friend or someone who is a real friend and yet also a rival—such as teammates on a sports team who are friends but competing for the same starting position. While people have dealt with frenemies throughout history, it's only been in the past decade or so that the term "frenemy" has become popularized.

Dictionary.com (2014) defines frenemy as a person or group that is friendly toward another because the relationship brings benefits, but harbors feelings of resentment or rivalry. *The Free Dictionary* (2016b) defines a frenemy as a person who is ostensibly friendly or collegial with someone but who is actually antagonistic or competitive; a supposed friend who behaves in a treacherous manner; and as a person who is considered as both a friend and a rival. The *Urban Dictionary* provides a variety of interpretations of what a frenemy is, including: fake friends you have for selfish purposes—a perspective that reminds us that while we may see others as potential frenemies, we too can be the frenemy and we would do so in order to gain something (a type of friend of utility); friends you know, but who you don't really like and don't really like you either; and friends you make that were once enemies because you're planning on stabbing them in the back.

The world of popular culture provided us with a great example of frenemies with the 2016 film *Captain America: Civil War*. In this film, superheroes who are supposedly friends took sides on a matter of public interest and fought against one another. Apparently, quite a few of these superheroes had their tights in a bundle as there existed a great deal of tension and animosity between the heroes. And, just like in real life, mutual friends of the frenemies (the viewing audience) were forced to take sides on who to cheer for. This idea made many fans of the individual superheroes very uncomfortable.

In our survey of college students, we asked participants if they had a frenemy. Nearly 32 percent of males and 24 percent of females responded "yes" (see Table 2.7).

Table 2.7: Do You Have Any "Frenemies?" by Gender and in Percent

Males (N=79)		Females (N=111)	
Yes	31.6	Yes	24.3
No	68.4	No	75.7

We also asked respondents, "If you have a frenemy, why do you hang out with this person(s)?" The most common response for both males and females centered on the idea of competition; usually friendly competition, and generally in the sports arena. In other cases, frenemies are tolerated because they are a part of a larger friendship group. A sampling of comments from male respondents included the following:

- To improve my skills and competitive spirit
- He is my cousin and I like competition
- Similar friend group
- Sometimes I hang out with him to keep the peace
- To be better than him
- I live with this person, we get along sometimes, other times we want to fight each other

Female respondents offered far more diverse comments than the males in our survey but they still included the ideas of competition and keeping the peace among a larger friendship group as key aspects as to why they hang out with frenemies. Here is a sampling of female survey respondents:

- Teammates are often frenemies
- There is a feeling of competition when we do something together
- She is my roommate
- To keep the peace
- We are in most of the same classes together so I cannot escape her and yet we do our homework together and study together
- Because my other friends are friends with her
- We were best friends as kids but all we've done since then is compete for boys
- We have fun together, I just can't trust her
- Because our moms are friends
- It's easier to be her friend than to be her full-time enemy
- We've known each other for a long time and the good out-weights the bad

Perhaps reflecting on the question "Why do you hang out with person(s) [frenemy]?" a bit more, one female respondent said, "I'm not sure."

Given that nearly one-third of males and one quarter of females in our survey admit to hanging out with a frenemy, this would seem to be a topic worthy of further future examination. While our survey involved college students only, we did speak with many non-college students about the topic of frenemies and found that some people tolerate frenemies because their school-aged children are friends. Many people are put in a situation where they have to associate with their co-workers because of employment requirements. Older adults often commented to us that it would seem odd to "break up" with a friend that they had for so many years but then acknowledged that the concept of a frenemy did indeed characterize their friendship. And, like college students, many adults told us that they maintain a relationship with frenemies because of the greater circle of friends in the friendship group.

While frenemies are people whom we consider to be friends but don't always enjoy hanging out with, the next category of friends we will examine are friends we really do enjoy spending time with because of the intimate benefits they provide us. This category of friends is known as "friends with benefits"; a category of friends that might fit Aristotle's concept of "friends of pleasure."

Friends with Benefits (FWB)

When we (the authors) were kids, "friends with benefits" might include someone with a swimming pool, a big backyard, or someone with the largest toy collection in the neighborhood. But "friends with benefits" is an adult category of friendship and as we all (presumably) know, we're talking about "sex buddies." Friends with benefits involves two friends (or perhaps more than two depending on the friends) who have a sexual relationship without being emotionally involved with other aspects typical of an intimate relationship such as monogamy and explaining their whereabouts or daily activities to one another. For single people, having friends with benefits is a great way to achieve happiness. Of course, as most people understand, whenever sex is involved in a relationship of any kind, things tend to eventually get complicated.

Gayana Sarkisova (2012) offers some advice to people who want to have a friends with benefits relationship via "10 Commandments to Being Friends with Benefits":

1. They Shall Not Fall in Love—Falling in love with a sex buddy will change the dynamics completely.
2. Thou Shall Not Text unless it's a Sext—Keep the conversations related to sex.
3. Thou Shall Not Go on a Date with a Friend with Benefits—Again, keep the activities related to sex only.
4. Thou Shall Not Introduce Them to Friends—Do not cross the line by introducing your sex buddy to your friends or family.
5. Thou Shall Keep the Door Open for New Relationships—A sex buddy is best kept as a temporary fix to fulfilling sexual needs until a "real" relationship begins.
6. Thou Shall Not Get Jealous—Remember, the relationship is based on sex only; if the other person moves on, let them go.
7. Thou Shall Know the Difference between a Back-Up and a FWB— A back-up friend is someone you have likely never slept with, you

are friends, your friends and family may know of them, and some day, you may end up in a relationship with them. But, this person is definitely not a FWB.

8. Thou Shall Not Cuddle—The beauty of a FWB relationship is that the normal relationship rules do not apply—keep it that way.

9. Thou Shall Not Be a FWB with an Actual Friend—This is a gray area because becoming friends with a FWB is a major step in changing the relationship.

10. Thou Shall Follow All of these Rules—Anyone who's been in a FWB relationship knows these commandments to be true!

The expression "best friend with benefits" was popularized by a line in Alanis Morissette's "Head Over Feet" song from her 1995 *Jagged Little Pill* album. The song is about best friends who are also lovers with Alanis thanking her sex buddy for his manners, love and devotion. The friends with benefits mantra has also been extended to the world of popular culture in other ways including a movie and TV show of the same name—*Friends with Benefits*.

Friends of Friends, or Secondhand Friends

Friends of friends are an interesting category of friends in that you may find such people to be just as cool as your original friend or you may find you cannot tolerate them and despise sharing your friend time together with "secondhand friends." Creedon (2001) adds that "when someone introduces you to someone else, supposedly because they think you'll hit it off, it could be a clever strategy to ditch you both. Which is good [as] secondhand friends are a better deal than new friends." You may find that you have more in common with a friend of the friend than with your actual close friend. Initially, you are likely to discuss the mutual friend but eventually it may morph into a true friendship and you both move on from the original friend (Friedlander 2014). In this regard, the original friend becomes an ex-friend.

Ex-Friend

As explained by the *Urban Dictionary* (2016b), an ex-friend is someone you were once friends with, but you are no longer friends with, usually due to some kind of an argument and/or betrayal of trust. The idea of ex-friends, or unfriending, is very relevant in the electronic world, especially Facebook (see Chapter 4). The nature of the reason for friends "breaking up" dictates the level of disdain ex-friends may have for one another. A best friend who stabs his friend in the back by "stealing" his girlfriend away via lies and other manipulations is the lowest of the low and the target of emotions that can include hate. Conversely, friends who simply drift apart from one another because each has developed interests that are no longer mutual are likely to hold no grudges against one another (a point, as we say earlier, that Aristotle would consider to be a natural progression).

If ex-friends who parted in less than pleasant circumstances cross paths with one another a great deal of emotion is likely to be let loose. After all, we expect far more from our close and best friends than we do from strangers. The ex-friend who feels betrayed is likely to experience feelings that are less than civil but it is best to either try to avoid talking to that person or, at the very least, try to be a bigger person. Being civil might be difficult, especially if you want to rip his/her head off, but in the long run, that is the best course of action. Ex-friends that you bump into that parted in a more civil manner should be treated accordingly. Sincere inquiries about their lives is a good course of action. Ideally, civil ex-friends will avoid slandering one another, kept long-held secrets, and if it is reaffirmed that the friendship is truly over, just move on.

Bromance Friends

The term "bromance" is a blend of bro (a slang term for males who are best friends) and romance (an interest in another person beyond the platonic). A bromance is a close nonsexual friendship between men (*Merriam-Webster Dictionary* 2016a). The *Urban Dictionary* (2010) has a variety of entries on the meaning and characteristics of a bromance including the following:

- A complicated love and affection shared by two straight males.
- A non-sexual relationship between two men that are unusually close that involves the act of wooing for the purpose of becoming closer; going to unusual lengths in an attempt to become closer with another male friend.
- A close relationship between two bros to such a point where they start to seem like a couple.
- A strictly non-sexual relationship between two completely heterosexual men that are close and enjoy each others company but still enjoy the company of women.

A bromance then, is a highly-formed friendship between male friends. And while such relationships have likely occurred throughout history (think of Meriwether Lewis and William Clark or John Adams and Thomas Jefferson), only recently has the term "bromance" come into existence. Whether or not Aristotle would consider "friends of the good" to constitute a "bromance" remains an open question!

Work Friends

We spent more awake time with work friends than we do with most of our close or best friends or spouses. If for no other reason then, it is important to have work friends as it makes the environment seem more pleasant. Employers tend to like work friendships too as it creates a sense of camaraderie and comfort (Sanacore 2014). "The key to the development of work friendships is the same as developing personal friendships. Allow the friendship to develop naturally and organically. Given the fact that so much of our time is spent with our coworkers, it's a natural development to recognize those folks you want to legitimately become friends with versus those with whom it's better to just remain friendly" (Sanacore 2014). Sanacore provides a few pros and cons of workplace friendships. Pros include:

1. They [coworkers] often see you at your worse (e.g., the breakup of a marriage, the loss of a family member).
2. They celebrate your birthday and anniversary (there's always cake at work!).
3. They share a common sense of purpose and truly understand what your work is all about (friends and family may not have a clear idea as to what your work entails).
4. They promote creativity (when it's easy to talk to your coworkers it's easier to brainstorm new ideas).

The cons of workplace friendships include:

1. Work can become unprofessional.
2. Backstabbing can happen (because coworkers can learn about your vulnerabilities).
3. Lack of work-life balance (friends at work may not get any work done if they spend too much time socializing with one another).

Because we spend so much time at work it is easy to confuse work friends with real friends. Alexandra Levit (2011) provides us with a list of some good questions to ask ourselves in order to determine whether a work friend is really a real friend. Here is a sampling:

- If your friend left the company, would you still be in touch with her in a year?
- If you had a personal emergency, would you consider asking your friend for help?
- Have you met your friend's significant other or her other close friends outside of the office?
- If your work friend received a promotion that you too were up for, would you be genuinely happy for her?

- If you ran into your friend in the grocery store, would you be able to talk to her for 10 minutes without mentioning work?
- Do you and your friend have anything in common besides your job?

Having friends at work is generally a positive experience and can help you attain overall happiness. However, most work friends are not good or best friends. They seem to fall within the category of what Aristotle would call "friends of utility."

Single-Modifier Friends

The single-modifier friend is a peculiar person in that they find the need to qualify a friendship with a modifier such as, "This is my gay friend Harry" or "This is my straight friend Paul." In most instances of friendship there is no need to add the modifier. If the person being introduced is indeed your friend, just introduce them as your friend. The use of the single-modifier is often equated to saying something like, "some of my best friends are..." in an attempt to inoculate oneself against negative labels such as being a racist. Most people begin to roll their eyes the moment they hear a sentence that includes the "some of my best friends are..." as it appears to indicate that the person really *is* a racist.

Nonetheless, using the modifier approach may have its benefits. In a study conducted on 450 Americans, it was revealed that the mere mention of minority friends can reduce how racist a person seems to be toward that minority group (Chokshi 2016). Research conducted by Thai and associates (2016) found that referenced minority friendships help to reduce the negative reactions from others when someone expresses prejudiced attitudes. The study involved "White and Asian participants being presented with a Facebook profile depicting a White target who posted an anti–Asian statement. Being depicted with Asian friends (Study 1) or even verbally claiming that they had Asian friends (Study 2) reduced attributions of racism irrespective of whether they were being evaluated by White or Asian observers. Furthermore, the presence of Asian friends made the conceivably racist comments seem relatively benign, and observers were less offended and upset by them. The data suggest that minority friendships can partially offset costs associated with expressing prejudice" (Thai, Hornsey and Barlow 2016).

There are other instances when using the single-modifier to introduce a friend may be appropriate. Consider for example, you are having a discussion with a group of people on the history of the American Civil War when your friend Chris, a history professor, enters the room and you say, "This is my friend, history professor Chris." Of if you are having a discussion on the wear and tear of playing football when your NFL friend Donovan joins the group and you introduce him by saying, "This is my friend, the football player, Donovan."

It is, perhaps, the friend who uses the single-modifier approach to introduce all types of friends that becomes truly annoying.

Special-Interest Friendships

A number of friendships are formed around a shared passion or interest, such as music, cultural heritage, sports, or shared experiences. This is understandable when we consider that our identities and sense of self are shaped by our passions. Music, for example, has the ability to draw people together simply by sound, a sound that is appealing to the listener. It makes sense that people who enjoy the same type of music then automatically have a connection. Followers of the Grateful Dead have long shared a kindred spirit. Research has been conducted that shows the connective bonding ability of music. Selfhout and associates (2009) found that similarity in music preferences is related to friendship formation and yet differences in music preferences was not related to friendship discontinuation. Thus, sharing a passion for similar music is enough to help created a friendship but formed friendships are generally not in jeopardy due to different musical tastes. Ariel Zambelich (2014) conducted a review of research on music and friendship and found that: (1) A 2007 study had strangers meet in a chat room with the only instruction being to learn about one another. After analyzing the transcripts, the researchers found the most common topic, by far, was musical preferences. (2) A 2003 study found that people link musical genres to their personality characteristics. (3) Several studies have found an agreement about various stereotypes of music fans (e.g., Top 40 fans are outgoing; heavy metal fans have bad moods; and classical music listeners are more likely to enjoy a glass of wine than smoke weed. (4) A 2011 study on dorm roommate preference among college students found that similar musical tastes help to make roommates closer. So, if you've noticed that your best friends like the same music as you do, you can attribute music to be a contributing factor. Then again, if your best friends do not share the same musical tastes, such a difference alone is unlikely to cause your friendship to dissolve.

People who share the same ancestry and find themselves being raised in a foreign country often bond with one another. Nearly every major city has a "Chinatown" or a "Little Italy." Ethnic neighborhoods such as "Little Odessa" in Brighton Beach, New York or "Little Saigon" enclaves in many American cities are just a few examples of ethnic neighborhoods that foster friendships based on traditional customs and behaviors. In 2007, the Syracuse newspaper *The Post-Standard* ran a feature column on how three girls from

South Korea—who nicknamed themselves SOY, which stands for "Souls of Yellow"—bonded together via various adoption support groups (there is not a large Korean population in Syracuse). One of the girls, Kasey Buecheler, was taking Korean dance classes because she hoped to attend college in South Korea. Another girl, Allie Leogrande, was a cheerleader. And yet, interestingly enough, they all shared the third girl's (Theresa Rutkowski) love for Korean pop music (Korean boy bands) (Lee 2007). Their heritage combined with music helped these three girls forge a solid friendship.

The adoption support groups that the three Korean girls shared to help forge a friendship is just one type of support group that helps people. The National Down Syndrome Society (NDSS), for example, helps students with Down Syndrome become more acclimated as such students are increasingly being taught in mainstream schools. Most schools work very hard to assure an educational experience of inclusion but support groups such as the NDSS help fill the voids. Successful inclusion in the schools will help children with Down Syndrome do better with their academic pursuits but also makes it easier to form friendships with other school children (Cuckle and Wilson 2002). The NDSS (2012) also supports parents of children with Down Syndrome and these parents in turn often become friends because of their shared special interest.

Surviving tragic events can help the survivors forge friendships with each other. The people of the greater New Orleans area, including parts of Mississippi, who survived Hurricane Katrina can recollect that deadly storm, the damage it caused, and share in stories of survival. One horrific story of survival involves the children, parents and teachers at the Resurrection Catholic School in Pascagoula, Mississippi. "Churning waters 4 feet high carried a mix of raw sewage and mud through the classrooms … ripping maps and posters off the walls and consuming shelves of textbooks as floodwaters rose" (Neus 2015). When the parents and teachers discovered the extent of the damage to the school after the roads reopened they described it as a surreal experience. But they were undaunted in their shared desire to reopen the school. Six miles away, the storm destroyed St. Peter the Apostle Catholic School, a historically black elementary school. The children from St. Peter joined the children at Resurrection following its renovation. Bonds of friendship centered on a commitment and a shared interest, and helped turn this tragedy into a success.

An interesting example of a friendship formed based on a shared interest involves the distinction between "drinking buddies" and "friends." *Drinking buddies* are those folks who, as implied, spend a great deal of time drinking at some bar. ("Drug buddies" is essentially the same thing as a drinking buddy, only these friends take drugs other than alcohol together.) These drinking buddies might not even recognize one another outside of the bar and do not meet most other qualifications to be considered friends. Drinking buddies can be dangerous as they can only relate to you over alcohol. They will attempt to coerce you into further drinking, especially when you start to suggest that it is time for you to "clean up" (Sober Bastard 2012). This seems closest to what Aristotle would call a friend of pleasure, the pleasure in this case being the shared love of intoxication. True friends will support your decision to quit drinking, or to at least sober up and dry out. When it comes to friendships and losing friends, one of the saddest things to witness is the close friend who needs to go to rehab but refuses to do so. One cannot help but think of the immensely talented, yet very troubled, Amy Winehouse who wrote a song called "Rehab" (on her critically acclaimed second album, *Back to Black*, 2006) during a dangerous period of taking drugs and alcohol, with song lyrics that included, "They tried to make me go to rehab. I said, no, no, no. Yes, I been black. But when I come back, you'll know, know, know. I ain't got the time. And if my daddy thinks I'm fine. He's tried to make me go to rehab, I won't go, go, go." Her management company had tried to get Winehouse to enter rehab but instead she dumped the company and wrote the song "Rehab." And according to the Academy Award-winning 2015 documentary *Amy,* her own father did indeed discourage her from going into rehab when she needed to do so. The singer died tragically in 2011, at the age of 27, from accidental alcohol poisoning.

Interestingly, if a person with a drinking problem attempts to clean up by attending a treatment program they may form friendships with others in the program. These are known as "Treatment Friends." The treatment friend may become as dependent on others as the drinking buddy but eventually are likely to experience the same fate, a passing friendship.

Other Friendships

We did not attempt to provide an exhaustive list of categories of friendships but we feel as though we have discussed the vast majority of the important ones. Friedlander (2014) in her listing of 21 types of best friends does include a few others worth, at the least, mentioning including: the free spirit best friend; the imaginary best friend; the best friend that's your twin; the best friend that's your opposite; the Debbie Downer best friend; the antisocial best friend; and, the know-it-all best friend. We would like to also acknowledge the numbers of college students who join fraternities and sororities as they find a closeness of friendship that leads them to using descriptions such as "brother" and "sister" to describe fellow members. The "Greek" system of fraternities and sororities is designed to create a "we" feeling and many participants find lifelong friends via such an association. There are also people who think they are your friends but they really are not your friends from your perspective. This confusion over the nature of one's relationship can cause much drama, which is yet another reason why having a good sense of where one stands in connection to another is so important.

Characteristics of Friendships

Throughout our discussion on the categories of friendships a number of positive characteristics of friends were provided. Among the key characteristics are: loyalty; intimacy; a shared "we" feeling; feelings of affection and caring; providing expressions of harmony, accord, understanding and rapport; showing support no matter the circumstances; trustworthiness; judgment free; will not deliberately hurt your feelings; kind and respectful; enjoys your company; makes you smile; sticks around when things get tough; listens; cries when you cry; would rather take your pain than see you in pain; a confidant of shared stories and experiences; and, shares similar passions. *Ellie Bean Design* (2013) published a list of 11 characteristics of a true friend, some of which we have already covered, but others which are worth mentioning here: dependable; honest; gives you space; always keeps in touch; does not gossip about you; supportive; and giving. The ability to keep a secret is another fundamental characteristic of a good friend as well. (Note: We will discuss secrecy within the context of the Facebook status "It's Complicated" in Chapter 4.)

Although it would seem unnecessary for true friends to need codes of behavior that involve the inclusion of many of the characteristics of friendship described above, a number of codes of friendships—especially those based on one's sex and the perceived corresponding expectations of behavior based on one's gender—have been created. Let's take a brief look at some of these codes.

Codes of Friendships

Codes of friendships, such as the "Bro Code," represent quasi-desperate attempts by friends (mostly single people) to hold on to their friendships, especially in light of the "threat" of that friend spending an increasing amount of time with a dating/marriage partner.

We begin our discussion on codes of friendships with the "Bro Code" as, presumably, most readers have heard of this unofficial doctrine of how men are supposed to keep their male friendships intact and as a top priority even when they are dating (or married). According to the *Urban Dictionary* (2013a), the "Bro Code" refers to a set of rules meant to be guidelines to live by between Bro's—the rules were originally unwritten but because it's been deemed that so many men no longer act like real men, the Bro Code now appears in written form. (Yes, it would seem as though the Bro Code is an attempt by reactionary men to maintain certain traditional ideals of how a man should act.) There are nearly 200 Bro Code rules with the #1 rule— "Bro's before Ho's." This #1 rule is specifically designed to keep male friendships intact and to reinforce the idea that a bro should put the needs of his follow bro ahead of that of a woman (Ho). Listed below are a few of the rules in the Bro Code that come from the "official" Bro Code (2016) handbook:

1. Bro's before ho's—A "ho" is any woman that is not your wife or any other direct family member.
4. Whether a Bro is into sports or not, a Bro picks a team and supports them until his dying breath.
8. Bros do not share dessert.
9. A bro never dances with hands above his head.
11. A bro will not sleep with another bro's sister. However, a bro is allowed to be vocal about her attractiveness.
14. When using urinals, a Bro stares straight ahead AT ALL TIMES.
20. A bro never applies sunscreen to another bro.
32. A bro ALWAYS enhances another bro's job description when introducing him.
43. A bro never wears socks with sandals.
63. No sex with your Bro's ex. It is never permissible for a bro to sleep with his bro's ex.
76. A bro always has his bro's back.
110. A bro does not cock-block another bro for any reason.
147. A bro never tickles another bro.
163. Bro's don't giggle.
184. Bro's do not keep a personal diary.

Fans of the TV show *How I Met Your Mother* (2005–2014) have undoubtedly heard of the character Barney Stinson (Neal Patrick Harris) and his constant usage of "The Bro Code," a variation of a code of conduct for bros described above. Harris, under the pen name Stinson, along with Matt Kuhn published a book titled *The Bro Code* (2008). The book mostly discusses bro code rules but introduces the idea of a "Chick Code" in Article 22—"There is no law that prohibits a woman from being a Bro." Among some of the rules expressed in the "Chick Code" are:

- A chick shall not sleep with another chick's ex-boyfriend, unless she does.
- A chick never pays for anything. Ever.
- If a chick hears a chick-empowerment song like "I Will Survive,"

she shall stop whatever she's doing, grab another chick's hand, and shriek the lyrics at the top of her lungs.
- If two chicks are wearing the same outfit, each retains the right to accidentally spill a drink on the other.
- A chick has a free pass to slut it up on Halloween.

Although not as popularized, or elaborate, as the bro code, there do exist female equivalents (other than the "Chick Code") to friendship codes for women. The *Urban Dictionary* (2013b) describes a "Broette Code" but that pertains mostly to women who hang out with guys and act like one of the guys. In this sense, a "broette" is a chick who is like a bro to you; she is the female equivalent of a bro who participates in bro-like activities. It would appear that the biggest concern among women who care about a female code of friendship is coming up with a term opposite of "Bro's before ho's." Among the examples we found: "chicks before dicks"; "sistahs b4 mistahs"; "bows before bows"; "locks before cocks"; "busts before thrusts"; "biscuit before brisket"; and "PJ's before BJ's" (Quora 2016). Writing for the website Pop-Sugar.com, Annie Gabillet (2009) asked readers "to come up with a woman's version of the douche bag rallying cry, 'bro's before ho's.'" Among the responses were: "lasses before asses," "Venus before penis," "dolls before balls," "hos before bros," "ladies before maties," and "besties before testes."

While some people might find these codes of friendships important, most are likely to place a higher value on the previously discussed characteristics of friendships.

The End of Friendships

Over the course of a lifetime we will lose many friends, including some good friends and some best friends. While we are enjoying close friendships with others it seems inconceivable that such a relationship will ever end. And yet, they do. This is explained, at least in part, by the realization that despite how important friendships are, they take a back seat to romantic partners, our children and, in many instances, close family members (especially those in need of a great deal of attention and assistance, especially if medical issues are involved). Romantic relationships, for example, alter friendships because far more energy is exerted on a romantic partner than on a friend. Thus, while it is possible to go months without ever seeing or talking to a good friend, we would not go that long without maintaining other voluntary bonds such as marriage or a romantic relationship. Research has found, however, that "individuals who are not in co-resident partnerships found that some actively decentered their sexual relationships in favor of friendships" (Cronin 2015).

We should recall the earlier discussion on our natural inclination to form groups and the role of socialization and especially the primary component of socialization that it is a life-long process of developmental changes. Whenever we speak of a process, we are speaking of something fluid and ever-subject to change. And that's what happens to us all. People come and go from our lives for a variety of reasons.

The introductory story of this chapter pointed out that children can lose a best friend because adults make decisions that children have no control over. Nikki and her former best friend did nothing wrong, they did not "fall out of friendship" like some people "fall out of love." Variables beyond their control intervened and cost them a trusted friendship. And yet, when the new family moved into the home of the former best friend, the children involved were able to become new best friends. The adults in this situation did not have as easy a job of a transitioning to best friends as such things are generally tougher for adults due to a variety of variables that may interfere (or assist) in friendship formation.

The voluntary nature of friendship also makes such relationships subject to life's whims in a manner that other relationships are not. Thus, one can choose to enter into a friendship relationship and one can just as easily choose to exit a friendship relationship (Beck 2015). We can choose to leave a friendship for a variety of reasons. The friendship of two close friends with the same political perspectives can be threatened when one of them changes and joins the rival political party. The behaviors (e.g., a "free spirit" when it comes to fidelity in a relationship; a constant flirt; getting drunk every weekend; or regularly taking drugs) of a friend once tolerated when they were both younger can now form a schism between the two.

Interestingly, revealing your insecurity about your relationship (friendship or romantic) to others, especially the friend/partner involved, has the potential to generate a whole new kind of insecurity—the concern that those individuals perceive you to be an insecure person. Insecurities, which also includes being passive aggressive, can contribute to a relationship breakup (Joel 2015).

From childhood, to high school, to college or the military, to starting a family and starting a career, to retirement, and any other major life event in between, we are constantly going through changes. It stands to reason that friendships will also have to adjust to these life changes as well. In short, when priorities and responsibilities change, so too do most friendships.

In our survey, we asked respondents to provide some reasons why they had a friendship(s) that ended (see Table 2.8). As the information in Table 2.8 reveals, friendships end for a variety of reasons including some of the classic explanations such as, the friends grew apart, issues of dishonesty and distrust arose, and because the friend betrayed them (e.g., slept with their significant other).

Table 2.8: Reasons Why Friendships End by Gender

Males

* He slept with my girlfriend
* We grew apart
* Attended different colleges
* Moved away
* Different hobbies
* Different social circles
* Different goals/interests
* Stopped liking each other, over time
* Started a family
* New job
* Neglect, did not work on friendship
* The other became a "jerk"
* Inconsiderate
* Self-centeredness
* Drugs/Alcohol use/abuse
* Untrustworthy
* Not genuine
* I'm hard to get along with
* Talked about me behind my back
* We both changed
* Different political stances
* Relationship became static
* Because of a girl
* Distance
* Disagreements
* Dishonorable actions
* Grew apart due to priorities changing
* Money
* Lack of communication
* Their morals changed
* Not enough time to hang out
* They got into drugs
* One of us said something we shouldn't have
* Life takes you in a different direction
* He got addicted to coke and used his friends instead of being a friend
* Different hobbies
* Different mutual friends

Females

* Disloyal
* Grew apart
* Changed geo location/Distance
* The friendship required too much effort
* Mutual changes in interests/ ideologies
* Dishonest
* She slept with my boyfriend
* People change
* Lost contact with each other
* Miscommunication/lack of communication
* Lying
* Not trustworthy
* Betrayal
* Selfish friend
* Being taken advantage of
* Rude behavior of friend
* Self-centered, friend became
* Too much drama
* She caused too many problems
* One person just stopped giving an effort
* Made new friends
* Different interests
* Someone else picked me to be her best friend
* Different schedules
* Other person changed for the worse
* An argument was never resolved
* Negative mindset, of the other
* Talks behind your back
* Friendship was toxic
* Too busy, to maintain friendship
* Back-stabbed
* They were haters, liars, two-faced, or dumb
* Because of boys
* My aspirations were not respected
* Hurt my self-esteem
* Rumors/gossip
* Jealousy
* Friend became mean

(Males)

(Females)

* Friend was too pessimistic for me
* Took advantage of me
* Mean
* Took too many risks
* They didn't put equal effort into the friendship
* Rumors that they believed
* They were bullies to me/other friends
* Boyfriend/girlfriend choices
* (From the one who said she had 11 best friends): I have lost a few friends because they got upset over time that I did not spend enough time with them (I was too busy), which made them feel as though I didn't care about them enough

---

Popular Culture Scenario 2: Best Friends on TV Shows and Movies

The popularity and commonality of having friends, and for most people, to have more friends than close family members, underscores the reality that friendship is a theme in nearly every television show or movie. When we look at television shows, then and now, we can see that a close buddy was an underlining theme in non-animated as well as animated shows. For example, in the 1960s, Fred and Wilma Flintstone had Barney and Betty Rubble as best friends on *The Flintstones* and Ralph and Alice Kramden had Ed and Trixie Norton as best friends on *The Honeymooners*. In the contemporary era, Peter and Lois Griffin have Joe and Bonnie Swanson as best friends on *The Family Guy*, while on *The Big Bang Theory*, Leonard, Sheldon, Howard and Raj are male best friends along with Penny, Bernadette and Amy as female best friends.

One of the more popular TV shows of the '90s and early '00s is *Friends*—a show so blatantly about friends they used "friends" as the show's title. *Friends* was centered on six main characters that were, of course, all friends—Rachel, Monica, Phoebe, Joey, Chandler and Ross. Limiting our discussion to "best friends" on TV shows and movies yields us the realization that such a subject area has been used in the title. On TV, there was a show entitled *Best Friends Forever*. This show lasted just one year—far less time than the typical BFF relationship. There have been a variety of film variations with "Best Friends" as the title including the 1975 film starring Richard Hatch, Susanne Benton, and Doug Chapin; the

1982 film that starred Burt Reynolds, Goldie Hawn and Jessica Tandy; the 2005 variation starring Claudette Mink and Megan Gallagher; and the 2016 *Best Friends Recycled* film starring Marcy Conway, Donald James Parker and Diana Lenska.

Undoubtedly, readers have their own favorite TV show or film featuring best friends. Writing for *Glamour* Magazine, Hannah Lyons Powell (2014) created a list of the Top 25 "Ultimate TV & Movie BFFs":

1. *Absolutely Fabulous*; Patsy and Eddie
2. *Boy Meets World*; Cory, Topanga and Shawn
3. *Bridesmaids*; Annie and Lillian
4. *Buffy The Vampire Slayer*; Buffy, Willow, and Xander
5. *Dawson's Creek*; Pacey and Dawson
6. *E.T.*; Elliot and E.T.
7. *The Fresh Prince of Bel-Air*; Will and Carlton
8. *The Gilmore Girls*; Rory and Lorelai
9. *Harry Potter*; Harry, Ron and Hermoine
10. *Now and Then*; Roberta, Teeny, Samantha and Chrissy
11. *One Tree Hill*; Brooke and Peyton
12. *Romy and Michelle's High School Reunion*; Romy and Michelle
13. *The O.C.*; Ryan and Seth
14. *Top Gun*; Goose and Maverick
15. *Toy Story*; Woody and Buzz Lightyear
16. *The X-Files*; Mulder and Scully
17. *Friends*; Monica, Chandler, Rachel, Ross, Phoebe and Joey
18. *Sabrina The Teenage Witch*; Sabrina and Salem
19. *Girls*; Hannah, Shoshanna, Jessa and Marnie
20. *Clueless*; Dione and Cher
21. *New Girl*; Jess, Cece, Schmidt, Nick and Winston
22. *Gossip Girl*; Serena and Blair
23. *Saved by the Bell*; Jessie, Lisa, Kelley; Slater, Screech and Zack
24. *Mean Girls*; Janice and Damian
25. *When Harry Met Sally*; Harry and Sally

What, no *Thelma and Louise* or *The Walking Dead*!? The authors would pick *Seinfeld* and the best friends of Jerry, Elaine, George and Kramer and *Boston Legal*'s best friends Alan Shore and Denny Crane as other excellent examples. Who would you pick as the best TV show or movie about best friends?

Summary

In this chapter we learned about the value of group formation and its role in the survival of humanity. The socialization process and theories of human development were also discussed to demonstrate how people form groups for both survival and social purposes. The agents of socialization and, in particular, primary groups were revealed as the key component in the development of friendship groups.

A number of categories of friends and friendship groups were discussed, starting with regular friends, good friends and best friends. A large number of subcategories of friends from these three major categories were revealed. A number of other categories of friends, including friends with benefits, friends of friends (or secondhand friends), ex-friends, bromance friends, work friends, single-modifier friends, and special-interest friends, were also discussed. In addition to the discussion of the types of friends was a presentation of the many character traits associated with friendships. The chapter concluded with some examples as to why friendships end. Throughout the chapter we presented data results from our own original research.

3

Cyber Socialization

The Transitional Step
Toward Electronic Friendships

Does it seem like the world is becoming increasingly impersonal? We are all being socialized by the various institutions of society, our peers and even our family members into conducting everyday activities online rather than through more personal ways such as face-to-face interactions and conversations. Consider these scenarios. Calling someone on the phone rather than texting them is likely to lead to an opening statement like, "Why are you calling me?" And if you leave someone a voice message they might snap and say something like, "I don't listen to my voicemails, what did you want?" Of course, at that point you will have to repeat yourself because they haven't listened to the voicemail. Send someone a text and they might interpret a "tone" in your message that simply was not intended and when you explain yourself they might respond by saying, "Well, use some emoticons next time and then I'll know."

Did you ever go shopping at a store and receive a receipt only to have the cashier say to you, "If you go online and fill out a survey you might win $1,000"? She assures you it will only take a minute or two. "Can't I just answer the survey now with you and you can let me know if I won the $1,000?" "Of course not," she replies. Now that you are thinking about money matters and making purchases, you may say to yourself, "I wonder what my credit/debit card balance is?" before you attempt your next purchase. To find out the answer to this question you must go online and communicate electronically with a machine rather than a live person. And trying to get a hold of a live person at most corporate headquarters is extremely frustrating and impersonal as you must go through a series of prompts that will connect you in the right direction. It might even be impossible to get a human being on the line rather than a human-sounding soothing machine voice. In fact, almost all basic information must now be attained online.

If your internet connection or WiFi stops working and you call the provider, you are likely to get a message that says something like, "For faster service use our website at...." Want to call for a cab, pizza delivery, or order tickets to a ballgame? Just do it online please. Walk into a bank to conduct some simple banking activity such as cashing a $100.00 check or making a simple deposit, and you are likely to wait at least 5 to 10 minutes to be served only to have the bank attendant say, "You know, you could've done this at the ATM outside." Reply by saying, "What, you don't want to see me?" and observe their confusion. View a commercial on TV by a drug company that purports to provide some potentially life-saving drug only to hear at the end, "Go to our website to learn more." I want to learn more *now*! Hear a news report during your favorite primetime TV show or while listening to the radio that warns, "A dangerous felon has escaped and may be lurking in your neighborhood. Tune in tonight at 11 p.m. or go to our website to learn more." Chances are, you will want to know more about this dangerous felon now and not at 11 p.m.

Just like every scenario described above, and countless more, if the information is important enough to you, you will indeed go online. We go online for so many things now because we are being socialized into a cyberworld that increasingly dominates our daily activities. Then again, if you need information on things as varied as how to tie a tie or how to fix a leaky faucet, you can go to YouTube and view a "How-to-Video." So, it's not all bad. Welcome to the machine, you are now a part of it.

In this chapter, we will learn about the cyber socialization process and how this relates to friendship. Cyber socialization developed for a number of reasons but especially because of the development of communications technology and the rise of the Internet and the changing cultural norms and values that encourage impersonal forms of communication.

The Development of Communications Technology and the Rise of the Internet

We have established that people have formed groups and friendships throughout the history of humanity. Primitive friendships were primarily centered on basic survival needs. By the time of Aristotle, humans had evolved enough to develop friendships for three primary reasons. As we learned in Chapter 2, the contemporary era is exemplified by many different categories and subcategories of friendships—and this does not include our yet to be discussed concept of electronic friendships (also known as e-friends). We are being socialized by both the traditional agents of socialization and by cyber (electronic) technology into accepting that the way of the world is now dictated by computers and impersonal forms of communications. And for the most part, people are willingly going with the flow.

The cyber socialization process is aided tremendously by the exponential advancements in technology. *Technology*—the branch of knowledge that deals with the creation and practical use of technical means to solve problems or invent useful tools—is stimulated by progressive, creative thought that allows for the invention of new skills and expertise in the many spheres of social life, including forms of communications. It is the area of advancements in communications that is of relevancy to us here as this branch of knowledge is important in the continued development of cyber socialization. But how did we get to this point wherein computers and electronic friendships have come to dominate our way to thinking? After all, for most of history nearly all friendships were limited to face-to-face relationships. The answer to this question, as you might have guessed, has a great deal to do with the development of advanced forms of communications that better assisted people in their attempts to keep in touch with one another despite their lack of close proximity.

We begin our examination of advancements in communications technologies by looking at the postal service and its role in helping to keep people in touch.

Communication via the Postal Service

In the United States, the postal service was established on July 26, 1775, by the members of the Second Continental Congress in Philadelphia. The formation of the U.S. Postal Service was deemed essential a couple of months earlier after the battles of Lexington and Concord as the colonists fought for independence from Great Britain. A committee chaired by Benjamin Franklin found that "the conveyance of letters and intelligence was essential to the cause of liberty" (The United States Postal Service 2012:6). The narrative of the Post Office quickly changed to the principle that "Every person in the United States—no matter who, no matter where—has the right to equal access to secure, efficient, and affordable mail service" (USPS 2012:2). Throughout its history the USPS combined to work with other forms of emerging technology including steamboats and rail cars. "In 1823, Congress declared waterways to be post roads. Use of steamboats to carry mail peaked in 1853 prior to the expansion of railroads" (USPS 2012:14). On April 3, 1860, the Pony Express began its run through parts of Missouri, Kansas, Nebraska, Colorado, Wyoming, Utah, Nevada, and California. On average, a rider covered 75 to 100 miles daily (USPS 2012).

The Pony Express was founded by William H. Russell, William B. Waddell, and Alexander Majors primarily due to the threat of the Civil War and the need for faster communication with the West (Pony Express National

Museum 2016). "The Pony Express consisted of relays of men riding horses carrying saddlebacks of mail across a 2,000-mile trail. The service opened officially on April 3, 1860, when riders left simultaneously from St. Joseph, Missouri, and Sacramento, California…. Eventually, the Pony Express had more than 100 stations, 80 riders, and between 400 and 500 horses. The express was route was extremely hazardous, but only one mail delivery was ever lost" (Pony Express National Museum 2016). The Pony Express only lasted nineteen months before being replaced by the Pacific Telegraph line.

For centuries, the USPS has played an important role in "strengthening the bonds of friendship, family, and community. Our system has encouraged civil discourse, disseminated information, and bolstered the national economy" (USPS 2012:2). One example of strengthening the bonds of friendship, family and community is the sheer volume of letters sent to military personnel during time of war (and peace) and their return mail correspondences. In 2006 alone, the Military Postal Service Agency delivered 70 million pounds of mail to men and women serving in Iraq (USPS 2012). Even in this, the digital era, the USPS still delivers a high volume of mail. In 2015, the postal service delivered 154.2 billion pieces of mail (USPS 2016).

Included in delivered pieces of mail throughout the years were letters sent by friends and family members to others. Among the more fascinating personalized pieces of mail designed to create and/or maintain friendships were pen pals. A pen pal is a person with whom one keeps up an exchange of letters, usually someone so far away that the likelihood of a personal meeting is highly unlikely. Throughout most of the 20th century it was fairly common for people to have pen pals, especially school-aged children who were encouraged to practice reading and writing in a foreign language, to improve overall literacy, to learn about the culture of others, to make new friends, to keep in touch with old friends, and to encourage military personnel fighting abroad. Some pen pals would continue writing to each other for years while others quickly gave up after just a few letters.

In popular culture, it is Charlie Brown of the *Peanuts* comic strip that is likely to spring to mind when looking for an example of a pen pal scenario. The first strip that had Charlie Brown write to his pen pal was on August 25, 1958. Reflecting the general idea of why school children were encouraged to send pen pal letters to other children in foreign countries—practicing penmanship and learning of diverse cultures—Charlie Brown, of course, initially fails at this chore. His penmanship is so poor that he is unable to use a fountain pen successfully. He tries repeatedly to pen a letter but he spills ink on the paper and onto his writing area and the floor below and the sentences he does form consist of ink running down the pages. Utilizing the underdog spirit that endeared him as good 'ol Charlie Brown to so many of us, he decides to establish "pencil pals" instead, with the same principle of pen pals only the writing is in pencil.

He explains this to his pen pal and correspondences between the two would reappear in the comic strips for decades. Interestingly, when Charlie Brown's nemesis Lucy van Pelt first learns of his pencil pal exchange she asks what they write about. Charlie Brown replies, "He tells me about his country, and I tell him about ours." Upset by this reply, Lucy states, "You sound like a couple of spies to me." For years we fans of the *Peanuts* gang were left to wonder who Charlie Brown's pencil pal really was. Charlie, who in all reality is suffering from depression, tells his pencil pal that "everyone hates me." He sees his pencil pal as his only friend. In September 1994, it is revealed that the pencil pal is a girl from Scotland named Morag. Naturally Charlie Brown fantasizes about a romantic future with her but alas in true Charlie Brown—crushing fashion, he learns that Morag has thirty other pencil pals.

On June 2, 2016, Muhammad Ali died at the age of 74. Tributes galore from nearly every media source ensued praising this former U.S. Olympic and three-time boxing champion. Born Cassius Marcellus Clay, Jr., on January 17, 1942, Ali was known for many things. His detractors would point out that he turned his back on his country for refusing to serve in the U.S. Army during the Vietnam War, claiming he was a "conscientious objector" and that war is against the teachings of the Holy Koran—a significant bit of information because he had recently become a Muslim and changed his name to Muhammad Ali. His supporters, of which there were legions that continued to revere him up to his death, praised him for taking a stand against what many deemed an "unjust war." Ever the biggest personality in any room, people loved his "trash talking" ways (he did this in an era when athletes, especially African Americans, were expected to "keep their place") and his poetic way of speaking. Ali was diagnosed with Parkinson's disease in the early 1980s and, once again, people marveled at how he kept a positive outlook on life and fought the good fight against this motor functioning attacking disease. Despite his lack of using social media and his avoidance of the cyber world, Ali was, without question, the most famous and beloved athlete in the world at the time of his death.

Many people know of the Ali described above but most people likely did not know that he kept a pen pal relationship for 30 years with a woman named Stephanie Meade. Meade first wrote to Ali when she was a ten-year-old student in Seattle, Washington. Meade recounts how everyone told her she was crazy writing the champ because he would never write back to her. Three weeks from the date of her first letter to Ali, she received a handwritten letter. It reads:

> Dear Stephanie, thanks for the sweet letter, one day I hope to meet you also. Tell all my fans I said "Hello," from me. Kiss Mother and Daddy for me and wish them my love. May Allah always bless you and guide you. Love from Muhammad Ali [Henderson 2016].

Meade explains how to the world he was an incredible athlete and humanitarian, but to her, "he was just my friend Ali." To Meade, Ali was her own personal superhero, only her superhero was real, unlike her school mates who had make-believe heroes like Superman. Meade sent Ali her report cards and told him her deepest secrets. And Ali, without fail, would reply to every single letter from his pen pal. Even during the early years of Parkinson's disease, he would write her back. She always told him how she wanted to meet him someday. In 1992, when Ali was at a function in Seattle she finally had her chance to meet him. She describes how she had to beg security guards to let Ali know she was outside hoping to meet him. As Meade states, "The next thing I knew, I was being escorted to the seat next to Muhammad Ali, right after Ali asked Mike Tyson to vacate his seat for me. I finally got to meet my hero" (Henderson 2016). They continued to exchange letters until eventually his wife Lonnie would reply on his behalf. Lonnie told Stephanie to keep writing because he loved her letters. Meade explained, "The world has lost the greatest athlete, champion, and humanitarian. I have lost the best friend I ever had" (Henderson 2016). Stephanie was a family guest at Ali's funeral.

The power of the pen pal and U.S. postal service helped to create and maintain a friendship between Meade and Ali. But most people during the era of this specific pen pal friendship had long turned to telephones to keep in touch with friends and family.

Communication via the Telephone

The invention of the telephone was hugely significant as an advancement in communication technology. Three days following the issuance of patent #174,465 on March 7th, 1876, Alexander Graham Bell spoke the first words into a telephone (Zigterman 2013; Old Telephones 2016). Bell filed his application at the patent office (February 14, 1876) just hours before Elisha Gray filed his Notice of Invention for a telephone. Nearly 600 lawsuits would be filed on behalf of Gray's Notice for the telephone patent but Bell would eventually win, or settle, all of them. Despite the controversy over the filing competition, the telephone would eventually become one of the most valuable patents ever issued (Old Telephones 2016). Interestingly, Bell, who was dealing with financial difficulties offered to sell his telephone patent rights to Western Union for $100,000. "In one of the greatest miscalculations in history, Western Union said no. Instead, Western Union believed that the telegraph, not the telephone, was the future" (Old Telephones 2016).

There were a number of attempts to incorporate the non-electric telegraph system first invented by Claude Chappe in 1794 and improved upon by Bavarian Samuel Soemmering in 1809 and American Harrison Dyar in

1828 (Bellis 2015). In 1835, New York University professor Samuel Morse proved that signals could be transmitted by wire via his invention of the Morse Code—a system that utilized dots and dashes. Until 1877, all rapid long-distance communication depended upon the telegraph (Bellis 2015). The telephone system would change any hope of the telegraph system to take significant hold as a mass form of communication.

The first phone call made by Bell was to his assistant, "Mr. Watson, come here, I want to see you." Ever since this call, people have made countless phone calls to business associates, family members and friends. The popular form of the telephone during the 1890s to the 1930s was the "candlestick" phone, a device separated into two pieces. The mouthpiece formed the candlestick part, and the receiver was placed by the ear during the phone call. This style died out in the 1930s when phone manufacturers started combining the mouthpiece and receiver into a single unit (Zigterman 2013). The rotary phone—to place a call you would rotate the dial to the number you wanted, and then release—was the popular form of telephone until the push-button phones gained popularity in the 1960s and '70s. The Touch-Tone phone, first introduced by AT&T in 1963, allowed phones to use a keypad to dial numbers and make phone calls via a frequency that corresponded with each number dialed (Zigterman 2013).

The invention of the answering machine, first popular in the 1960s, represented a relatively huge development in communications as people were free from waiting around the phone all day to receive an important phone call (or not to miss any potentially important phone calls). With the answering machine, people could go about their business and if someone called while you were not home, the machine would record the message. Most people today, of course, do not use answering machines for their home phone— if they even have a landline phone—they just use cell phone voicemail. The development of portable, or cordless, phones represented another big advancement in telephone history. These 1980s phones became the forerunner of cellphones as you could talk on your phone anywhere in your house and in some cases out on decks or yards. The first commercially available mobile phone was released in 1984 by Motorola (the Motorola Dyna TAC 8000X). Younger folks today might be alarmed to learn that these phones weighed nearly 2 pounds, had just 30 minutes of talk time, and first cost nearly $4,000 (Zigterman 2013).

The continued development of the telephone would lead to smaller, lighter, longer-lasting versions of mobile phones that would continually add new features such as Caller ID (which allowed phone users the opportunity to screen out certain callers). In 2003, the Sanyo SCP-5300 became the one of the first phones to include a camera. The Palm Treo became the first smartphone. In 2009, the Treo was replaced with the Palm Pre, a failed response to the iPhone that was first introduced in 2007 by Apple. Android became the iPhone's leading competition (Zigterman 2013).

The telephone represents an unbelievable advancement in the evolution of communications technology. Everywhere you look people are on their phones glued to tiny screens ("screen sniffers") to send and receive electronic messages from friends and family and a variety of other folks while, ironically, rarely actually using phones to talk to someone. And while the advancements in telephone technology have assisted cyber and electronic communications and socialization, it is slowly destroying face-to-face interactions and inter-personal skills. The future of telephones is limitless, at least for as long as we have a power grid. The discussion of the potential (or inevitable) collapse of the power grid is reserved for other publications (see Delaney and Madigan's *Beyond Sustainability*) as this book is about friendships and happiness and, for most people, the collapse of the power grid would put a major damper on most of their relationships and their overall quality of life.

Communication via the Mass Media

The trademark of the mass media has been providing news, information, and entertainment. According to Real (1996), "The term *media* refers to all communication relays and technologies" (p. 9). The term "media" is the plural of medium. The word "mass" refers to the large size of the media's audience (Ryan and Wentworth 1999). Put together, the mass media collectively become the vehicle by which large numbers of people are informed about important events in society. "[The] most narrow view of the mass media refers precisely to the technological apparatus that literally carries or trans-mits information. That is the strictest sense of the word *medium*: a means of communicating information" (Ryan and Wentworth 1999:10). Real (1996) concurs and states, "Any device that relays messages is a medium. Any tech-nology that ritually structures culture is a medium in the broadest sense" (p.9).

The massive scale of the mass media leaves some people befuddled in their attempt to describe it. Jennifer Akin (2005) states, "'Mass media' is a deceptively simple term encompassing a countless array of institutions and individuals who differ in purpose, scope, method, and cultural context. Mass media include all forms of information communicated to large scales of peo-ple, from a handmade sign o an international news network. There is no standard for how large the audience needs to be before communication becomes 'mass' communication. There are also no constraints on the type of information being presented. A car advertisement and a U.N. resolution are both examples of mass media."

While Akin is correct, the mass media is nearly omnipresent and since nearly anything directed to the public could be considered the mass media, let's simplify the traditional mass media and examine the cyber mass media later in the chapter. The mass media consist of television, radio, motion pictures, newspapers, books, magazines, and sound recordings. Generally, the media are divided into two major categories: print media, which includes newspapers, magazines, and books; and electronic media, which includes television, radio and motion pictures, and the Internet. Traditionally, the mass media have been viewed as forms of communication that permit a one-way flow of information from a source to an audience (Ryan and Wentworth 1999). However, as Delaney and Wilcox (2002) indicate, with the increased use of the Internet, the development of interactive television, and the ability to text-message votes on TV shows while the show is airing and with the older interactive medium of cal-in radio programs, and the ability of readers to write a letter to the editor of a newspaper, describing the mass media as a one-way form of communication would be inaccurate. Bryant and Bryant (2003) speaking on entertainment research specifically and of the changed role of the mass media in general, concur with Delaney and Wilcox by stating, "With the advent of newer forms of mediated communication, in which the end is both producer and consumer and assumes considerable agency over media content through interactivity and other means of selectivity and control, the potential for productive entertainment research is almost unlimited" (p. 213).

The overwhelming size and influence of the mass media cannot be understated. "Through its various formats, the mass media can reach most people on earth. This is an incredible opportunity for communication and education among the peoples on the planet. As these technologies become cheaper, they are becoming ubiquitous and closing the technological divide that exists between the rich and poor. As the technology necessary for mass communication becomes cheaper and more widespread, the planet will indeed become smaller as news travels even faster among all people of the world" (*New World Encyclopedia* 2008). It is the advent of the computer that has spearheaded the spread and power of the mass media as an agent of socialization and as a major form of communication.

Communication via Computers

A computer is a machine, or device, usually electronic, used for accepting information and processing data according to a set of instructions or programs. Complex computers will also possess the means for storing data for some necessary time or duration. Programs built into the computers are generally viewed as microprocessors, an integrated computer circuit that performs all the functions of a central processing unit (CPU). Computers have changed quite a bit over their history and take numerous physical forms. Early computers were the size of a large room and consumed as much power as several hundred modern personal computers. Today, computers can be made small enough to fit into a wristwatch and be powered by a watch battery. Many people carry around with them laptops or iPads or some other equivalent as a means of always having access to information. Cellphones are deemed a necessity by nearly all people including children. "However, the most common form of computer in use today is by far the embedded computer. Embedded computers are small, simple devices that are often used to control other devices—for example, they may be found in machines ranging from fighter aircraft to industrial robots, digital cameras, and even children's toys" (*New World Encyclopedia* 2013).

It is difficult to define any one device as the earliest computer as the very definition of a computer has changed over the years and it is therefore impossible to identify the first computer. In fact, many devices once called "computers" would no longer qualify as such by today's standards. Consider, for example, that originally, a computer referred to a person who performed numerical calculations (a human computer), often with the aid of a mechanical calculating device. With this realization in mind, the abacus, a slide rule, would arguably be among the first computers (*New World Encyclopedia* 2013). What most of us think of as computers were developed in the 1930s and 1940s, gradually taking on the features of many modern computers. The defining feature of modern computers which distinguishes them from all other machines is that they can be programmed via a list of instructions (programs). Computer programs might include anywhere from a dozen instructions to many millions of instructions like a word processor or a web browser. A typical modern computer can execute billions of instructions every second and nearly never make a mistake over years of operation. (Errors in computer programs are called "bugs.") Computers have four main sections: the arithmetic and logic unit (ALU), the control unit, the memory, and the input and output devices (collectively termed I/O). As nearly any user can tell you today, a computer is great at multitasking—running many programs simultaneously (*New World Encyclopedia* 2013).

Of greatest relevance to us is how computers assist in communication in an organized fashion. In the 1950s, computers were used by the U.S. military to create a defense system (the Semi-Automatic Ground Environment, or SAGE) that consisted of numerous large computers and associated networking equipment that coordinated operations at a single place while interpreting data from multiple radar sites. In the 1970s, computer engineers at research institutions throughout the U.S. began to link their computers together using telecommunications technology. Shortly afterwards, the network spread beyond academic and military institutions and became known as the Internet. In the 1990s, the spread of applications like email and the World Wide Web, combined with the development of cheap, fast networking technologies like Ethernet and ADSL saw computer networking become almost ubiquitous (*New World Encyclopedia* 2013). The Internet allows users to gain immediate access to a communications system that allows for long-distance social interactions through a series of networking sites that further allows for the maintenance of existing friendships—those originally formed via face-to-face contact—and for the creation of new friendships—electronic friendships—wherein those involved in this type of relationship have not necessarily ever met.

The Internet is a relatively new, but very influential and prevalent aspect of human life in contemporary society. To underscore the importance of the Internet it might be helpful to think of it as the electronic nervous system of the planet. The Internet was created in an effort to speed communication between people separated by long distances. While there might be some debate as to who exactly created the Internet (remember, Al Gore told CNN's Wolf Blitzer on March 9, 1999, that he created the Internet), many people have contributed to its creation and growth. Al Gore, for example *did* help pass legislation that advanced the information technology highway, but he was *not* the person who "created" it.

According to Leiner and associates (2014), "the first recorded description of the social interactions that could be enabled through networking was a series of memos written by J.C.R. Licklider of MIT in August 1962 discussing his 'Galactic Network' concept. He envisioned a globally interconnected set of computers through which everyone could quickly access data and programs from any site." Thus, the Internet was intended to be a widespread information infrastructure designed to help speed up communication, especially among intellectuals conducting scientific research. And while the Internet still helps intellectuals conduct research, its everyday usage is far removed from such lofty endeavors.

Today, some of us use the Internet to conduct research; it sure does make it easier to write papers and books. Most people, however, use the Internet for its social component, especially via social network sites that allow us to engage in such cyber social interactions as sharing photos (including "selfies") and videos, wishing people a "happy birthday," and bragging about our latest vacation or favorite sports team victory. In some instances, people have used the Internet to achieve more ambitious goals such as organizing flash mobs, protests, or revolutions. In brief, nearly everyone uses the Internet and we use it so regularly the term "digital diet" has been created as a way to describe the regular intake of electronic data via the Internet (e.g., playing video games, watching television or going on social media) that so many of us consume every day. At least there are zero calories and zero fat grams associated with the digital diet. Conversely, researchers are looking into the effects of the digital diet on the brain as the lure of the Internet is similar to the siren's song. As one might suspect, scientific research has shown that Internet addiction (Internet Use Disorder) may lead to impaired brain structure and function. (See for example: Cash et al. 2012.)

Changing Cultural Norms and Values

The world of communications has certainly changed quite a bit over the past couple of centuries and especially the past few decades. These changes have had a profound effect on the formation and maintenance of friendships in particular and on culture in general.

Culture and Social Structure

All societies have both a culture and a social structure. Analyzing a society's culture and social structure is a cornerstone of sociology. After all, sociology is literally the study of society.

Let's begin by quickly reviewing some key aspects of culture. Culture may be defined as the shared knowledge, values, norms and behavioral patterns of a given society that are passed down from one generation to the next, which help to form a way of life for its members (Delaney 2012a). Viewed as the set of ideas shared within society, culture becomes the social determinant of behavior. That is to say, culture serves as a script for acceptable behavior as it gives order to our social lives. A society's culture is present prior to our birth; consequently, we are born into a system filled with behavioral expectations. Most aspects of culture change only in gradual increments and as a result it helps to provide social stability and social control. This last point is emphasized by the realization that culture does not change every time a child is born in order to meet his or her needs as that would be incongruous.

While culture helps to provide stability within a society it is subject to change. Social change involves the alteration of mechanisms within the social structure and significant changes in cultural norms and values. Technology, for example, can stimulate changes in a society's culture. The previously discussed changes in communications technology have allowed people easier access to their significant others but they have also changed the way in which most of us go about our daily business. Consider for example, people used to walk and drive with their heads up keeping an eye out for obstacles that could cause harm or for stimuli that could cause joy and happiness. People used to dine at restaurants and talk to those at the same table; now they are glued to tiny screens reaching out to those not at the table. The authors, as professors, have noticed in their time as teachers in the classrooms that prior to the start of class students used to converse with their classmates or maybe their professor; now they are texting people not in the classroom. It is eerie to enter a classroom full of students, none of whom are conversing with each other, and all of whom have their eyes glued to their iPhones instead.

With such technology as cellular phones, people are generally communicating with others outside of their immediate physical environment instead of within it. In short, one of our fundamental values of interacting with others has changed dramatically in the past decade. Cellular phones are, of course, just one example of a technological change that has altered the behavior of a massive number of people. Rather than fighting this change, society has enacted new rules and policies to adapt to the emerging culture that consists of the need for instant communication with those not in close proximity. Society has passed laws to discourage driving and texting (and talking on a phone that is not hands-free) and yet it has also set up free WiFi zones so that people can use their cell- phones and other electronic devices while they are away from their home or their office. The self-absorption of some people to communicate with others outside their immediate environments has led to a number of violations of basic protocols of etiquette. For example, it has become increasingly common for people to use their cellphones at movie theaters, at plays, in the classroom, at business meetings and while dining. Often, the agents of socialization in these locales are left to make announcements that remind violators of protocol that the use of cellphones is prohibited at movie theaters, in the classroom, and so on.

The astute reader has undoubtedly noticed the repeated use of the word "society" in relation to the description of culture. It is important to note that the terms "culture" and "society" are related to one another but have different meanings. Whereas culture refers to a shared way of life, society pertains to a group of persons (the largest collection of people in group form) who interact with one another as members of a collectivity (who share a common heritage and culture) within a defined territory and a highly structured system (and subsystems) of human organization. This system helps to shape the social structure of a society.

A society's social structure consists of a prevailing social organization— the groups to which people belong—and its prevailing social arrangements, or institutions (Delaney 2012a). As Juette and Berger (2008) explain, "Sociologists use the concept of social structure to refer to patterns of social interaction and relationships that endure over time and that enable and/or constrain people's choices and opportunities. Social structure is, in a sense, external to individuals insofar as it is not of their own making and exists prior to their engagement with the world" (p.4). However, Juette and Berger go on to point out that "people are not mere dupes or passive recipients of social structures; they are thinking, self-reflexive beings who are capable of assessing their circumstances, choosing among alternative courses of action, and consequently shaping their own behavior" (p.7). As thinking humans, we possess free will and are capable of choosing from a wide variety of courses of action. Nonetheless, these choices are influenced by our social group memberships and the institutions of the social structure in which we live.

Consider this example of the role of the social structure and its ability to affect culture and influence people's behaviors. On June 4, 1989, an incident known as the "June Fourth Incident" occurred in Tiananmen Square, Beijing, China that involved government troops mass murdering protesting students. The Chinese government forcibly suppressed the protests after declaring martial law. The number of civilian deaths has been estimated at anywhere from hundreds to thousands. This event was filmed live as it occurred and was made available to viewers across the globe. The next day, on June 5, 1989 "an iconic image that defined courage and defiance for a generation around the globe" (Shin 2014) was also filmed. This image was of a man (protester) who blocked the path of a column of tanks rolling down Chang'an Avenue near Tiananmen Square.

The video shows the lead tank moving back and forth, going left and right, trying to go around the man, but the man kept in front of the lead tank, blocking its path. The man then climbs up on the lead tank and appears to talk to one of the soldiers inside the tank. The man was eventually led away by his arms by two men. It remains unclear if those men were police or security forces, or just bystanders who were concerned about the man. The identity and the whereabouts of this man are still unknown (Shin 2014). Following the violent military response and the scale of the bloodshed that ensued, the Chinese government arrested protesters across the nation, expelled foreign journalists, censored media coverage of the event, and banned the image of the Tank Man who was dressed in a white shirt and held onto a shopping bag (Saul 2014).

The authors were in Tiananmen Square in 2016 just prior to the 27th anniversary of the massacre and learned first-hand that, officially, the incident never occurred. We had both witnessed it on the news from different parts of the United States in 1989 and like most adult Americans today, we have the image engraved in our memory banks. And yet, the social structure of present-day China insists that such an event never happened. The authors also noticed that on many occasions during their trip to China in 2016 that various news stories—especially anything that referenced the Tiananmen Square incident—that aired on CNN (or other foreign news agencies) were blocked out (e.g., a live news broadcast would suddenly turn to a blank screen and then seconds later resume). We had been warned ahead of time not to make gestures similar to that of the Tank Man when we were in Tiananmen Square and certainly not to take a photo of ourselves making such gestures.

Today, like Americans or Westerners in general, Chinese people all have cellular phones (with many sites such as Facebook officially blocked, but still easy to access via a Virtual Personal Network), thus reflecting a change in culture; but they cannot find news reports of the June Fourth Incident or of the "Tank Man." The lesson learned here is, the social structure of China allows only certain aspects of their culture to change even in the face of advancements of technology in communications.

Gestures, Symbols, Language and Emoticons

Regardless of how one communicates with others, a system of symbols and words that make up a language are utilized. Even the old "Morse Code" had a system of dots and dashes that made up a language for those who could understand it. Thus, whether we communicate with people electronically or via face-to-face interactions, we rely on gestures, symbols and language to convey our thoughts, meanings and messages to others.

George Herbert Mead believed that language has its origins in gestures (Thayer 1968). The most important characteristic of the gesture is its social properties, that is, how it affects and coordinates behavior between two or more individuals (Thayer 1968). Gestures represent the most basic form of communication. Gestures are a form of non-verbal communication or non-vocal communication in which visible body movements convey a feeling or emotion. A gesture occurs when a person uses limbs, body parts, or facial expressions to convey a thought, intention or attitude. An extended, upturned palm is one of the oldest and most widely understood signals in the world. It can symbolize a general request for help, such as a homeless person reaching out with an upturned palm in hopes of receiving a donation from a passerby. A homeowner using a lawnmower only to have it mysteriously shut down may hold an upturned palm toward the lawnmower as if to say, "What do you want from me?" Gestures are very commonplace in society and often taken for granted. However, we do become keenly aware of the importance of gestures when someone misinterprets them. For example, students, alumni and faculty at the University of Texas at Austin employ a greeting consisting of the phrase "Hook 'em Horns" while using the "horn" gesture created by extending the index and pinky fingers while grasping the second and third fingers with the thumb. This gesture is meant to symbolically look like a Texas Longhorn steer. However, many people who are not affiliated with the University of Texas might misinterpret the gesture as devil worship as fans of heavy metal use the same symbolic gesture as a sort of tribute to Satan.

Symbols are somewhat similar to gestures but a bit more advanced as physical items, rather than gestures, come to signify ideas and qualities of a culture (or subculture). These items possess meaning and represent something else to people in a society. Symbols, again like gestures, are very common in a particular culture. Important symbols are to be respected as they represent cultural ideals of importance. For example, a nation's flag is not simply a piece of cloth and important religious symbols such as a cross are not simply two pieces of wood nailed together; instead they are representations of values held by people. Realizing that the letters of an alphabet are symbols that have meaning to people, we can say that symbols are the building blocks of language.

Language, as implied above, is an abstract set of symbols but these symbols can be strung together in an infinite number of ways to express ideas and thoughts. Some languages, such as English, are spoken nearly everywhere in the world, while others, such as many Native American languages, are far more localized and specific to their own cultures. Within a given society, such as the United States, different dialects of the same language may be spoken. Language tells us a great deal about what is important and relevant to a culture. For example, as technology alters the world in which people live, it also changes their perceptions, thoughts and symbolic interpretations of the world (Krug 2005). Changes in technology, as well as changing cultural values, often lead to the creation of new words. This helps to explain why hundreds of new words are added to dictionaries with every new edition (Pyle 2000).

If the total number of words spoken by a culture of people is an indication of changing cultural values and norms, then English-speaking people are on the forefront of social change. According to the Global Language Monitor (GLM), the English language, as of June 2009, contained over 1 million words. GLM estimates that the millionth English word, "Web 2.0," was added to the language on June 10, 2009. Web 2.0 refers to the second, more social generation of the Internet (Shaer 2009). The year 2009 was a banner year for the impact of cyber socialization on the changing culture via the addition of new words to the English language as "unfriend" (to remove someone as a "friend" on social networking sites such as Facebook) was named the 2009 Word of the Year by the *New Oxford American Dictionary*. Oxford lexicographer Christine Lindberg says "unfriend" has "real lex-appeal." Other finalists for the word of the year in 2009 had connections to the cyber world as well: netbook (a small laptop with limited memory) and sexting (sending sexually explicit texts and pictures by cell phone) (*The Post-Standard* 11/17/09). Other words added to the dictionary in 2009 included: hashtag (a # sign added to a word or phrase that helps search engines); intexticated (distracted because of texting on a cellphone while driving a vehicle); and paywall (a way of blocking access to a part of a website which is only available to paying subscribers).

Interestingly, there was a bit of controversy over the use of the word "unfriend" as some people, including Facebook co-founder Chris Hughes, prefer the word "defriend" (Moriarty 2009). Whether you unfriend (according to Oxford, a verb meaning to remove someone as a friend) or defriend (the term Hughes and his friends use) the meaning is the same—you have dropped someone from your acknowledged list of friends.

Among the many other words that have been added to the dictionary that have their primary usage in the cyber world is "ghosting." Ghosting refers to withdrawing or avoiding contact with your partner, friends or electronic friends, by not answering texts, posts or calls (Borgueta 2015; Sakaluk 2012). The expressions used could include, "Why are you ghosting me?" or "Where you been, you ghost?!"

Despite our love for creating new words, many people on social network sites prefer to use emoticons to express their feelings. Emoticons are text gestures that take on meaning for the sender and the receiver. They are tiny pictures used to add a little flavor to text messages and tweets. Emoticons developed from emoji, which means "picture character" in Japanese (Keyes 2014). A variety of hearts and smiley faces are the most popular emojis. In 2013, the top ten emojis used on Twitter were: Hearts (342m); Joy (278m); Unamused (135m); Heart Eyes (124m); Relaxed (110m); OK Hand (109m); Heart (106m); Kissing Heart (100m); Blush (99m); and Pensive (88m) (Chalabi 2014). A study released by Rice University in 2012 revealed that women are twice as likely as men to use emoticons; however, men used a larger variety of emoticons to express themselves (Ruth 2012). In 2012 alone, more than 8 trillion emoticons were used in conjunction with text messages (Ruth 2012).

There are many good reasons to use emoticons. For one thing, consider all the electronic messages (e.g., text messages, emails, cyber posts) you receive and think of how many times some of these messages were hard to understand/interpret because of the lack of visual signs from the sender, such as gestures, that allow the reader to understand the emotion behind the message. As a result, the reader sometimes imposes a "tone" to the message that may be inaccurate as they, for example, misunderstand a joke for a serious comment (e.g., "I don't like the tone of your text. Are you mad at me?"). To avoid possible misunderstandings, it has become commonplace for people to use emoticons to express feelings. Thus, if the message was meant as a civil, nonconfrontational, or humorous comment people add some variation of a smiley face. People also use emoticons to express themselves and there certainly are more than enough to choose from; in fact, there are so many emoticons available today that they represent a type of language. A number of messages are sent with just emoticons and if you are not fluent with emoticons you will be lost. And yet, sociologists would point out, emoticons are simply symbols that help to form a language just like every other language.

Changing Norms and Values

We have alluded to norms and values already in this chapter but let's take a closer look at both terms. Norms are socially defined rules and expectations regarding human behavior. They are generally enforced by sanctions (punishments). Norms can range from the conventional rules of everyday life (folkways) that people follow almost automatically (e.g., basic mannerisms), to more serious norms that constitute basic moral judgments of a society (mores) that result in outrage when violated (e.g., abuse of children, and cruelty to animals), to those norms which are so important that they have been written down by a political authority (laws) wherein their breach entails designated punishments that officials have been empowered to enforce.

Values are those aspects of culture, perhaps the most deeply rooted of all social expectations, that reflect the things we cherish and place high importance on. Examples of values would include equality, loyalty, success via hard work, sacrifice, and respect for human dignity. Social values provide general standards of societal expectations reflecting entrenched principles of a society. Without such evaluating standards as those provided by a society's values, it would be difficult to judge individual behavior or social action. While certainly related to social norms, values are generally not specific while norms are explicit. Because of their idealistic principles, values help to bring legitimacy to social norms. In other words, norms are rules of behavior that we have to follow but sometimes wonder why; however, if there is a value component added to the norm it makes following the rules seem like a moral obligation rather than a legal obligation.

A clear indication of a changing culture is the general acceptance of emerging norms and values that are quite different from those of which older generations abided by their entire lives. Consider, for example, the social network site Facebook was once reserved for college students only. However, once Facebook was opened to non-college members, parents, and eventually the grandparents, of college students were soon on Facebook as well. The presence of older folks and non-college students on Facebook has become so dominant that many college-aged students avoid Facebook today in favor of other social networking sites. Still, it is the general acceptance of social networking sites, via the cyber socialization process, by people of all ages and backgrounds that speaks volumes about a general willingness to accept changing cultural norms and values. Furthermore, older people are just as likely to check their cellphones while dining out at restaurants with friends and family as are younger people.

Presentation of Self, Dramaturgy, Narcissism and Taking Selfies

Perhaps the most famous work of the noted sociologist Erving Goffman (1922–1982), and his first major publication, is *The Presentation of Self in Everyday Life* (1959). Goffman believed that the individual (expressed as "the actor") is an active and reflective self capable of making a vast number of choices in determining how the self should be presented in the varied social situations in which they must perform a role. People attempt to present themselves in a manner in which they wish to be perceived in an attempt to neutralize the possible negative reviews put forth by others.

Utilizing the dramaturgical approach (dramaturgy is a method of examining social interaction as a series of small plays, or dramas), Goffman viewed society as a stage where humans are actors giving performances for audiences. "While acting, individuals attempt to present themselves according to their identity constructs. The 'self label' is an identity that one presents to others in an attempt to manage their impression of him or her. Individuals deliberately give off signs to provide others with information about how to 'see' them. This information helps individuals to define situations and direct courses of action. Picking up on signs and clues provided by others allow the acquainted and the unacquainted alike to proceed with their interactions" (Delaney 2014:262). Individuals who are with unacquainted persons can present themselves as they want others to see them and they may be successful in this presentation because the audience has no past knowledge of them and they therefore cannot be discredited. Acquaintances and friends of individuals who attempt to present themselves in a certain manner may discredit those who put on a false presentation of self.

In Chapter 2, we stated that the socialization process is responsible for taming narcissism. While it is normal, up to a point, to want to be admired and to admire one's own accomplishments, when the self-directed admiration becomes excessive, narcissistic behavior is, at the very least, annoying to others, it has also been described as "evil" by the famous philosopher Bertrand Russell (1930). Russell, of course, lived in an era long before social media and if he were alive today he might be more forgiving in his disdain for narcissism; if not, he would likely "blow a mental gasket" at the level of narcissistic behavior in today's cyber social media world.

Annoying or evil, or somewhere in-between, the agents of socialization have often not only failed in taming narcissistic behavior, they have encouraged it. In his discussion on "princess parenting" Delaney (2012a) describes how some parents, mostly mothers, dress their baby girls in "princess" outfits and treat their children as if they are royalty. Because the "princess" has been pampered throughout her childhood and placed on a pedestal, she comes to think of herself as overly special and develops a delusional sense of self enti-tlement. The delusions of grandeur generated by princess parenting also lead to the development of narcissistic traits. Based on their research findings, Jean Twenge and W. Keith Campbell, coauthors of *The Narcissism Epidemic Living in the Age of Entitlement* (2009), found that college-age women today are developing narcissistic traits at a rate four times that of men. The authors attribute this high rate of narcissism only in part to the princess syndrome, given that a generation of young women have been socialized by parents and the media (especially Disney) to embrace the princess fantasy. Among the characteristics of the princess in adulthood are extreme insecurity, the urge to be the center of attention (drama-queen behavior), wanting everyone to know she is a princess, failure to take responsibility for things, and a desire to be waited on.

Twenge does not solely blame the princess syndrome for this rise in nar-cissism. In her book *Generation Me* (2006), Twenge describes the younger generation of the 2000s as the "GenMe" generation. Twenge, who presents a great deal of data to support her claim, argues that young people don't care as much about making a good impression or displaying courtesy as their par-ents and grandparents did when they were growing up. Citing Twenge's research, Sharon Jayson (2006) writes, "Among kids today, 62 percent of col-lege students say they pay little attention to social conventions. In 1958, an average of 50 percent did. Among ages 9–12, the difference was even greater: 76 percent in 1999, compared with an average of 50 percent in 1963" (p.4D). Twenge and Campbell (2009) compiled additional compelling statistics, charts and studies in an attempt to support her theory that the current gen-eration is the most narcissistic in American history.

We believe that it's not a coincidence that narcissism has been increasing during the past couple of decades, as this phenomenon has coincided with the rise of popularity in social networking. Social networking sites such as Facebook, Twitter, Instagram, Snapchat and others have been socializing users to share all sorts of private moments for the public (or a select group of friends). Among the most obvious forms of narcissistic behaviors being encouraged in the cyber socialization era is the taking of "selfies." The exces-sive use of posting selfies on a social networking site is a sign of narcissism. *Groupies*—selfies taken by an individual within a group context—are not as narcissistic as they promote friendship group behavior.

Sociologists and psychologists alike are interested in the link between narcissism and the prevalence of people to take selfies and post them on social network sites for a variety of reasons including the realization that self-ies are an aspect of the presentation of self. It seems impossible that anyone does not know what a "selfie" is but just in case, a "selfie" is a self-portrait photograph usually taken with a digital camera or camera phone held in the hand or supported by a selfie stick with the intent of sharing in the cyber world by uploading to a social network site. In this regard, the photographer is both the object and the subject of the photo. Based on data collected on taking selfies, millions, perhaps even billions, of people have been socialized by the social media into believing that this form of narcissistic behavior is acceptable in the contemporary era. (And certainly those who take a large number of selfies think that is acceptable.) Listed below is a sampling of data available on the act of taking selfies:

- In 2013, *The Oxford English Dictionary* announced that its new word for the year was "selfie." The announcement included the following quote, "[T]he decision was unanimous this year, with little if any argument. This is a little unusual. Normally there will be some good-natured debate as one person might champion their particular choice over someone else's" (*The Oxford English Dictionary* 2013).
- *The Oxford English Dictionary* defines "selfie" as: "A photograph that one has taken of oneself, typically one taken with a smartphone or webcam and shared via social media: occasional selfies are acceptable, but posing a new picture of yourself every day isn't necessary." Thus, taking a selfie once in a while, but less than once a day, would be considered acceptable but taking a selfie everyday, and certainly more than one a day, would be not be considered normal, from the *Oxford English Dictionary* perspective.
- Millions of selfies are shared every day across all the major social media platforms (Bennett 2014).
- According to data from Samsung, selfies make up almost one-third of all photos taken by people aged 18–24, with Facebook, WhatsApp, Twitter, Instagram and Snapchat leading the way (Bennett 2014).
- Men (50 percent) and women (52 percent) are nearly equally likely to take selfies; 14 percent of all selfies are digitally enhanced; 36 percent of people have admitted to altering their selfies; and, 34 percent of males state they retouch every selfie, while just 13 percent of females state they retouch every selfie (Bennett 2014).
- Nearly half (48 percent) of all selfies taken end up Facebook followed by 27 percent on WhatsApp and Text, 9 percent on Twitter, 8 percent on Instagram, 5 percent on Snapchat, and 2 percent on Pinterest (Bennett 2014).
- The top ten cities with the highest percentage of people who take and post selfies are: Makati City, Philippines (258 selfie-takers per 100,000); Manhattan, NY (202); Miami (155); Anaheim and Santa

Ana, CA (147); Petaling Jaya, Malaysia (141); Tel Aviv, Israel (139); Manchester, England (114); Milan, Italy (108); Cebu City, Philippines (99); and George Town, Malaysia (95) (Wilson 2014).

- Taking selfies has increasingly been linked to mental health conditions that focus on a person's obsession with looks. According to psychiatrist David Veal, "Two out of three of all the patients who come to see me with Body Dysmorphic Disorder since the rise of camera phones have a compulsion to repeatedly take and post selfies on social media sites" (*True Activist* 2014).
- Writing for *Psychology Today*, Pamela Rutledge (2013) states, "Selfies frequently trigger perceptions of self-indulgence or attention-seeking social dependence that raises the damned-if-you-do and damned-if-you-don't spectre of either narcissism or very low self-esteem."
- Researchers in Thailand found that selfie addicts may be suffering from loneliness, are vain, or have a need "to seek approval from others" on a constant basis. Taking selfies, the researchers conclude could be a sign of relationship trouble or mental health problems (CNN 2016).
- A popular meme about selfies appeared on many people's Facebook newsfeed in 2017 that read: "They call it a 'selfie' because 'narcissistie' is too hard to spell."

The narcissistic tendencies that often accompany the act of taking selfies has led many people to think that they are more important than the events occurring in their immediate environment and background. Consequently, an increasing number of people are taking selfies in very inappropriate places. Examples include taking a duckface selfie at the Vietnam Memorial, or any memorial site; in jail; in front of a burning house; while rushing the field of play and being chased by security guards; in front of a casket at a funeral home during calling hours; hospital personnel in the surgery room during a surgery; while lying on a stretcher being escorted to the hospital following an accident; while on the toilet; crying and looking for sympathy; after being pulled over by the police and showing the officer your license; taking a sexy selfie with your small child in the background; while people are fighting behind you; while someone is drowning or threatening to jump from a building ledge; and, while running with the bulls in Pamplona. These are just a few examples ill-advised selfies we found online that clearly show how self-absorption (narcissism) has become a growing social problem due to cyber socialization and a lack of basic etiquette.

It is also worth noting that selfie fatalities are becoming increasingly common. Putting it into perspective more people died from selfie fatalities in 2015 than by those attacked by sharks (Hughes 2015). During the years 2014 and 2015, 49 people died while attempting to photograph themselves; the average age of the victims is 21 years old, and 75 percent of them are male (Crockett 2016). The leading causes of selfie-related fatalities are: fall from heights, drowning, train, gunshot, grenade, plane crash, car crash and animal. The leading country for selfie-related fatalities is India followed by Russia and the USA (Crockett 2016).

Still, the prevalence of selfies is not entirely bad. Even Pope Francis has weighed in on the subject. When queried why young people often ask him to take a selfie with them, he replied: "What do I think of it? I feel like a great-grandfather! It's another culture—I respect it." Who are we to criticize the selfie when the pope himself voices respect for it?! (Delaney and Madigan 2016).

As demonstrated in the previous pages, there are many examples of a changing culture that has been greatly influenced by the forces of cyber socialization. As of yet, we have not actually defined cyber socialization so let's take a closer look.

Cyber Socialization

Today, people of most ages spend a great amount of time communicating with one another in the cyberspace (the electronic world) rather than in face-to-face interactions. This process is called *cyber socialization*, and its influence on our lives is increasing. The amount of time spent in the cyberworld generally comes at the cost of less time spent with personal relationships in the real world. The "cyberworld" refers to a world that involves computers, inter-computer communication, and computer networks such as the Internet; it is a place where humans go to communicate electronically. It has become so common for people to spend time in the cyberworld that socializing and conducting business online is an expected form of behavior. Consider, for example, that Americans aged 18 and older use electronic media on average 11+ hours per day (Richter 2015). The average time American adults (18+) spent with electronic media during the 4th quarter of 2014: live television (4 hours and 51 minutes); radio (2:43); smartphone (1:25); internet on a PC (1:06); time shifted TV (:33); game console (:13); DVD/ Blu Ray (:09); and multimedia device (:07) (Richter 2015). In a study conducted in the UK, it was revealed that young people aged between 16 and 24 spend more than 27 hours a week on the internet (Anderson 2015). This figure is an increase double from 10 years ago and is fueled by the increasing use of tablets and smartphones. The biggest increase has been among young adults, with time spent online almost tripling from ten years ago (Anderson 2015). Younger people are watching television programming, but they are increasingly watching it streamed online rather than on television.

The most popular websites accessed from mobile phones among young people in the UK is Facebook, Twitter, Google+, Linkedin, and MySpace (Anderson 2015). Almost 70 percent of internet users in the UK report that they feel comfortable giving away personal information on the Net, including their home addresses, and a quarter say they don't read website terms and conditions or privacy statements at all. Two-thirds of internet users use the same passwords for most or all websites (Anderson 2015). Such lax attitudes contribute to the high frequency of cyber crime and cyber deviancy (to be discussed later in this chapter).

Our fascination with the cyberworld and the utilization of cyber socialization did not develop overnight. For nearly two generations now, people have been increasingly raised in an electronic world. As alluded to in this chapter's introductory story, the use of computers is no longer a fascination, it has become a necessity and their use is treated as a given. Herbert Spencer, a philosopher and sociologist who coined the term "survival of the fittest" would likely say that those who embrace the cyberworld are "fitter" and therefore more likely to survive and flourish. Today's children and young adults have used computers their entire lives. Socializing online is a norm for them and social networking in cyberspace fulfills the purpose of staying connected. Perhaps the best attraction of the cyberworld is the instant access people have to each other's lives.

The power and predominance of the cyberworld is illustrated in many ways but perhaps one of the best ways to put things into perspective is to realize that even when governments block out certain websites, there is always a way to access it. For example, in China, as mentioned earlier, the government blocks people from accessing Facebook and some other social media sites. When the authors visited China we were told to download a Virtual Personal Network (VPN) app to our phones while still in the U.S. We chose the "Private Tunnel" as our VPN and it worked great. From time to time we got bounced off our sites but we just switched our VPN to pick up a signal from some other part of the world that does not block apps. Even in democratic societies the governments may block any number of websites, generally claiming that illegal activity is conducted at such sites. People can still access these sites by going on the "dark web." The dark web "is a small portion of the deep web that has been intentionally hidden and made inaccessible" and allows for the provision of anonymity (*The Globe and Mail* 2015). In relatively liberal and democratic countries such as the United States, the dark web tends to conceal criminal activity but in highly repressive regimes, it is often a place for activists and freedom fighters to meet.

Mentioning the dark web provides us with the opportunity to point out that despite all the good things in the cyberworld—news, information, sports, weather, and an opportunity to socialize with friends in the cyberworld—there are a number of negative by-products to cyber socialization. In the following pages we will take a brief look at some examples.

Some Negative Effects of Cyber Socialization

The cyber socialization process has been going on for generations now. Nearly everyone, including the elderly who grew up in an era mostly devoid of socialization via the cyberworld, has access to the cyberworld via an electronic device and feels comfortable being a part of it. And yet, there are many who still feel that communication with friends and family and relationship maintenance via cyber socialization is impersonal and dehumanizing. Sure, we can Skype and FaceTime people, but it's not the same thing as being able to hug or shake hands with someone. There are also many people who find the cyber narcissistic tendencies of celebrities (such as the Kardashians), and regular folks alike, very annoying. But, in the grand scheme of things and with the state of the world as it is, are increased narcissistic behaviors such as taking selfies really that bad? Aren't they really just a reflection of the current times?

Still, it could be argued that there is a slippery slope involved when accepting certain forms of unconventional, deviant or criminal behaviors as the norm as the acceptance of certain activities may only encourage people to stretch the boundaries of social decorum to the point wherein cyber activities can cause great harm to people. Count the Rev. Cedric Miller of New Jersey as among those sounding the alarm of cyber evil. In 2010, the Reverend Miller declared that Facebook was a "portal to infidelity" and told married church leaders to delete their accounts or resign. He said his edict came about because much of the marital counseling he has performed over the past year and a half has concerned infidelity stemming from the social-networking website (*The Post-Standard* 11/24/10). While social network sites can contribute to infidelity, the "sin" of infidelity has been occurring long before the creation of the cyberworld. It is also interesting to note that the Reverend Miller himself had testified in a 2002 criminal case that he had a three-way sexual relationship with his wife and a male church assistant (*The Post-Standard* 11/24/10).

The comfort that many people find residing in the cyberworld after years and years of cyber socialization *has* led to the transformation of a number of deviant and criminal activities once reserved for the world of face-to-face interactions to the cyberworld. These activities range from the relatively harmless (e.g., drunk shamings and catfishing) to the more serious (e.g., cyberstalking, cyberbullying cyber porn, and revenge porn). In the following pages we will discuss these activities as they pertain to friendships.

Drunk Shamings

One of the authors of this text, Tim Delaney, has conducted a great deal of research (e.g., he interviewed and surveyed many college students) on drunk shamings and made it a primary topic in his 2008 book, *Shameful Behaviors*. Drunk shamings are still quite popular today. What is a drunk shaming, you might be asking? A drunk shaming is an example of an informal degradation ceremony designed to shame and embarrass the targeted drunk person. Degradation ceremonies represent attempts by others to alter one's identity by means of embarrassment and shame. Drunk shamings represent a rather unique type of contemporary degradation ceremony as they are generally not planned (Delaney's research found that 95 percent were not planned and the 5 percent that were planned were in retaliation for previous shaming victimizations) and spontaneous that arise when situations present themselves.

A drunk shaming occurs when people become too drunk to defend themselves from a private or public shaming. (Note: Nearly all drunk shamings are caused by young people typically of high school or college age.) A drunk shaming is an example of a quasi-degradation ceremony because it is conducted informally; and, usually by close friends and/or family members. Often, the drunk person will have his or her picture taken and usually posted online. Many people film the shaming process and upload the video on YouTube. Drunk shamings entail a four-step process:

Step 1: A person(s) drinks excessively (in the company of a group of other people) to the point where he or she passes out drunk.
Step 2: Someone from the group of people needs to take action. That is, he or she needs to start the drunk shaming process.
Step 3: Some application of a method(s) of drunk shaming must be conducted.
Step 4: The drunk shaming is captured for posterity via photo and/or video; which may then be posted in the cyberworld.

As stated in Step 3 of the drunk shaming process, some sort of drunk shaming method must be initiated. And there are a number of drunk shaming methods from which the shamers may choose. The most common method involves drawing (usually with a permanent black marker) on the victim's skin (especially derogatory and obscene messages). This type of drunk shaming was demonstrated in a scene from the movie *Garden State*. The character Andrew Largerman, played by Zach Braff, is on an MRI machine after a night of partying (drinking alcohol and taking other drugs) and he has drawings of male genitalia and other obscene things drawn on his body. (Male drunk shamers seem to have a preoccupation with drawing homo erotica images, such as penis, on their passed-out friends.)

Other shaming methods include: putting objects on/near the victim (e.g., clothing, beer bottles, sex toys, food products); exposing the victim by taking his/her clothing off; shaving eyebrows and/or hair; duct taping a shamee to toilets, walls, chairs, beds, and so on; wrapping the shamee in plastic wrap; and rearranging the victim's body into embarrassing positions. In some cases, perpetrators of a drunk shaming may employ shaming techniques known as "antiquing" and "tar and feather." (These two methods are sometimes combined.) There are various was to "antique" someone including the most popular, wetting the shamee's face with a washcloth and then throwing flour on them. The flour will stick because of the wet face. Baby powder, flour and powdered sugar may also be used instead of, or in addition to, the flour. The tar and feather technique does not involve actual hot tar, of course— remember, these are friends shaming friends—but does involve pouring a sticky substance (e.g., honey) on the shamee and then dumping pillow feathers (or some other related type of object) on the shamee.

Some participants of drunk shamings insist that there are rules involved. For example, any person who drinks excessively is a potential victim of a drunk shaming. Although most drunk shamings are administered by friends (71 percent based on Delaney's research), complete strangers (3 percent based on Delaney's research) or family members (26 percent) may also victimize a drunk person. Because drunk shamings are meant to be "good natured" fun, the victim is not to be physically harmed (e.g., no beatings, stabbings, or sexual acts committed against the shamee). It is important to note, that drunk shamings are designed to embarrass the victim, to draw attention to the victim, not to injure the person. Nearly all drunk shaming participants recognize that the host of a party is not to be shamed—it is a sign of respect to the person for hosting a party. Related to this rule is the idea of "house rules"— meaning that the host can dictate if or how a shaming will occur. Perhaps the most golden rule of drunk shaming is: if the drunk person is asleep in his or her own bed, they cannot be shamed—this is because he or she was at least able to make it home safely. Some people believe, however, if a person passes out with their shoes on, no matter the circumstances, they are fair game. Despite these generally adhered to rules, there are always some friends—and you know who you are!—that feel rules do not apply to drunk shamings.

While it has been common to shame drunk people who pass out at parties for (one assumes) centuries, only with the advent of modern technology did drunk shamings become public. Because of the age of the authors of this text, we can recall people shaming their drunk friends at college parties and maybe taking photos, especially Polaroids, but there wasn't a cyberworld where one could post such photos. So clearly, with the rise of cyber technology, drunk shamings are now available on all sorts of social networking sites, including Yik Yak and YouTube. (Note: In an article by Jesse Nickles appearing in *CollegeTimes.com,* Yik Yak is referred to as "the anonymous 'shaming' app.") To learn more about the research on drunk shamings conducted by Delaney see his book *Shameful Behaviors.* To see photos of present-day drunk shamings go to YouTube, Google Images, or do a Google search. There are plenty of photos and videos of young, drunken people online and interesting enough, in this era of narcissism, many of the so-called "victims" see such postings as a "badge of honor" or a testament to their popularity and high level of fun they engaged in while young and foolish. As Delaney recommended in 2008, future research in the area of drunk shamings should involve longitudinal studies where the long-term effects of being victimized by a drunk shaming are reexamined. In this manner, it would be possible to ascertain whether any permanent damage to one's self-esteem, sense of identity, employment and family life, is caused as a result of being victimized by a drunk shaming.

Catfishing

A drunk shaming is an example of a prank among friends. Generally, drunk shamings are good-natured and most of the people involved, even the "victims," laugh it off. Catfishing is another type of prank. Sometimes friends may set up one of their friends in an attempt to convince them that someone from the cyberworld has a crush on them. However, other motivations for catfishing may be far more sinister and include revenge, loneliness, curiosity, boredom and blackmail. The *Urban Dictionary* (2015) defines *catfishing* as "The phenomenon of internet predators that fabricate online identities and entire social circles to trick people into emotional/romantic relationships over a long period of time." The person who pretends to be someone they're not and who creates false identities on Facebook or other social networking sites for deceptive purposes is known as the "catfish." Catfish was added to the *Merriam-Webster Dictionary* in May 2014. (Note: See Popular Culture Scenario 3 for a discussion on its origin and its connection to the 2010 film *Catfish.*)

People who are victimized by a catfishing scheme feel embarrassed, angry, upset and a number of other emotions when they learn they were duped into thinking they had a relationship with someone who turned out not to be real. A well-documented case of catfishing involves current NFL, and former Notre Dame, football player Manti Te'o who believed he was involved in a "real," albeit, electronic relationship (e-relationship) with a girl named Lennay

Kekua in 2012 while he was a senior in college. As it turned out, Te'o was deceived by a man, Ronaiah Tuiasosopo, the "catfish" who sent photos of Kekua (they were photos of a different young woman that Tuiasosopo found online—thus creating another victim) to Te'o to keep the prank going (Goodman 2013). Te'o has since explained that he met a woman online with whom he maintained what he thought was an authentic relationship through frequent phone calls (Tuiasosopo disguised his voice to sound like a woman) and online conversations and fell in love with her. "He called himself the victim of 'someone's sick joke'" (Brady and George 2013). To be kind, Te'o was naive; to be blunt he was foolish to think he was in an actual relationship with a young woman, Lennay Kekua, someone he never met. The young woman who was used in the catfishing scheme was Diane O'Meara and she claims that her pictures were stolen and that she never met Te'o (Goodman 2013).

Popular Culture Scenario 3: *Catfishing*: The Movie and the TV Show

"Catfishing" is a slang term that refers to the deceptive activity of internet predators that create false online identities in order to trick someone into thinking they are involved in an emotional and/or romantic relationship. The illusory relationship is generally extended over a long period of time which has the intended consequence of hurting the targeted victim all the more. While the fake romance, when revealed, is bad enough for the duped victim, it can be compounded if the catfish (the person who runs the scam) attempted and was successful in gaining access to the victim's bank accounts, credit cards and so on.

The origins of "Catfishing" are attributed to the 2010 film *Catfish*, a "pseudo-documentary that chronicled a young man's online friendship with a woman that turned out to be very different from her Facebook profile" (Palmer 2013). (The film was a critical and commercial success and would lead to the MTV reality TV series called *Catfish: The TV Show*.) In the film *Catfish*, young Manhattan (NY) filmmakers, Yaniv "Nev" Schulman, Ariel Schulman and Henry Joost document the budding online friendship and romance of Nev with a young woman named Megan and her family living in rural Ishpeming, Michigan (Ebert 2010). Nev and Megan send each other posts online and after a while, Megan sends him MP3s of song covers she performs for him (that he later discovers were lifted from other performers on YouTube). They talk on the phone with one another. Nev marvels at her beautiful Facebook photos. They have entered into a cyber romance, a type of romance that is achieved without having met the other person face-to-face. Nev thinks that Megan could be the girl of his dreams. Driving home from their shoot of a dance event in Vail, the three videographers decide to take a detour to Ishpeming so that Nev can surprise and meet with Megan. And that's when the catfishing story of the film takes a surprising turn. No spoilers here, you will have to watch the film yourself to see what happens.

The TV show *Catfish* was inspired by the film of the same name. The MTV series brings together couples who've interacted solely through their LCD screens over the course of months or years to see what happens when these romantics who have become smitten meet in real life for the first time (MTV 2016). The first episode of *Catfish: The TV Show* aired November 12, 2012. New episodes were still airing at the time of this writing (2016). Each episode involves stories of people who are having trouble with their online dating relationships and the videographers documenting the pre-story and the meeting of the electronic lovers in an attempt to determine whether the cyber relationship is legitimate or whether a "catfish" is involved. If you like to peek at other people's relationships or are fascinated by the catfish phenomenon, this is the show for you.

Being a victim of catfishing is a contemporary phenomenon as the key elements necessary for catfishing have only existed in recent years. These elements include the existence of social networking sites. Second, there has to be people who are willing to consider strangers as "friends," something that is often the case on Facebook. Third, there has to be someone willing to victimize another person. And fourth, there has to a willingness among people to think that it is possible to have a dating relationship with someone strictly in the cyber world. These four elements combined explain why catfishing is possible today but was never possible in the past as previous generations would say it's only possible to have a relationship with someone with whom you have met (we will discuss this topic in Chapter 4).

The prevalence of catfishing would appear to be minimal at this point. In our own research we asked college students if they knew what the term "catfishing" meant. The vast majority of respondents (nearly 78 percent of males and 90 percent of females) reported that they did (see Table 3.1). Interestingly, only three respondents of the 184 total participants that answered this question reported any personal experience with catfishing. Of these three, just one was an actual victim of catfishing—via chat room conversations only, she said—while the other two reported that they caught on pretty quickly when they were electronically approached (one on Snapchat and one on Facebook) in a devious manner.

Table 3.1: Do You Know What the Term "Catfishing" Means? by Gender, in Percent

Males (N=76)		Females (N=108)	
Yes	77.6	Yes	90.0
No	22.4	No	10.0

The discussion of catfishing serves as a nice transition to the topic of cyberbullying as, according to the CyberBully Hotline (2013), catfishing is an example of cyberbullying.

Cyberbullying

Cyberbullying is the act of harassing someone online by sending or posting embarrassing photos/videos or mean-spirited messages, including spreading rumors/gossips, about a person, often done anonymously. Catfishing is considered an example of cyberbullying because someone had to create a false identity online and they did so for bullying purposes (CyberBully Hotline 2013). Teens suffering from angst may be susceptible to catfishing schemes because they often turn to websites that foster connections with strangers. The bullying form of catfishing has been increasing over the past few years. "Several teens have committed suicide after a 'catfish' in their school or community targeted them for abuse. Many more have experienced the pain of being deceived, abused, and teased after falling for the deceptive moves of a 'catfish' (CyberBully Hotline 2013). The CyberBully Hotline provides three suggestions to parents to help keep their teens safe from catfish cyberbullying:

1. Know all of the websites and mobile apps that your teen is using to network with others.
2. Encourage your teen to connect only with people they know in real life.
3. Keep your teens from disclosing personal information on social media sites.

As described by StopBullying.gov (a website managed by the U.S. Department of Health and Human Services), cyberbullying is different than face-to-face bullying, and emphasize these points:

- Kids who are being cyberbullied are often bullied in person as well
- Kids who are cyberbullied have a harder time getting away from the behavior as it can happen 24 hours a day, 7 days a week
- Cyberbullying messages and images can be posted anonymously and distributed quickly to a very wide audience. It is often difficult to trace the source
- Deleting inappropriate or harassing messages, texts, and pictures is extremely difficult after they have been posted or sent (StopBullying. gov 2015).

StopBullying.gov (2015) points out that cyber technology (e.g., smart phones and computers) is not to blame for cyberbullying, as social media sites are often used for positive activities; but, they warn that these same tools can be used to hurt other people. The effects of cyberbullying can be devastated to young people [and adults]. Kids who are cyberbullied are more likely to:

- Use alcohol and drugs
- Skip school
- Experience in-person bullying
- Be unwilling to attend school
- Receive poor grades
- Have lower self-esteem
- Have more health problems

Cyberbullying is quite common. According to the National Center for Education Statistics (NCES) (2014), approximately 9 percent of students ages 12–18 reported being cyberbullied in 2011. More girls than boys reported being cyberbullied. The 2013 Youth Risk Behavior Surveillance Survey found that 15 percent of high school students (grades 9–12) were electronically bullied in the past year (StopBullying.gov 2015). Trying to eliminate cyberbullying is as difficult of a challenge as trying to stop face-to-face bullying— something that has likely occurred throughout humanity. Cyberbullying does not end in high school or in one's teens. Cyberbullying occurs in college, outside of college and after college years of age. One must be careful about their social networking as many sites and apps perpetuate cyberbullying, even when it's their intent to simply foster sociability. Consider, for example the Yik Yak app. In October 2013, two Furman University students launched the popular app Yik Yak in an effort to connect people through anonymous location-based posts. While the Yik Yak app rules allow for communication of almost any kind, they specifically state that there is a zero tolerance policy on bullying. Nonetheless, the site is a place where the trend of cyberbullying exists alongside the proper usage of sharing ideas, having fun, and meeting people (Inguaggiato 2014).

Cyberstalking

The cyberworld provides people with an opportunity to communicate with a wide variety of people including friends, family, business associates, acquaintances, and long lost people from our past. Conversely, it provides a series of networks that allow people an opportunity to track others who may not want anything to do with specific others. This negative aspect of tracking down others leads us to cyberstalking, or cyberharassment. The repeated act of following, watching, harassing, or trying to communicate with someone who does not want your attention is known as stalking. When stalking is done in the cyber world it is known as cyberstalking. *Cyberstalking* involves the use of electronic forms of communication (e.g., social networking sites, email, or smart phones) to track or harass a person. Cyberstalking can be combined with traditional forms of stalking and either deviant instance is a criminal offense. While the terms of *cyberstalking* and *cyberharassment* are fairly similar there are differences. According to the National Conference of State Legislatures (2015b), *cyberstalking* is the use of the Internet, email or other electronic communications to stalk, and generally refers to a pattern of threatening or malicious behaviors. Depending on the credible threat of harm, sanctions against cyberstalking may range from misdemeanors to felonies. Cyberharassment differs from cyberstalking in that such actions do not involve a credible threat. Cyberharassment usually pertains to threatening or harassing email messages, instant messages, or to blog entries or websites dedicated solely to tormenting an individual.

In a 2011 poll, thirty-two percent of respondents said that they had used a social-networking site to spy on an old flame (*Parade* 2011). There are a number of ways to keep track of your current friends and loved ones by using SpyBuddy software. SpyBuddy allows you to spy on website visits (it lets you know what websites people visit that use your various electronic devices); spy on IM and online chats; spy on emails; spy on passwords; spy on files downloaded and printed documents; emails sent/received; Twitter messages and updates; YouTube Videos watched; Skype chats; external USB file transfers; and capture screenshots. In sum, SpyBuddy (2016) promotes themselves as a reliable, stealthy and easy way to spy on others.

In 2011, a 12-year-old Washington girl was sentenced to probation and community service for a cyberstalking incident in which she and another 11-year-old girl hacked an ex-friend's (and classmate's) Facebook account and filled it with explicit photos and solicitations for sex. The victim was going through therapy following the revelation of her doctored Facebook account. The mother of the victim wanted, at the least, for the convicted cyberbully to be banned from access to social media for the full term of probation. The judge however, felt that it would be fine for her to go online with parental supervision (Riparbelli 2011).

Revenge Porn

Remember when we suggested that longitudinal studies should be conducted on the long-term effects of being victimized by a drunk shaming in order to ascertain whether there were any negative effects to the shamee based on a cyber posting of their questionable behavior? Well, the same concern applies to the topic of "revenge porn" as the posting of photographs/videos of one's past indiscretions, or maybe lack of better judgment, can come to haunt people who allowed their friends/lovers to take sexual ("porno-graphic") photos of them. As with drunk shaming photos, revenge porn photos can compromise one's self-esteem, self-concept, sense of identity, and private and public lives.

What is revenge porn? Revenge porn involves the cyber sharing of sexually explicit photos/videos of another person (generally an ex-lover or ex-friend) by an angered ex-partner without the consent of the person(s) in the photo/video for the purpose of spiteful humiliation. (Note: Posting photos/videos of non-consenting adults and minors engaged in sexual acts are not examples of revenge porn as they would fall under a different category of crime, such as rape.) The process of revenge porn begins innocently enough via sexting or posing in a sexual manner. The photos are meant to be shared only between the immediate persons involved. Sexting and posing sexually brings excitement to a relationship. When one sends a sext or allows themselves to be photographed or video recorded they are caught up in the moment of flirting or romance. Such persons work with a sort of assumption that the photographs or videos are going to be kept private and because there is trust involved, people may lose their inhibitions and allow photos to be taken that would otherwise be reserved for porno magazines or video recordings.

While sexting or posing seductively or while performing a sex act involves a leap of faith, such trust is often violated. This is especially the case if the lover/friend who was "dumped," feels jilted and wants to get some sort of revenge. With sexually explicit photos/videos at their arsenal, they upload the electronic images to the cyberworld. Once in the cyberworld, the material is readily available. It is surprisingly easy to find revenge porn photos or videos on such mainstream sites as Google Images and YouTube.

Because revenge porn is a relatively new development, it has taken various judicial systems a while to catch up with this cyber activity. Consider for example, that a man who posted nude photos of his ex-girlfriend without her consent on her employer's Facebook page became the first person to be convicted under California's "revenge porn" law in late 2014 (O'Connor 2014). The UK began introducing revenge porn laws in 2015. In April 2015, a new law went into effect forbidding people from sharing sexually explicit images without the subject's consent (Barrett 2015).

While we would like to think we can trust our friends—and certainly people with whom we have sexual relations should be considered friends in addition to a romantic partners—anyone who has, or is thinking about, sexting or sexually posing for another should consider revenge porn as among the potential devastating conclusions. This is especially true when we realize that the vast majority of romantic relationships anyone has over their lifetime is likely to end up in failure (or break-up, if you prefer).

This concludes our discussion on some of the negative effects of cyber socialization. There are, of course, many other negative aspects of cyber socialization including cyber porn, identity theft, and large-scale hacking of commercial and financial institutions but we have kept our discussion limited to those that involve friendship relationships.

Summary

In this chapter we learned how the development of communications technology and the rise of the Internet combined with the changing cultural norms and values of society contributed to cyber socialization. We also learned how the cyber socialization process itself developed and expanded to become the powerful force in our lives that it is. While cyber socialization has many positive aspects, it also has some negative effects as well.

The development of communications technology began in earnest with the creation of the postal service, which also involved the short-lived pony express and telegraph wire service; the evolution of the telephone from its modest beginnings to its now mini computer status; the role of mass media communications; and the omnipresent role of the computer. All of these developments have assisted in the maintenance of friendships while also serving as aspects of cyber socialization. The development of communications technology could not have evolved as it did without changes to the prevailing cultural values and norms of society. Many aspects of culture have changed that have led to the general acceptance of a world dominated by cyber socialization. The cyberworld has, much to the chagrin of many people, amplified the audience of people who might be able to judge us when we make mistakes. In an effort to counteract such things as drunk shamings, catfishing, cyberbullying, cyberstalking and revenge porn, many people have turned to a trusted way of trying to maintain a positive sense of self-identify via a controlled presentation of self. This preoccupation with self, however, has led to an increase in narcissistic behaviors.

4

Electronic Friendships

Facebook, often referred to as "Big Brother" because the entity has so much information on so many people that it concerns some of us (and should concern everyone), seems particularly intrusive when it suggests to us people we should invite to be our friends. In many instances we have no friends in common, or just one or a few mutual friends in common, with Facebook's suggested friend (to be fair, in other cases, we do have multiple friends in common). Surely, anyone on Facebook sometimes wonders why it thinks specific people would make good friends for us. Count Victor Van Rossem, a 24-year-old student from Belgium, among those people who wonders why he should send a friend request to an unknown person just because Facebook suggested it. Van Rossem received a friend request suggestion from Facebook for 49-year-old Neal D. Retke, a person with whom he had one mutual friend. Van Rossem browsed through Retke's photos, hobbies, likes and posts and found him to be "a very eccentric person" (White 2015).

Possessing a curiosity, and apparently with a great deal of time on his hands, Van Rossem and a real-life friend decided to travel 5,000 miles to meet Retke in person. Upon their arrival in Retke's Texas home city, the two Belgians searched for a week, putting posters up on many streets and asking people if they knew Retke. (They also made a short documentary chronicling the trip.) The two Belgians also made shirts that read "Neal D. Retke for President!" in order to get the word out to passersby. They eventually found Retke at a book signing and nervously approached him—"We didn't know how he would react," Van Rossem said. "But after we explained the whole thing he just laughed and said, 'Well, you found [me],' as if he was expecting us" (White 2015). The three men ended up spending three weeks together. Retke said that he may visit the two students the following summer in Belgium.

Among other things in this chapter, we will examine the concept of electronic friendships and the growing number of online friendships and also compare and contrast real friends with virtual friends.

Spending an Increasing Amount of Time in the Cyberworld

The cyber socialization process discussed in Chapter 5 has assisted in ushering in electronic worlds filled with electronic friendships and virtual forms of realities that people choose to spend a great time of time to reside in. The cyber socialization process, among other things, indoctrinated us into accepting the fact that an increasing number of social interactions once done in person could, and would, now take place in the cyberworld. Following our acceptance for the need of a cyberworld we have become further drawn into virtual worlds where an escalating number of social interactions take place.

Not Now, I'm Online

It will not come as a surprise to anyone that the amount of time people spend using the electronic media and communicating with one another in cyberspace rather than in face-to-face interactions has increased dramatically over the course of the past few decades. The amount of time spent in the cyberworld generally comes at the cost of less time spent with personal relationships in the real world. In a 2008 study, 65 percent of Americans were found to spend more time with their computers than with their significant others (Kelton Research and Support 2008). *USA Today* declared 2010 "the year we stopped talking to one another" in light of the unprecedented use of technology (Cafferty 2011). In 2010, it was estimated that 93 percent of Americans used a cell phone or wireless device; about one-third of those people used smartphones which allow users to browse the Web and check email on their phones. From June 2009 to June 2010, cell phone subscribers sent 1.8 trillion text messages; up 33 percent from the year before (Cafferty 2011).

Citing data provided by ZenithOptimedia (a marketing firm that prioritizes "Return on Investment," or ROI for its clients), Jason Karaian (2015) reports that Americans spend a little more than 8 hours per day consuming media. Television is still the king, followed by internet use. Karaian states that average daily internet media consumption has doubled over the past five years, up from 13 percent in 2010 to an estimated 30 percent in 2017. Latin Americans spend the most time (13 hours per day) with some sort of media and Asian-Pacific residents the least amount of time (a little more than 5 hours) (Karaian 2015).

Statista (a leading statistics company that compiles quantitative data, statistics and related information for business clients and academics since 2008), however, reports that in 2014, Americans aged 18 and older spend more than 11 hours a day watching TV, listening to the radio or using smartphones, and other electronic devices (Richter 2015). Richter (2015) further reports that when we factor in that most people are awake 16 to 18 hours a day, 11 hours per day of electronic media represents a high percentage of our waking activity. To be fair though, people can still socialize with one another while watching TV, listening to the radio, or using electronic devices. Perhaps underscoring the idea that people multi-task while they use electronic devices, Richter's article on Statista's data provides links that allow readers to share his article on Facebook, Twitter, LinkedIn and Google+. Richter also reports that the use of Tablets and Smartphones has increased the most from 2010 to 2014 while television viewing has remained relatively steady (a slight increase during this time period) and reading newspapers and magazines has dropped a bit from its already relatively low share of people's time.

According to a report by Common Sense Media (their website states that Common Sense Media is an independent nonprofit organization dedicated to helping kids thrive in a world of media and technology), American teens spend about nine hours a day using media for their enjoyment; with some 13-year-olds checking social media 100 times a day (Wallace 2015). Putting that into perspective, nine hours spent on social media is more time than teens typically spend sleeping, and more time than they spend with their parents and teachers—and these daily nine hours of usage do not include time spent using media at school or for their homework (Wallace 2015). Tweens, identified as children 8 to 12, spend about six hours, on average, consuming media. "When it comes to consuming media on screens, including laptops, smartphones and tablets, teens, on average, spend more than six and a half hours on screens and tweens more than four and a half hours" (Wallace 2015).

As previously described by Richter in his analysis of Statista data, Wallace found that tweens and teens believe that they can effectively multi-task while using electronic devices. More than 60 percent of tweens and teens, for example, report that they text and more than 75 percent say they listen to music while working on schoolwork at home. Nearly two-thirds say watching TV or texting makes no difference and more than 50 percent feel the same way when it comes to social media (Wallace 2015). Research studies, such as the one conducted at Stanford, however, reveals that there are dramatic differences in cognitive control and ability to process information between heavy media multitaskers and light media multitaskers. The Stanford study, conducted by Ophir, Nass and Wagner (2009) found, among other things, that:

- When intentionally distracting elements were added to experiments, heavy media multitaskers were on average 77 milliseconds slower than their light media multitasker counterparts at identifying changes in patterns.

- In a longer-term memory test that invited participants to recall specific elements from earlier experiments, the high media multitaskers more often falsely identified the elements that had been used most frequently as intentional distracters.
- In the presence of distracting elements, high media multitaskers were 426 milliseconds slower than their counterparts to switch to new activities and 259 milliseconds slower to engage in a new section of the same activity (Ophir et al., 2009; Wihbey 2011).

Wallace (2015) reports that there are gender differences when it comes to multitasking for tweens and teens as 62 percent of boys say they enjoy playing video games (i.e., Xbox) "a lot" versus 20 percent of girls; while 44 percent of girls say they enjoy using social media (i.e., Instagram) "a lot" versus 29 percent for boys. Socioeconomic status (SES) also plays a role in the amount of time tweens and teens spend online as only 54 percent of youth in households making less than $35,000 a year have a laptop in their home versus 92 percent of youth in households making $100,000 a year or more. Despite the many proclamations that TV is dead, the favorite media outlet for tweens and teens is watching television, followed by listening to music. And yet, 53 percent of tweens have their own tablet and 67 percent of teens have their own smartphones. Mobile devices account for 41 percent of all screen time for tweens and 46 percent for teens (Wallace 2015).

In the UK, young people aged between 16 and 24 spend more than 27 hours a week on the internet and people of all ages are spending twice as much time online compared to 10 years ago, fueled by increasing use of tablets and smartphones. Young adults are especially responsible for this increase in the UK as the time spent online has almost tripled from 10 hours and 24 minutes each week in 2005 to 27 hours and 36 minutes in 2014 (Anderson 2015). The average person spends 2.5 hours every week "online while on the move"—away from their home, work or place of study. This is a five-fold increase from 2005, when the figure was just 30 minutes. Overall, the proportion of adults using the internet has risen from six in ten in 2005 to almost nine in ten in 2015 (Anderson 2015). A similar trend is occurring in the UK as in the U.S.; while people are still watching a great deal of TV and films, they are increasingly watching this programming online. Many people will be reluctant to give up TV because of the large screens as, let's face it, any show, movie, or sporting event looks a lot better on a 55-inch screen than a 5-inch screen, especially in high-definition.

As documented above, people are spending an increasing amount of time online. While online sites and viewing has become a norm in society, there are some people who have a real problem, a compulsive problem, with their need to use the internet.

Internet Use Disorder

Along with the increased dependency that so many people have with being online comes the expected growing number of people who have become, or risk becoming, addicted to the Internet. Recognized as an addiction for over a decade now, internet addiction is "characterized by excessive or poorly controlled preoccupations, urges or behaviours regarding computer use and internet access that lead to impairment or distress" (Shaw and Black 2008). In their 2008 published research results, Shaw and Black reported:

- Just 0.3 to 0.7 percent of the US population suffered from internet use disorder
- Internet disorder occurs worldwide, but mainly in countries where computer access and technology are widespread
- Their results also showed a male preponderance to internet use disorder with onset generally occurring in their late 20s or early 30s age group

Among the symptoms of internet use disorder are dimensionally measured depression and indicators of social isolation. Psychiatric co-morbidity is common, particularly mood, anxiety, impulse control and substance use disorders. Aetiology is unknown, but probably involves psychological, neurobiological and cultural factors. Shaw and Black (2008) were unaware of any evidence-based treatments for internet addiction.

When addictions are particularly intense the term "compulsive" becomes applicable. Compulsive behaviors are characterized by a strong, obsessive urge or desire to do something. Compulsive internet use disorder is characterized by such behavior as people having an "inability to stop themselves from using computers, rising levels of tolerance that drive them to seek ever longer sessions online, and withdrawal symptoms like anger and craving when prevented from logging on" (Fackler 2008: A9). While deemed a mental health issue in many countries as recently as 2013, the American Psychiatric Association's (APA) Diagnostic and Statistical Manual of Mental Disorders (DSM)—the diagnostic bible for mental health professionals—had not listed internet use disorder as a mental health problem in its manual. The 2013 manual did, however, recognize Internet Gaming Disorder in its appendix as requiring further study (Steiner-Adair 2015).

In 2008, researchers in South Korea believed that internet addiction was a big problem in their country. Ahn Dong-hyun, a child psychiatrist at Hanyang University in Seoul, led a government-financed survey on the problem and found that "up to 30 percent of South Koreans under 18, or about 2.4 million people, are at risk of internet addiction" (Fackler 2008: A9). South Korean youth spent at least two hours a day online, usually playing games or chatting, and in extreme cases users have started dropping dead from exhaustion after playing online games for days at a time. A growing number of South Korean children are skipping school to stay online (Fackler 2008). To address this social problem, the South Korean government established a number of Internet-addiction counseling centers in addition to nearly one hundred treatment programs at local hospitals. Fast-forward to 2015 and research estimates put the number of South Korean children between the ages of 10 and 19 addicted to the internet at roughly 10 percent (Steiner-Adair 2015).

In 2008, Jerald J. Block, a psychiatrist at Oregon Health and Science University, estimated that up to nine million Americans were at risk for internet use disorder, or what he called pathological computer use. Block reported that only a handful of clinics in the U.S. specialized in treating the disorder (Fackler 2008). A 2014 study indicates that a much higher percentage of young adult Americans may be suffering from internet addiction disorder than warned by Block just six years earlier (Steiner-Adair 2015). A survey of 1,300 young adults (18- to 25-years-old), conducted by marketing agency Digital Clarity found that 16 percent displayed symptoms of net addiction—with nearly of al them admitting to spending over 15 hours a day online (*BBC News* 2014). This survey looked at five signs of possible net addiction:

- Spending hours online on a daily basis
- Becoming irritable when interrupted during web use
- Feeling guilty about how much time is spent online
- Isolation from family and friends due to excessive online activity
- A sense of euphoria when online and panic when offline

Perhaps reflecting the reluctance of the APA to classify internet use disorder as a legitimate mental disorder, a number of psychiatrists believe the effects of internet addiction are just symptoms of other psychological conditions (*BBC News* 2014).

Whether or not excessive internet use is an addiction, a mental disorder, or simply a reflection of our changing times, it is clear that people are spending a great deal of time online.

Most Popular Social Network Sites

People spend about a quarter of their time online social networking. Global Web Index polled 170,000 internet users about their internet habits and found that average usage times for social media sites rose from 1.66 hours per day in 2013 to 1.72 hours per day in 2014 (Bennett 2015). Micro-blogging, which includes Twitter, is also up slightly to 0.81 hours per day, and now accounts for about 13 percent of total time spent online (Bennett 2015). The average person has five social media accounts (Davidson 2015). At one hour and 20 minutes per day, Britons spend less time than Americans on social networking sites (Davidson 2015). The importance of social network sites is very important in the study of friendship and happiness, as this is where electronic friendships reside.

So, where do people go when they social network? Is Facebook the most popular social network site? Has Facebook always been, and will it always remain, the most popular social network site? The exploration of Facebook is quite enlightening as its history provides us with a glimpse into the changing nature of social networking in the cyberworld.

At the beginning of 2008, MySpace maintained about 72 percent of the social-networking market, while Facebook held about 16 percent. MySpace was so popular that only two other websites enjoyed higher total cybermarket shares in January 2008: google.com (5.27 percent) and mail.yahoo.com (4.91 percent), with MySpace.com at 4.49 percent (*Hitwise U.S.* 2008). Facebook, which was reserved for college students only at that time, hardly registered as a significant social networking site. Everything changed once Facebook allowed nonstudents to use its social-networking site as the number of subscribers increased dramatically, and by mid–2008 Facebook had surpassed MySpace. By August 2010, Facebook's membership neared 600 million and many wondered whether MySpace could survive. The number of Facebook users would continue to skyrocket for the next four years until 2015 when it became the only major social network to see a decline in active users; overall growth in new members would continue to increase, however (Davidson 2015).

That the number of active Facebook users did not increase in 2015 is understandable when we consider two very important factors: (1) Its total number of users is still far ahead of any other social network site, and (2) the realization that younger people are more active on other sites, such as YouTube and Snapchat, even though they maintain a Facebook account. According to statistics provided by Facebook (2016), the total number of monthly active Facebook users was 1.44 billion in June 2016. At nearly one and half billion users, Facebook was the most popular social networking site in 2016.

Conducting research on the top social networking sites provides interesting contrasts in statistics. For example, eBiz (which bills itself as the eBusiness) acknowledges Facebook as the most popular social networking site (as of June 2016) but claims that there are "just" 1.1 billion estimated unique monthly visitors. Below are the "Top 15 Most Popular Social Networking

Sites/June 2016" and the estimated unique monthly visitors as compiled by eBiz (2016):

1. Facebook, 1.1 billion
2. YouTube, 1 billion
3. Twitter, 310 million
4. LinkedIn, 255 million
5. Pinterest, 250 million
6. Google+ (or Google Plus), 120 million
7. Tumblr, 110 million
8. Instagram, 100 million
9. Reddit, 85 million
10. VK, 80 million
11. Flickr, 65 million
12. Vine, 42 million
13. Meetup, 13 million
14. Ask.fm, 37 million
15. ClassMates, 15 million

In February 2016, "trends expert" Elise Moreau, writing for *About.com*, compiled a listing of "The Top 25 Social Networking Sites People are Using" and, of course, Facebook was ranked #1. Let's take a look at their list and you can compare it to the one generated by eBiz four months later (Moreau 2016):

1. Facebook (interestingly, About.com states there are 1.59 billion monthly active users)
2. Twitter (public microblogging)
3. LinkedIn (social networking for professionals)
4. Google+ (emphasis on "Communities and Collections" features)
5. YouTube (owned by Google but with its own identity as *the* place to watch or post videos)
6. Instagram (very popular photo sharing social network)
7. Pinterest (social shopping, among other things)
8. Tumblr (social blogging popular with teens and young adults)
9. Vine (owned by Twitter and featuring short videos)
10. Snapchat (totally mobile-based, instant messaging, very popular with tweens and teens and young adults)
11. Reddit (social networking with friends and celebs and public figures)
12. Flickr (Yahoo's photo-sharing network)
13. Swarm by Foursquare (social location discovery tool)
14. Kik (free instant messaging app poplar with teens and young adults)
15. Yik Yak (anonymous posting social network site popular with teens and young adults)

16. Shots (photo and video sharing social network site that young kids love to use)
17. Periscope (live web video broadcasting)
18. Medium (the best social network for readers and writers)
19. SoundCloud (most popular social network for sharing sounds)
20. Tinder (a location-based dating app that matches you up with people in your area)
21. WhatsApp (instant messaging social networking site)
22. Slack (communication platform for collaborative teams; essentially a social network site for the workplace)
23. Musical.ly (social networking app for sharing short music videos)
24. Peach (launched in 2016, trying to find its true niche)
25. Blab (live streaming social network site)

In our own research, we asked college students to identify the social media sites they used most often (see Table 4.1). Instagram was much more popular in our survey—reflecting the general age of our respondents who were mostly between 18 and 24 years old—than in the other two lists previously described. Facebook remains popular with our surveyed college students but it does not possess exclusivity with many of our respondents. As shown in Table 4.1, Instagram, Snapchat, Facebook and Twitter are the four most popular social network sites used by our survey participants.

Table 4.1: Most Commonly Used Sites by Gender, Number and in Percent

Males (N=76)			Females (N=108)		
Social Media Site	#	Percent	Social Media Site	#	Percent
Facebook	54	71	Instagram	89	82
Instagram	51	67	Snapchat	83	77
Snapchat	41	54	Facebook	80	74
Twitter	37	49	Twitter	59	55
YouTube	4	5	Tumblr	12	11
Reddit	3	4	Pinterest	4	4
Tumblr	3	4	Yik Yak	2	2
LinkedIn	2	3	YouTube	2	2
Steam	1	1	BuzzFeed	1	1
Beme	1	1	Reddit	1	1
Yik Yak	1	1	Messenger	1	1
Twitch.tv	1	1	Tinder	1	1
None	3	4	VSCO	1	1

We can see that most of the same popular social network sites appear in each of the three research studies cited here, although not necessarily in the same order. Despite the competition of an ever-increasing array of social network sites available to internet users, Facebook remains, for now, as the overall most popular social network site.

Facebook is, perhaps, the most important of all the social network sites for our discussion on friendship as its basic public mission is to help people maintain and "add" new friends. Facebook *is* a friendship social network. We will discuss Facebook again later in this chapter when we discuss electronic friendships but right now it is helpful to analyze the social network site a little more closely to see how it works and what makes it so popular. First, let's look at some other data provided by Facebook (2016):

- Total number of mobile Facebook users at 874 million
- Increase in Facebook users from 2014 to 2015 at 12 percent
- Total number of minutes spent on Facebook each month at 640 million
- Percent of all Facebook users who log on in any give day, 48 percent
- Average time spent on Facebook per visit, 18 minutes
- Total number of Facebook pages, 74.2 million
- Number of fake Facebook profiles, 81 million
- Average number of friends per Facebook user, 130; and, average number of pages, groups and events a user is connected to, 80
- 48 percent of 18–34-year-olds check Facebook when they wake up and 28 percent check Facebook before they get out of bed
- The number of languages available on Facebook is 70
- Three out of four Facebook users live outside of the United States
- Every 20 minutes on Facebook there are 1 million links shared, 2 million friends requested, and 3 million messages sent

It is worth noting that, officially, Facebook is not allowed in China (but as we described in Chapter 3 in our discussion on Virtual Personal Networks, it is accessible), but if it were to be allowed to operate in the open, their user numbers would surely increase tremendously.

What is the appeal of Facebook? For many, the answer to that question is relatively simple. People like to keep up with their friends, they like to add new friends, and they like to let their friends know what is going on. For some people, Facebook is their source for news, and for others, it's a great way to follow their favorite sports teams. Yet for others, Facebook provides an opportunity to control their presentation of self via the select posts they make and the photos they share. What many users may not be aware of is the positive experience Facebook can provide people in their *nucleus accumbens*, which is a very small but critical structure located deep in the center of the brain and which is responsible for the reward system of the brain (Meshi, Morawetz and Heekeren 2013). The nucleus accumbens is the part of the brain that's associated with motivation, pleasure, and addiction—sometimes called the brain's "pleasure center." Meshi and associates (2013) found that positive feedback on Facebook in the form of "likes" and positive feedback to comments made via posts can stimulate the nucleus accumbens. The researchers found that brain scans taken while someone received positive feedback could be used to predict that user's intensity of Facebook use. The results suggest that people may be driven to use Facebook by a desire to monitor their reputation (Meshi et al. 2013; Mohan 2013). The triggering of the reward system can transform social networking use into an addictive behavior which needs further stimulation. However, an opposite experience on Facebook—the lack of positive feedback (few or no likes and favorable comments to posts)—can make social networking a bummer and lead to a less active status. This negative experience on Facebook can also lead to a drop in immediate mood and long-term outlook according to Meshi and associates. There is a lesson to be learned by this: if you want to create a successful app, make sure it makes people happy—that it stimulates the nucleus accumbens.

Facebook is certainly aware of the idea that if they make users happy on their social networking site people will continue to use it. Facebook is, after all, a business. They weren't always a business but they have been for a few years now. Thus, Facebook uses programs designed to find out what people "like" and then shares it with advertisers who will then target their products to specific users (consumers) who are most likely to want them. Thus, if you "like" political messages from one party or specific candidate, you are likely to get targeted message from that source. If you "like" a particular sports team, expect to receive messages from them via advertisements.

In 2016, political conservatives accused Facebook of disproportionately labeling liberal news items as "trending topics" so that its users would be influenced by particular political leanings. In an article appearing in *The Post-Standard*, the Rev. Michael Meath went so far as to claim that Facebook is unwittingly intensifying and accelerating polarization of our society and therein may be fostering bigotry and intolerance. Meath (2016) states, "By surrounding ourselves with like-minded opinions, we as a society are becoming more fractured and losing our connection to the common ground and goals that bind us together as a nation" (p. A-14).

The idea that Facebook has sinister plot designs to separate people into like-minded categories based on their "likes" leads to other complaints. (We should bear in mind that Facebook seems to be the primary target of various complaints and accusations of conspiracies because of its large number of users.) For years now, as the popularity of social networking has increased, primarily at the expense of face-to-face interactions, a number of people—health organizations, academics and parents among them—have begun to mockingly refer to social networking sites like Facebook as

"antisocial networking." "Children used to actually talk to their friends....
But now, even chatting on cell phones or via e-mail (through which you can
at least converse in paragraphs) is *passé*. For today's teenagers and preteens,
the give and take of friendship seems to be conducted increasingly in the
abbreviated snatches of cell-phone texts and instant messages, or through
the very public forum of Facebook walls and MySpace bulletins" (Stout
2010:C-2). (It should be noted that Facebook forums can be limited to specific
friends or groups and posts are not necessarily public.)

Novelist and columnist Stephen Marche (2012), writing for *The Atlantic*,
argues that Facebook may be making us lonely rather than helping to maintain friendships. Marche was inspired to write his article following the discovery of the body of Yvette Vickers, a former *Playboy* playmate and B-movie
star, best known for her role in *Attack of the 50 Foot Woman*. At age 82, Vickers's body lay dead for a better part of a year before a neighbor and fellow
actress, Susan Savage, noticed cobwebs and yellowing letters in her mailbox
and eventually pushed her way through an unlocked door and piles of junk
mail and mounds of clothing that barricaded the house. Vickers' lonesome
death became the subject of over 16,000 Facebook posts and 881 tweets. As
it turns out, Vickers had slipped into loneliness because she did not have
contact with any close relatives (she did not have children), no religious
group, and no immediate social circle of friends. There exists an accelerating
contradiction: the more connected we become in the cyberworld, the lonelier
we are as people become transfixed by the glare of a screen, awaiting responses
from others (Marche 2012). Eric Klinenberg, a sociologist at NYU, writes:
"Reams of published research show that it's the quality, not the quantity of
social interaction that best predicts loneliness" (March 2012). It is estimated
that about 60 million Americans are unhappy with their lives because of loneliness. Thus, while social networking has its place, it does not replace face-
to-face interactions with family and friends. To be fair, it may not be that
Facebook makes someone lonely, but rather, perhaps lonely people are
attracted to social networking. Among the things that almost all mental health
advocates agree on is that loneliness (or social isolation) can have a serious
detrimental effect on one's mental and physical health (*Psychology Today*
2016).

There are those who have predicted the demise of Facebook. For example, in 2014, researchers John Cannarella and Joshua Spechler at Princeton
University using publicly available Google data, cited the downfall of
MySpace, and incorporated a modified SIR model (S = Susceptible individuals; I = infected individuals; and R = recovered individuals), the Infectious
Recovery SIR model (irSIR) used to measure the spread of infectious diseases,
and determined that Facebook would undergo a rapid decline (via a type of
infectious disease analogy) in the coming years, losing 80 percent of its peak

user base between 2015 and 2017. As the data provided in this chapter indicates, Facebook is not dying off, it is thriving. We guess that it is time for these researchers to go back to the drawing board and perhaps use a different model.

In June 2014, YouGov research suggested in its "Social Media 2014" report that Facebook and Twitter would lose substantial numbers of users over concerns about privacy and advertising fatigue. Again, as we know, in mid–2016 Facebook is still going strong (we will look at Twitter next). Facebook has stayed viable by evolving with the needs of users (Williams 2014). Time will tell if and when Facebook and other social networking sites may collapse but it seems safe to say that Facebook will be around for at least a few more years, or for as long as people prefer cyber connections and electronic friendships over face-to-face ones.

It is true that MySpace, the once dominant social networking site, lost its lofty position atop the cyberworld, having been replaced by Facebook in mid–2008, but we do not foresee Facebook falling off its haughty perch any time soon. In 2010, Twitter, another social networking site predicted to collapse, surpassed MySpace for the first time with a marginal advantage of 96 million users versus 95 million. Twitter, a microblogging service, remains quite popular (ranked #2 and #3 in the data provided previously in this chapter). Data provided by eBiz (2016) indicates that Twitter had 310 million users in mid–June 2016. Twitter (2016) itself, however, claims more than 645 million registered users with 289 million active users and 115 million active users every month. Twitter also reports an average number of tweets per day at 58 million and approximately 2.1 billion Twitter search engine queries every day.

Twitter is known as the real-time, public microblogging network where news breaks first. Most users loved it for its iconic 140-character limit and unfiltered feed that showed them absolutely everything. Twitter has changed dramatically over the years, and today it's criticized a lot for going the way of looking and functioning almost exactly like Facebook—people can share all sorts of multimedia content in tweets and can expect to see algorithmic timelines soon (Moreau 2016).

There are apps designed to help people accomplish almost anything information-related including those that help you follow your favorite sports teams, find restaurants and gas stations, and receive the latest weather information and traffic delays. There are also apps that are designed to make it easier for you to find someone to hook-up with (i.e., Tinder) or to have an affair (i.e., Ashley Madison). Tinder is a dating profile site that allows people to search for other like-minded people who want to meet with others to date, or more bluntly, to have sex. Tinder is also known as the heterosexual version of Grindr, an older hook-up app that identifies available gay, bisexual, or "curious" partners in the vicinity (Chamorro-Premuzic 2014).

Launched in September 2012, there were an estimated 50 million Tinder users in March 2015 (Smith 2016a). Tinder users can set up for a brief profile that mainly highlights their photo, and then anyone who's matched up to them can anonymously swipe right to like their profile or left to pass on it as a match. If someone who liked a profile is liked back, then it's a match, and the two users can start chatting privately with each other through the app and decide from there what to do next. Tinder is free, but there are premium features that allow users to connect people in other locations, undo certain swipes and get more "Super Likes" to let another user know they're special (Moreau 2016). Doesn't this sound like a "friends with benefits" scenario?

Romantics do not turn to Tinder, they go to EHarmony or Match.com, even if many are still embarrassed to admit to using such dating sites. Tomas Chamorro-Premuzic, a professor of business psychology at the University College London, states that Tinderers (as Tinder users are known) are proud to be on Tinder and that they find it cool that the social network site eliminates time lags and distance between their desire to avoid dating and gain instant sexual gratification. Chamorro-Premuzic (2014) states, "In our technosexual era, the process of dating has not only been gamified, but also sexualized, by technology. Mobile dating is much more than a means to an end, it is an end in itself. With Tinder, the pretext is to hook-up, but the real pleasure is derived from the Tindering process. Tinder is just the latest example for the sexualization of urban gadgets: it is nomophobia, Facebook-porn and Candy Crush Saga all in one." (Note: Nomophobia refers to the intense, irrational fear of being out of mobile phone contact with others.) Summing up the Tindering experience, Tinderers would rather judge 50 pictures in two minutes than spend 50 minutes assessing one potential partner in a traditional face-on-face dating environment. As expected, Tinderers are pretty shallow as their matching process is based 90 percent on looks and second dates are decided by whether the hookup was deemed equally attractive or worthy of each other's looks (Chamorro-Premuzic 2014).

The last social network site we will highlight is Snapchat. Launched in Venice, CA, in September 2011, Snapchat is all about the last 24 hours—it required that photos and videos shared with friends be taken in the moment—as the app focused on the here and now. Snapchat grew in popularity very quickly and had 100 million daily active users in May 2015 (Smith 2016b). By June 2016, there were approximately 150 million daily active users (Statista 2016a). In the United States, 23 percent of Snapchat users were aged between 13 and 17 years of age and 37 percent were between the ages of 18 and 24 (Statista 2016b). In July 2016, Snapchat was valued at $16 billion (Dave 2016). About.com had Snapchat ranked #10 in their top 25 listing of top social networking sites but surprisingly, it did not show up in the eBiz ranking. Snapchat is a social networking app that thrives on instant messaging and is totally mobile-based. It is one of the fastest growing apps and has built its popularity on the idea of self-destructing "snaps." A snap is a photo or short video message that is sent to a friend which automatically disappears a few seconds after they've viewed it. Youth of all ages enjoy the app because it is different from "traditional" social networking sites (Moreau 2016). The signs of Snapchat following the lead of Facebook had become increasingly noticeable by July 2016 as evidenced by the fact that a growing number of people over 25 were using the app and by the company's announcement that they would introduce a "Memories" feature that allowed users to create a camera roll of past photos and make posts "from camera roll" much like Facebook's nostalgic "Moments" app offers. There are limitations to "Memories" as searches can only pull up saved Snaps, whereas "Moments" can include all stored photos (Dave 2016). Both "Memories" and "Moments" allow friends an opportunity to relive past memorable moments together; thus, reinforcing the bonds of friendships.

On June 19, 2016, *Today* (a show airing on NBC) provided a news feature discussing the demise of shopping malls. Shopping malls were *the* place for young people to meet their friends in the 1980s and 1990s. Young people (mostly tweens and teens) had a place to hang out away from their parents, they were out of the house, and they could dress in the latest "hip" and "cool" styles. It was a great place for girls to gossip about boys and where boys went looking for girls. Reflecting the changing cultural norms and values that helped to assist cyber socialization (see Chapter 3), the children of these "mall dwellers" want, and have, nothing or little to do with shopping malls today. A *Today* reporter conducted a type of focus group interview with a group of teens and asked them about going to the mall. They all looked puzzled. The mall? Why would we go to the mall? When asked if they found it lame that their parents went to the mall for quality time with friends, these youngsters responded by saying such a notion is "whacked." When asked what they do to be seen, they all responded that they used and relied on Snapchat. Snapchat is the new mall experience for today's youth. As one group member said, if you have a nice outfit and want to show it off you can take a photo of yourself and post it on Snapchat (*Today* 6/19/16).

It is no small wonder why so many long-term friendships are maintained online and why so many others originate from the cyberworld when people, especially younger folks, have the attitude that spending time in the cyberworld instead of participating in face-to-face endeavors is just as rewarding.

Electronic Friendships

Philosophers and sociologists alike have long been interested in the behaviors of others. Georg Simmel (1858–1918), a famous German thinker, was especially interested in human interactions, what he called "sociation." Although he died long before the introduction of the cyberworld and electronic friendships, he would have, undoubtedly, been fascinated by them. Simmel was especially interested in "sociability"—the play form of sociation (Martindale 1988). Sociability is an important aspect of relationships. In the following pages we will take a closer look at what Simmel means by sociability, connect his thoughts to Goffman's ideas on "encounters," and add our own insights as we attempt to answer the ultimate question, "Are electronic friendships real friendships?" We will also examine the idea, introduced by Aristotle long ago, that there is a quantitative limit as to how many friendships we can successfully maintain.

Sociability in the Electronic Age

Spending time with friends in the cyberworld is a type of social interaction; it is within the realm of Simmel's concept of sociability. Sociability involves the association of people for its own sake and for the delight of interacting with others. The character of the gathering is determined by personal qualities and personalities of the participants. Interaction always arises on the basis of certain drives or for the sake of certain purposes (Delaney 2004). In this manner, people who find enjoyment socializing in the cyberworld are participating in aspects of sociability. Simmel categorized many characteristics of sociability including "sociability thresholds." Simmel believed that humans are a totality of dynamic complex ideas, wants, desires, and possibilities. As a result, each person develops their own tolerance toward socializing with others—creating different sociability thresholds (Delaney 2004). In this regard, individuals set their own limits as to how much interaction they can handle with others. Thus, some individuals can feel comfortable in large crowds (e.g., attending professional football games or festival concerts) while others prefer to distance themselves from such gatherings and reside within a much smaller grouping (threshold) of people. People with low sociability thresholds can find comfort in the cyberworld.

Another aspect of sociability is the idea of *artificiality*. Simmel wrote that the world of sociability is an artificial one, maintained only through voluntary interaction. Because of the harsh reality of one's real life, it is easy to understand why persons often prefer the deceptive social world they have created and work so hard at maintaining (Delaney 2004). While Simmel was certainly not talking about the cyberworld or virtual forms of reality and friendships, the concept of creating an "artificial" world is certainly applicable. Simmel and Hughes (1949) write, "This world of sociability ... is an artificial world, made up of beings who have renounced both the objective and the purely personal features of the intensity and extensiveness of life in order to bring about among themselves a pure interaction, free of any disturbing material accent" (p. 527). Cyber friendships are free from materialism, are personal, and can be as intense as face-to-face friendships.

In 2012, Tim Delaney applied Simmel's concepts of *coquetry* (flirting) and secrecy to the study of Facebook's relationship status feature, most specifically to the "It's Complicated" status. As depicted in the 2010 Academy Award winning film *The Social Network*, it was the relationship status of persons that intrigued Facebook founder Mark Zuckerberg's schoolmates at Harvard to check profiles of friends and fellow students as they wanted to know who was single (and presumably "available") and who was in a relationship. The relationship status of other users still intrigues people. This is especially evident whenever someone updates their status and the change indicates something significant is going on in that person's life. For example, if someone who has been married for a decade suddenly changes her status to "single" that will make people inquisitive as to what is going on. If a longtime single person suddenly posts that they are in a relationship, their friends will be very curious. As of mid–2016, Facebook acknowledged the following relationship statuses: single; in a relationship; engaged; married; in a civil union; in a domestic partnership; in an open relationship; it's complicated; separated; divorced; and widowed. The relationship status is an interesting feature on Facebook as most users volunteer to share that information, making it available to any one granted access. This is a big advantage for people seeking certain types of friends, such as a single person looking for another single person, or someone in an open relationship looking for hookups with others who share that same feature. In the conventional world, we do not know the status of others and if you were thinking of approaching someone to ask out on a date it would be easier if you already knew their relationship status.

Delaney (2012b) was specifically interested in the "It's Complicated" Relationship (ICR) as the very idea of a relationship being complicated seems redundant—aren't *all* relationships complicated? So why a specific category of "It's Complicated?" Delaney interviewed 15 people in an ICR and concluded that there were four primary reasons why someone would claim this Facebook status:

1. The person is dating more than one person at a time, but not necessarily hiding it;
2. The person is not dating anyone but wants the appearance of dating. The ICR status does not require identifying a name, so this option works well. Also, such a person may desire drama and attention;
3. There is forbidden love as the result of such things as lack of parental approval; boss-subordinate; or professor-student;

4. The desire for secrecy; they want to tell everyone but they cannot because it must remain a secret.

Although dating someone secretly can be the result of forbidden love, Delaney (2012b) proposed that one person in the ICR is already involved with someone else while the ICR identifier is not. Furthermore, only the ICR identifier will use the ICR status; after all, if the other person is in a committed relationship of some sort (e.g., engaged or married) changing her Facebook status to ICR will lead to a ripple effect of needed explanations. This type of ICR is a variation of secret dating, or having an affair.

The dynamics of an ICR, or secret/forbidden relationship, are quite fascinating. First, we have two individuals who share feelings about each other and feel compelled to let them surface. The best way to do this is via flirting, or what Simmel called "coquetry." Coquetry, according to Simmel, involves the two individuals playfully teasing an "offer" while countering with a "refusal." The refusal is never too strong as to scare off the other while the offer always has some strings attached, limiting the process prior to its climax (Simmel and Hughes 1949; Delaney 2012b). While people flirt for a variety of reasons (e.g., flirting with a bartender for a free drink; smiling at strangers to make them happy; or daredevils that flirt with disaster), coquetry involves flirting with an end goal of sex. In the contemporary era, we can add "cyber flirting" as a distinctive category of flirting. Monica Whitty (2003), among the early academics to study cyber flirting, wrote that "online flirting should be considered as a form of play" (p. 339). In this regard, cyber flirting would be an updated example of Simmel's sociability (the play form of sociation). In the cyberworld, such flirting is generally conducted via sexting (see Chapter 5). Cyber flirting can be the first step toward developing a relationship and the first step in cheating if the flirter is already in a relationship. There is a debate as to whether or not online flirting is really cheating. In some ways, the answer to this question depends on whether or not you consider electronic relationships as "real" relationships or not (a topic to be addressed later in this chapter). Cheating is typically viewed as someone who is in a committed relationship and breaks the trust of his/her partner by getting physically and/or emotionally involved with another person. A strictly online relationship forgoes the idea of physical cheating but certainly the emotional aspect can be real and thus a form of cheating. Thus, cyber cheating is a real thing as it involves emotional infidelity and, may or may not, cause harm to existing relationships and the individuals involved. A simple way to analyze whether or not online flirting is a type of cheating or not involves answering this question: Does your partner know you are flirting electronically with another person? If the answer is "no," then it's likely cheating (Neuman 2002).

Returning to the topic of the development of an ICR, following initial flirtations, continued flirting is either rebuffed or escalated. Moving onward leads to the development of a relationship and whether it should eventually involve face-to-face meetings, maintain solely online meetings, or a combination of both. Like any couple who date, those in a secret relationship can expect outcomes with very high levels of joy, or outcomes that end in dissolution and pain. That is to say, someone may get emotionally hurt and have their heart broken; or, if the ICR does involve one partner cheating on another in an established relationship, all hell can break loose.

Choosing to move on in an ICR with someone already in a relationship implies entering into a world of secrecy. Secret relationships can certainly be fun and exciting, especially at the beginning, but before long, the "complicated" part of the ICR really comes into play as both people have to maintain the secret and the one already in a relationship risks losing both partners. Simmel was an admirer of the secret as he argued that secrecy is one of humanity's greatest achievements as the ability to hold onto a secret represents an advancement from one's childish stage in which every conception is expressed at once, and every undertaking is accessible to the eyes of all to a point where one learns to hold back certain bits of information for the good of others or self (Delaney 2004).

While Simmel valued the concept of secrecy, he also celebrated the value of faithfulness. He described faithfulness as a significant sociological form because it is such an important feature of the sustainability of social relationships. Faithfulness promotes loyalty, social autonomy, reaffirming affective interests and the strengthening of psychological bonds. Faithfulness is applicable to the "It's Complicated" relationship that involves a cheating partner for many reasons, including the realization that the person secretly dating the "cheating" other will always have to consider the reality that he/she may fall victim to the other's cheating in the future (Delaney 2012b). Furthermore, while any breakup can be messy and the lover scorned may find it necessary to inform others of the cheating ways of the ex, the number of people that can be reached is generally much higher when it involves people who use social media—especially those who make posts in a public forum on Facebook. In this era of social networking, the scorned lover has a number of significant avenues by which to exert their anger. In general, these avenues can include making multiple posts on multiple social network sides; while specifically, it could involve revenge porn (see Chapter 3).

Roser Beneito-Montagut (2015) describes how internet users of today have an unprecedented collection of tools to interact with others and refers to these options as "modes of online sociability" that "allow users to pursue social encounters with variable levels of involvement, attention, and activity" (p.537). Beneito-Montagut expands on Erving Goffman's concept of "encounter" while connecting it to Simmel's ideas on sociability. What is an "encounter" you might ask. Goffman (1961) himself was vague in his explanation stating, "Encounters are everywhere, but it is difficult to describe sociologically the stuff they are made of" (p.19). The concept of "encounters" is not really that difficult to explain as they involve a face-to-face meeting, generally by chance; in other words, they are often unexpected experiences. This idea could be expressed as, "I met a very interesting and intelligent person at my conference last week; she seemed to know a great deal about sexting."

Goffman's ideas on encounters are a continuation, of sorts, of his concept of the "presentation of self" (see Chapter 3). Beneito-Montagut (2015) extents Goffman's theoretical framework on the presentation of self to explain how identities are constructed symbolically online. She also further develops Goffman's concept of encounters to "online encounters" with a focus on emotions. "*Encounters* is one of the most instructive works for understanding and analyzing emotions in social interactions and my proposal is to expand this notion to online 'encounters'" drawing upon "Goffman's theoretical foundations to scrutinize how conversational encounters are structured and to expose how people perform and manage emotions online. In other words, it focuses on social interactions on the social web" (Beneito-Montagut 2015: 538–539). There is a growing body of research centered on examining the role of emotions in online relationships (Castells 2009; Holmes 2011; Maloney 2012; Thelwall 2010) and Beneito-Montagut has added to this literature by focusing on emotional body expressions that are implicated although may not be visible to others. This idea is similar to our earlier discussion on the use of emoticons (see Chapter 3) to help eliminate the guess work between online exchanges and whether or not there is a "tone" to a correspondence.

Beneito-Montagut (2015) also introduces the term "focused encounter" for online interactions. A focused encounter is one that is directed toward a specific person and not the entirety of one's friends on the social network. She states that the focused encounter is a fundamental unit of interaction in social networking and found that in many ways it is similar to a face-to-face interaction. "This similarity particularly concerns the structure of encounters in one-to-one communications, in which at least two persons agree to have a conversation and share some time together, although this does not necessarily happen synchronously and with undivided attention" (Beneito-Montagut 2015: 549). Beneito-Montagut's data was based on a very small sample size (6 subjects) so generalizations are tenuous at best. Still, the study is a worthy starting point and the results indicated that frequent internet users derive distinctive meaning from online encounters and develop management strategies. We would add that online encounters with focused others are initiated and will continue if those individuals involved have shared beliefs, values and norms and if the encounters with others are positively reinforced via "likes" and "shares."

Are Electronic Friendships Real Friendships?

Earlier in this chapter we promised to answer the question, "Are electronic friendships real friendships?" Questioning the legitimacy of electronic friendships came to the forefront (in earnest) following years of persistent claims by millions of people that *all* Facebook friends, whether known in the real world (on a face-to-face basis) or not, do indeed count as "real" friends. But, is it truly possible to be "friends" with thousands of people? And, don't we have to have a face-to-face interaction with people in order for them to qualify as friends? One of the authors of this book is active in social networking and admits to having hundreds of Facebook friends he has never met (in addition to hundreds of friends he knows on a face-to-face basis). Referring to them as Facebook "friends" is easy because they are "counted" as friends on his home page. Nonetheless, he too questions the notion of counting people known only in the electronic world as "real" friends. Nonetheless, some of these electronic friends (known only in the domain of Facebook) have become special as it is fun to keep up with their exploits. In some cases, we get to know our electronic friends' family members (via their posts), where they have traveled, and many of their other trials and tribulations—just like "real" friends. We click "like" to their posts and occasionally make comments and they reciprocate. So, if we change the traditional parameters of the definition of "friend" and the idea, implied or stated, that a friend is a person with whom we must have actual face-to-face contact (a criterion of "primary groups" as defined by Cooley in Chapter 2), to those with whom we communicate with regularly, then these electronic friends may be considered "real" friends.

Academics and laypersons alike have been pondering this notion of whether or not electronic friendships are "real" friendships for a number of years now. Alia Dastagir, writing for *USA Today*, cites William Rawlins, a professor of communication studies at Ohio University, who said that all friendships have the same basic ingredients: voluntary, mutual, personal, affectionate and equal (which, as seen in Chapter 1, corresponds well with Aristotle's criteria for friendship). Rawlins writes: "The voluntary part is key. Reciprocity is one of Facebook's central tenets. I can't friend you unless you accept me. This isn't the case for all social networks. On Twitter and Instagram you can follow without being followed back, creating a more impersonal network" (Dastagir 2016). On Facebook, however, one must be accepted as a friend, and you can always be unfriended. The affectionate (emotional) component of friendship is an interesting variable, however, when applied to electronic friends. As mentioned in Chapter 1, a study conducted by Oxford University psychology professor Robin Dunbar (2016) resulted in his conclusion that, on average, only about 14 (13.6) of your Facebook friends could be counted on for emotional/social support in time of crisis.

The Dunbar study (2016) also points out another similarity between electronic friendships and face-to-face friendships, namely that they are all subject to natural decay in the absence of contact (what Aristotle would call "not sharing salt together"). It appears that social media can function to slow down the decay of friendships but face-to-face relationships require some face-to-face contact to prolong themselves. Electronic friendships do not need face-to-face interaction; instead, they need to be maintained electronically.

As we stated in Chapter 2, there is a positive correlation between real life friendships and subjective well-being and happiness. However, as Helliwell and Huang (2013) point out, there is no such correlation with subjective well-being for individuals when analyzing the number of electronic friends (Helliwell and Huang 2013).

Tanya Hollander, a Facebook user, was wondering if her Facebook friends were real friends so she decided to track them down, all 626 of them. As a photographer, she decided to go on a quest to take all of their photographs. Some of these friends she knew in real life, some were old friends from high school (over 20 years prior), and others she only knew as electronic friends. She started her journey with low expectations, "There's no way these people will give a sh— about me" she told Claire O'Neill who wrote an article about Hollander for NPR. As it turned out, her friends, whether "real" or "electronic," were enthusiastic about the project. One electronic friend let Hollander crash with her for over a week as she looked for other electronic friends to meet in person and photograph. Hollander concluded that there is a thin line between electronic friends and real friends and that all it takes for the cross-over is to actually meet electronic friends and they may easily become real friends. Hollander stated, "I have been so surprised at how generous people have been. Apparently, all it takes is some face time to make Facebook friendships real" (O'Neill 2012).

In an interesting cross-media example of our analysis on whether electronic friendships are real or not consider this letter from a 20-year-old woman written to "Dear Abby" inquiring about grief and electronic friends. The woman wrote that her boyfriend ("my very first boyfriend") committed suicide and that she felt absolutely destroyed. The woman continued that while they lived several states apart and that they never met face-to-face, they did talk every night and video-chatted many times. "My feelings for him are real." She wrote that she broke down after hearing the news and that she was in great distress. Her heartache was made worse by her family's reaction to her loss. "My family thinks I'm overreacting. They can't understand how a relationship with someone online can be serious." The woman wanted help from Abby in making her family recognize how much pain she was in. Abby replied by first offering sympathy for the loss of "someone you cared about so deeply." Abby also wrote that it was sad that her parents minimized her feelings; mentioned how many serious relationships have now started online; and suggested that she seek emotional support elsewhere (e.g., a clergyperson, if she had one, or look online for a grief support group) (Dear Abby 2015).

So, what is our answer to the question of whether or not electronic friendships are real friendships? Here it is: The electronic world is real, in that it exists, albeit in cyber form. Real people access the electronic world in real ways via electronic devices, which exist in reality. All the mechanisms (e.g., smartphones, computers, satellite feeds) needed to access the electronic world are real. Within the electronic world are a number of electronic/virtual relationships including devious variations such as catfishing (see Chapter 3) and people who are cyber friends but have never had a face-to-face meeting. People involved in catfishing schemes include real people setting up other real people into believing that they are involved with a real person who has actually been fabricated with false stories substantiated by photos of real persons (who are not the real persons portrayed in catfish schemes). In some instances, real people from the real world meet other real people in the cyberworld and establish electronic relationships that happen to be devoid of real life interactions. To the folks involved, these virtual relationships are real even though they were created, maintained, and reside in the cyberworld. There are those who have established electronic romantic relationships in the cyberworld and consider themselves "together" in a real sense even though they have not met in the real world. Did you follow all that? We were being real! And, just as the words on this page are real, people also believe that electronic relationships are real and, in that sense, that makes them real.

In our research, we asked survey participants, "Is it possible to be in a relationship with someone strictly electronically (no physical interactions)?" There was a statistically significant difference between male and female responses with just 45 percent of males saying "yes" but 64 percent of females saying "yes" to the question is it possible to have a strictly electronic relationship without physical interactions (see Table 4.2).

Table 4.2: Is It Possible to Be in a Relationship with Someone Strictly Electronically (No Physical Interactions)? by Gender, Number and in Percent

Males (N=74)			Females (N=105)		
Yes or No	#	Percent	Yes or No	#	Percent
Yes	33	45	Yes	67	64
No	41	55	No	38	36

We asked respondents to explain their answer to the question "is it possible to be in a relationship with someone strictly electronically (no physical interactions)?" and listed below is a sampling of responses from males in support of electronic relationships:

- Relationships are vague and subjective; anyone who communicates with someone has a relationship with that person. Still, I couldn't do a strictly electronic relationship, but that's just me.
- As long as there is a similarity between both parties, a friendship can form.
- It's hard not being near someone you are close with, but it doesn't mean it can't happen.
- Yes, social media has created e-relationships.
- Yes, but it's weird.
- Yes, but it's an incomplete relationship.
- Yes, but only if both people are being true—no Catfish type situations.
- Yes, I am an avid gamer and have many friends that I only speak to electronically.
- Maybe, but I don't think it's sustainable. But, then again, the digital age is changing things.

Among the female responses in support of the validity of electronic relationships are the following:

- Yes, you don't need physical contact to have a relationship with someone (some variation of this comment was the most common).
- Yes, it's still someone to talk to.
- It is possible but not for me.
- Friendship yes; romance, no.

Among the male responses who disagreed with the validity of a relationship strictly electronically-based are the following:

- I don't believe in that. Social media is a mask for some people.
- You can't have a real relationship unless you have met that person.
- No, I must have physical contact (most common answer).
- No, in order to have a complete connection you must have some face-to-face/in-person contact.

Female respondents who did not support the notion of a purely electronic relationship offered comments such as these:

- No, you can only truly know someone if you are physically with that person (most common answer).
- No, I need to see/fee/hear the emotion in their voice and read their body language.
- No, electronics are a disconnect from emotion and gestures.
- How can you really know someone if you have never met them in person?

- No, it's like a modern-day pen pal.
- No, why would anyone do that?
- And from the respondent that was victimized by a catfishing scheme, "Never trust someone online. The people you think are real are not real."

Based on our research and the data revealed by our survey, it would seem that there is some debate about the validity of purely electronic relationships (e-relationships). On the one hand, electronic relationships *are* relationships; they're just not face-to-face relationships. They are as real as people make them. With electronic relationships, communication, even if limited to electronic communication, seems to be the key variable when describing e-relationships as true friendship or romance relationships. On the other hand, many people believe that face-to-face interaction is the key determinant in establishing a relationship. Either way, we all still value friendships. Thus, while the methods of securing friendships may change, the desire for friendship has not. We would ask that you consider a newspaper editorial that one of the authors possesses from 2009, the year *Sesame Street* celebrated its 40th anniversary. In this cartoon are two panels. The first panel is labeled "1969" and there is a photo of Big Bird holding up the letter "F" with a thought bubble that reads, "Friend." In the second panel, labeled 2009, Big Bird is holding up the letter "F" with a thought bubble that reads, "Facebook Friend." The two panels both display Big Bird trying to teach children the alphabet and the value of friendship but the 2009 panel reflects the electronic generation and the 1969 panel reflects the reality that social networking sites and the concept of electronic friendships did not exist.

Enough Is Enough, I Already Have 150 Friends

In this chapter's introductory story we described how a Belgian and his real life friend decided to travel 5,000 miles before sending a friend request to a stranger as suggested by Facebook. Natural curiosity or not, Van Rossem and his friend clearly had enough time on their hands to spend "interviewing" a prospective new friend, so apparently Van Rossem had room for at least one more friend. (The news report did not indicate how many real or electronic friends Van Rossem had.) The idea of prescreening new friends is an interesting one and serves as a nice transition to the question, "Is there a limit to how many friends we can handle, or should have?"

To answer the question above we must consider a number of things. For example, why is someone using a social network site such as Facebook in the first place? Is it for professional purposes? Is it to stay in touch with face-to-face friends known in the conventional world? Or, is it an attempt to acquire as many friends as possible as a type of mechanism to improve one's self esteem (as in, "I am very popular, I have 3,500 friends" and "I'm followed by over 2,200 people")? This great contrast in why people use social network sites is a good starting point in trying to ascertain whether there is a limit to the number of friends our respective brains can handle. In a letter to "Dear Amy" (yet another advice column in the fashion of "Dear Abby"), a woman in her mid–20s wrote that she and her sister (also in her mid–20s) have such different outlooks on how to use Facebook that it has created a schism between them. The letter writer, "Social Network Awkwardness (SNA)," wrote that her sister wants her to add all of her Facebook friends to her account; and, that the sister is "furious" that she deleted one of her friends over a year ago. The sister claims that "SNA" is "mean" and "rude." SNA wrote that she only has about 40 connections and that they're all people she knows personally. SNA asked "Dear Amy" if it is a "social faux pas not to 'friend' people you've only met once or twice?" (Dear Amy 2015). And there we have it, the changing cultural norms and values of some people have led others to question whether it is now the norm to "friend" a person with whom you have only a causal knowledge of, or a person you don't know at all.

The "Dear Amy" letter writer "Social Network Awkwardness" introduces some of the many issues that many people on Facebook have about "friending" others. For some, there is anxiety in asking someone to be their friend, especially if they would feel awkward to do so in a face-to-face situation. What about people you were not friends with in high school? In fact, maybe you didn't like each other at all, and they ask you to be Facebook friends. Do you accept? One of the authors of this text experienced this when he first got on Facebook and was immediately inundated with "friend" requests from people he barely remembered or didn't even know, from a high school he had only attended for one year after his original high school had closed (he still maintains close friendships with several people from the original school, but didn't bond at all with those at the second school).

If we return to the quantitative aspect of friending, Facebook, as most of us know, permits each account holder 5,000 friends. How did Facebook come up with this number? Did they conduct scientific research to determine that number? Do they really think we can keep in touch with 5,000 people and maintain a meaningful relationship with all of them? Recall that Aristotle said we can only handle at best a handful of friendships of the good, and even the other two types—utility and pleasure—are limited in number, due to the time and effort necessary to maintain them.

If Facebook had conducted scientific research on how many friends our brains can handle they would have set the bar at, or below, 150; that is, if they took the advice of evolutionary anthropologist Robin Dunbar. As mentioned previously, Dunbar, who has been conducting research for decades on the number of stable relationships that individuals can maintain, determined in 1993 that individuals' social circles—of close friends and relatives, and frequently seen acquaintances—consist of about 150 people (*The Economist* 2016). This "150" figure has become so significant that Dunbar has been immortalized with the distinction of the "Dunbar Number." "Not many people have a number named after them, but Robin Dunbar lays claim to the Dunbar Number" (Krotoski 2010). Dunbar was studying primates in the early 1990s and found a correlation between the average size of each species' neocortex (the most recently evolved part of the cortex) and that of the size of their social groups. He also found that from the time of Neolithic villages through the centuries of Roman rule, humans seem to have organized themselves into groups of 100–200 (*The Economist* 2016). This nicely corresponds with Aristotle's observations on the limited number of true social relationships any one person can naturally maintain.

Yet things have changed quite a bit since Ancient Times as people live in significantly larger sized cities and many of us have hundreds or thousands of Facebook friends. Still, our brain can still only process so much information from so many people. Dunbar notes that even those who have 1,500 friends on Facebook will only manage about 150 friends on a regular basis. In his recent research—which consisted of two surveys, one of which contained 2,000 regular social-network users; and a second group of 1,375 which contained full-time employment adults that may or may not be social networking users—Dunbar found that regular social-network users (Facebook) had 155 friends while full-time employed group members had an average of 187 friends. As we reported earlier in this chapter, Facebook itself states that the average number of friends per Facebook user is 130. Once again, the Dunbar Number comes into play. Seemingly, Facebook could set their friends limit to 10,000 and still the average user would have a Dunbar-expected number of friends. If you are now concerned that you might have too many friends, especially electronic media friends, you can always delete a large number of them on "National Unfriend Day"! (See Popular Culture Scenario 4 for a description of National Unfriend Day and other national friendship days.)

Popular Culture Scenario 4: National Friendship Days

Have you noticed that every day of the year now has attached to it "National … Day"? If you don't hear about specific designations from your friends and family you will learn about them via the mass media or the social media (especially Facebook). There are calendars you can look up online to let you know the "National … Day" too. For example, January

1st is "National Hangover Day" as well as "New Year's Day." The following day, January 2nd has less predictable designations: "National Buffet Day," "National Cream Puff Day," "National Personal Trainer Awareness Day," "National Science Fiction Day," and "National Thank God It's Monday Day" (for the 1st Monday of January) (National Day Calendar 2016).

Some national days seem quite worthy of acknowledging, like "New Year's Day," while others, like "National Buffet Day," seem overly trivial. Various "Friendship Days," perhaps, fall somewhere in between, as friendships themselves are far more than trivial, but in most cases not at the same level as more honored days such as "Independence Day" or "Labor Day." It should come as no surprise, then, that there are a number of specific days reserved for the realm of friendship, including the obvious starting point, "National Friendship Day." According to National Day Calendar (NDC) (2016), "National Friendship Day" is to be celebrated the first Sunday in August and we are to "observe this day in an appropriate manner, in accordance with the culture and other appropriate circumstances or customs of their local, national and regional communities, including through education and public awareness-raising activities." Based on this description provided by NDC, national friendship day has far loftier goals than to take a friend to lunch!

Not to be outdone by a mere *national* friendship day, the United Nations, in 2011, created the "International Day of Friendship" of July 30th. This special day promotes the role that friendship plays in promoting peace in many cultures. "The UN encourages governments, organizations, and community groups to hold events, activities and initiatives that promote solidarity, mutual understanding and reconciliation" (Time and Date 2016).

The importance we place on our closest, best friends is acknowledged on June 8th as "National Best Friends Day," a day "to honor that one special person you call your 'best friend.' This day is a time to show them how much you appreciate them, how special and important they are to you and how you cherish their friendship" (NDC 2016). If you are your own best friend, as demonstrated by a preoccupation with posting selfies, there is a day for you too! That's right, there is a "National Selfie Day" although there seems to be lack of a specific annual date. "The first time we detected Selfie Day was 5th of April 2015" and in 2016 it was June 21st (What National Day Is It 2016). There is a "Make a Friend Day" celebrated every February 11 that promotes the idea that the more friends we have the greater our wealth will be because "friends are one of life's valuable assets" (Holiday Insights 2016). We have also heard of a national "New Friends Day" on the news (*CBS This Morning*, July 19, 2016) but the internet does not provide too much information other than the obvious link to "make a friend" day. Apparently, on July 19th you are encouraged to make a concerted effort to make a new friend!

If anyone knows something about creating new friends and maintaining old friendships, it's Mark Zuckerberg, the man who became a multi-billionaire by creating a social networking site based on the ideas of "friends." It took him a while to capitalize on the national day phenomenon but in 2015 he created "Friends Day on Facebook Day." Via a post he made on Facebook, February 4, 2015, Zuckerberg (2015) wrote: "Today is a day to celebrate friends. It's also Facebook's birthday, but today isn't about celebrating us. It's about friendship…. Friendship isn't a distraction from the meaningless things in life. Friendship is what gives meaning to our lives."

There is one other day worth acknowledging with regards to friendships and that is "National Unfriend Day" held on November 17th. As the title of this day implies, this is the day we get rid of non-friends on Facebook by "unfriending" them. "Comedian Jimmy Kimmel founded Unfriend Day in 2014 to combat the growing trend of social media profiles collecting 'friends' like Pokemon cards, amassing a ridiculous amount of 'friends' they barely know at all in short periods of time. Getting rid of distant acquaintances on Unfriend Day can help you streamline your internet experience, allowing you to use your profiles to keep in touch with people you really care about, and preserving the true definition of 'friend'" (Days of the Year 2016). To see Kimmel's criteria of people you should "unfriend" view his YouTube video "Jimmy Kimmel's National Unfriend Day Warning."

Popular culture provides many valuable life lessons and the lessons learned about national friendship days is: keep your real friends close to you and cherish time with them and clean out your closet by unfriending those people who are not really your friends.

If our suggestion of taking advantage of "National Unfriend Day" and evolutionary anthropologist Dunbar's research on the number of friends our brains can handle haven't bummed out the readers with hundreds or thousands of electronic friends yet, wait until you hear what evolutionary psychologists Norman Li and Satoshi Kanazawa have to say about life satisfaction and well-being in relation to friendships. These researchers state that people who live in more densely populated areas tend to report less satisfaction with their lives overall; in other words, the higher the population density of the immediate environment, the less happy people are (Ingraham 2016). In contrast, living in less dense areas, like a savanna, would make people happier. This idea led to Li and Kanazawa penning the term "the savanna theory of happiness." (Note: See Chapter 7 for a closer look at the "savanna theory of happiness.")

Li and Kanazawa (2016) also present a theory that smart people are better off with fewer friends. They conducted a survey of adults aged 18 to 28 (15,000 respondents) and found that "More intelligent individuals experience lower life satisfaction with more frequent socialization with friends" (Li and Kanazawa 2016). Thus, smart people have fewer friends but are happier for it.

Virtual Reality

Our socialization into the cyberworld and compliance with spending an increasing amount of time in electronic relationships leads to the next step in the transformation process of friendships; one that involves further heading away from face-to-face interactions to friendships that can only exist in virtual realities. Virtual reality, among other things, allows people to create personas (the virtual self) that are real only in virtual worlds. Thus, virtual relationships become a distinctive sub-category of electronic friendships previously discussed.

Distinguishing the Cyber Self from the Virtual Self

The "cyber self" is a merging of aspects of the cyberworld and one's presentation of self (see Chapter 3 for a description of both aspects). The cyber self is created by people online who create profiles to represent themselves. Online users decide what information to share with the knowledge that other people (either one's online friends or the social network's public depending on user settings) are going to be able to access that information and form judgments based on this information. When choosing what kind of information to put into a profile, individuals are consciously choosing how they wish to represent themselves and their cyber identity. Laura Robinson (2010) believes that the creation of a cyber self is "formed and negotiated in the same manner as the offline self" (p. 94). We would disagree and modify her claim by saying that the norms and values of the face-to-face world are somewhat carried over into the cyber community. In the cyberworld, people *can* control their own profiles and profile photos and the posts they choose to make and respond to, but they *cannot* control the text and photo postings of others. Thus, their identity can still be shaped by others.

As an example of how someone's cyber self can be compromised by others online consider an American Facebook user who makes a post ranting against socialism. This is likely to get a large number of "likes" (assuming this person has active followers and is otherwise well liked online) as the concept of socialism is generally lowly regarded in the United States. However, this person risks being "called out" by real friends who know him in the real world and can reveal this anti-socialism poster as someone who is on unemployment, has a father that is collecting veterans benefits, a mother that is collecting disability benefits and both parents are collecting social security benefits and Medicare, making them beneficiaries of a system filled with socialist ideals and thus a system they do not really want to get rid of because of their own dependency on this socio-economic system. To be completely against socialism as the cyber persona person stated would mean that the real self would have to pay his own way through life (as well as his dependents) and not rely on government assistance. It may indeed be popular to condemn socialism in a society that loves its representative form of democracy but the reality is, the U.S. is a highly socialized nation in many ways, as evidenced by more than 75 examples of socialistic entities including, for example, the military/defense; highways/roads; public libraries; police/law enforcement; fire department; postal service; garbage collection; public landfills; farm subsidies; social security; public schools; jails and prisons; veterans health care (VA); sewer system; Medicare; judicial system; Medicaid; and so on (Daily KOS 2012).

While the cyber self is somewhat like the offline self, the "virtual self" is a sort of alter ego and an identity hidden from others. Definitions of "virtual" include such notions as "being in essence" (e.g., a virtual dictator), "existing in essence or effect though not in actual fact" (e.g., the virtual extinction of the buffalo), "existing in the mind, especially as a product of the imagination" (e.g., "I have followed the career of Christina Applegate so closely that I feel as though I know her"), and "as created, simulated, or carried on by means of a computer or computer network" (e.g., "I have over 2,000 Facebook friends") (*Merriam-Webster* 2016b; *The Free Dictionary* 2016a). It is this last notion of the concept of "virtual" that is of greatest relevance to our study of friendship (and happiness) as an increasing number of people have established all sorts of relationships ranging from romance to friendship entirely online making them subject to analysis of authenticity.

The "virtual self" then is not who we are in reality but rather a persona we use for the virtual world. Virtual selves exist to interact with others who have escaped into a realm that only exists in the virtual world (e.g., Second Life or World of Warcraft). In these fantasy worlds, participants can create a whimsical version of themselves through such mechanisms as avatars. The word "avatar" comes from Hindu mythology and refers to a Hindu deity in reincarnated form and is an embodiment or personification, as of a principle, attitude, or view of life (*Dictionary.com* 2016a). In the fantasy escapism world of virtual reality, individuals can essentially create a "virtual self" via avatar implementation. Individuals can also carry on friendships with people they have never met. We will discuss the virtual self in virtual world scenarios following our discussion of some of the practical developments and uses of virtual reality.

Developments and Uses of Virtual Reality (VR) and Augmented Reality (AR)

Virtual and augmented reality applications represent a growing characteristic of contemporary society. "Virtual reality" (VR) refers to technology that allows users to interact with a computer-simulated environment in a three-dimensional space. Users can explore different spheres of VR via equipment such as VR helmets. Closely related to virtual reality is "augmented reality" (AR), "a live direct or indirect view of a physical, real-world environment whose elements are augmented (or supplemented by computer-generated sensory input such as sound, video, graphics or GPS data" (Mashable.com 2016). AR is related to a more general concept called mediated reality, in which a view of reality is modified (possibly even diminished rather than augmented) by a computer, resulting in the enhancement of one's current perception of reality (Mashable.com 2016). The broadcasts of American football games, for example, are augmented by a great deal of computer-generated sensory input such as providing data information (e.g., the score, downs and yards) and the imposing of the first down line on the screen as a digital (usually yellow) line. Clearly this line does not exist in reality, but it does exist virtually on TV and computer screens. The popularity of Augmented/Virtual Reality is demonstrated by its financial impact, expected to hit $150 billion by 2020 (Digi-Captial 2016) and its application in a wide variety of settings to be discussed below.

In light of the fleeting popularity of "Pokemon Go," an AR game that was released on July 6, 2016, by Nintendo, the estimates of the financial impact of the AR industry cited above may have to be adjusted upward. In less than two weeks, the value of Nintendo stock doubled and the number of stock shares increased 25 percent, resulting in a nearly $9 billion increase in its market value (Pleasant 2016). In less than one week, the game had 15 million downloads and 21 million active daily users that spend an average of 33 minutes a day playing (Farren 2016). With Pokemon Go, gamers use real world locations to make cartoonish creatures (Pokemon) appear on their phone screens, giving users a chance to catch them. Immediately following its release, millions of screen sniffers were off their couches and out in the real world interacting with one another in an augmented fashion all in an attempt to find Pokemon characters. Many of the users praised the social aspects of the game because groups of friends can use the app together and roam the streets, shops and parks in surrounding neighborhoods. Of course, there were some immediate negative aspects of the app revealed such as people walking into streets with moving traffic unaware of their surroundings and in one early case, a user driving his car into a tree, making national news from the hometown (Auburn, New York) of one of the authors.

Virtual reality is different from AR in that the environments are completely simulated. Simulated environments, accessible as visual experiences via display technology, are utilized by a variety of social institutions, organizations, groups and individuals. The healthcare community uses virtual reality in a wide variety of methods including how to train surgeons for surgery and to experiment, virtually, with new radical procedures before subjecting humans to potentially harmful and untried techniques of treatment. Virtual robotic surgery—surgery that is performed by means of a robotic device controlled by a human surgeon—reduces time and risk of complications. The growing field of remote telesurgery—in which surgery is performed by a surgeon at a separate location to the patient—is a beneficiary of virtual reality (Virtual Reality Society 2016a). Other examples of virtual reality applications in the healthcare include the areas of dentistry, nursing, therapies, phobia treatment, treatment for PTSD, treatment for autism, and for the disabled.

The military uses virtual reality to train pilots, parachutists, and combat soldiers. VR can be used to train soldiers for combat situations or other dangerous settings without risk of harm or death. Other military uses of virtual reality include flight simulation, battlefield simulation and reenactment, medic training, vehicle simulation and virtual boot camp (Virtual Reality Society 2016a). Soon, they may add cloned personnel to their drones.

The field of education is another area that has adopted virtual reality for teaching and learning situations. Virtual environments enable large groups of students to interact with each other as well as within a three-dimensional world. Astronomy students, for example, can learn about the solar system and how it works by virtue physical engagement with the objects within. They can move planets, see around stars and track the progress of a comet. VR has also been increasingly used in the field of scientific visualization as a means of expressing complex ideas and scientific concepts (e.g., molecular models and statistical results) that would otherwise be beyond the grasp of most people's understandings (Virtual Reality Society 2016a). In addition to students studying planets via VR, NASA can implement flight simulations to train its astronauts how to handle adverse situations in space and how to react to things like sandstorms on Mars.

The entertainment industry is one of the most enthusiastic advocates of virtual reality, especially with gaming. Hollywood has increasingly employed virtual reality with filmmaking. Among their newest tricks is "digital cloning." Digital cloning was used in the blockbuster film *Maleficent* to affix "pixie-perfect" human faces on tiny fairies. Virtual museums with interactive exhibitions, art galleries, interactive theatre performances, virtual theme parks, and discovery centers (e.g., virtual reality heritage sites that allow users to visit famous monuments, Stonehenge, sculptures, caves, historical buildings, and archaeological digs) are among the subfields of the entertainment industry increasingly utilizing virtual reality (Virtual Reality Society 2016a).

There are numerous applications of virtual reality being used or developed for the world of business. Among the many ways in which VR is implemented are: virtual meetings with large numbers of employees in remote locations, virtual tours of a business environment, training of new employees, a 360 view of a products, and product design (Virtual Reality Society 2016a). Virtual reality tools are helping home owners envision new ways to redecorate their homes and assist real estate agents in selling property sites by using an app to show clients how an empty home or apartment could look once it was furnished. Wayfair.com, a company that sells furnishing, "is digitizing its catalog and testing augmented reality and virtual reality apps as well as 3D models of its products" (D'Innocenzio 2016: A-11).

Engineers use virtual reality in a wide variety of designs to test their functionality before proceeding to implement their construction in the real world. The use of a virtual environment in construction can cut down on the high amount of inefficiency and low profit margins and allow organizations an opportunity to view the structure in 3D and experience them as they would in the real world. Technology that allows engineers to virtually view their designs in a 3D manner help to spot flaws or potential risks before implementation. Virtual engineering design techniques are increasingly being used in rail construction for planning, prototyping, construction purposes, and costs projections. Car manufacturers can benefit in the same manner as rail designers (Virtual Reality Society 2016a).

Sports represent another obvious consumer of VR applications as they can measure athletic performances; analyze techniques (e.g., help a golfer with their swing), design clothing (e.g., athletic wear that helps keep athletes cool or warm depending on specific needs) and equipment (e.g., shoes, hockey and lacrosse stick design), and help improve the viewing audience of sporting events by allowing them to walkthrough a stadium and 3D broadcasts (Virtual Reality Society 2016a).

The media and telecommunications have been utilizing VR applications for some time now. VR has inspired many past movies and TV shows (i.e., *The Matrix*, *The Lawnmower Man*, and *Vanilla Sky*) and undoubtedly, many more in the future. There have been many books written on VR including Orson Scott Card's 1985 work *Ender's Game*. Virtual reality in the music industry includes experimental sound displays and sound installations but there are also apps that allow users to interact with instruments during performances or to create new compositions. Traditional forms of communications such as the telephone are being superseded by video conferencing, Skype and live chat. These communication mediums are used on the internet and other similar systems as they are deemed cheaper and more flexible (Virtual Reality Society 2016a).

Dmitri Williams, president of Ninja Metrics, an advanced data science company that works in gaming and retail, states that despite virtual reality's fun, vibrant niche, it will never become mainstream, whereas augmented reality will absolutely become mainstream. Williams states, "The reason is

VR separates you from people, while AR augments your interactions with people" (Lien 2016). VR and seemingly especially AR affords people a post-modern way of maintaining friendships ... so how can that be a bad thing? Depending on your outlook on life, time will provide the answer to that question.

Beyond the developments in the AR and VR worlds described above are a number of applications that allow people an escape into a virtual world separate from the real one. It is in this context that the virtual self comes into play, as well the formation of virtual friendships.

Residing in a Virtual World

In order for VR to be truly effective, it must have a good sense of realism and that comes at the cost of many resources, from hardware performance to the intellectual ability of the implementor of the system, to a highly efficient processing speed (Virtual Reality Society 2016a). If all these ingredients come together the experiences one can enjoy in VR are nearly endless. Let's say, for example, you have a fascination for dinosaurs. Unless you have a time machine to go back in time more than 65 million years or so, you will only encounter them on a screen wherein they have, of course, been created by a computer simulation (or in cheesy, older reproductions of dinosaurs on screens using plastic or rubber toys/puppets). In Japan, there was a virtual dinosaur revival at Dinosaur Expo 2009. Technology provided from Japanese camera maker Canon allowed visitors to view virtual recreations of dinosaurs and get a feel for their size and scale. The technology behind the simulation blends virtual reality with the real world. Users viewed the images through a hand-held viewer (YouTube 2009).

Michio Kaku, an American theoretical physicist, futurist and popularizer of science, described on *CBS This Morning* (5/13/16) his experiences with the *Science Channel* placing him in a virtual reality room with dinosaurs. Kaku "placed" his head in that of a T-Rex with the assistance of a type of VR monitoring glasses while standing in the middle of a room with 3D images of dinosaurs. Asked about the potential negative side effects of such experiences Kaku's first response was "motion sickness." He explained, what you see does not match what you feel in your inner ear, leading to brain confusion (motion sickness). A second concern was the lack of a sense of touch—you cannot walk for long before walking into a wall in the virtual reality room. To alleviate that problem, many VR simulators have users walk on an omni-directional treadmill with the user attached to a tether.

A large number of people enjoy interacting with others in virtual worlds. It is in the virtual world where the virtual self is allowed to roam and interact with others. Goffman's work on dramaturgy (see Chapter 3) is relevant to the utilization of the virtual self. When a person makes an online profile, she is presenting her front-stage persona—an attempt to control how others view her. One's backstage persona is the offline, or real, self. Participation in online virtual worlds like Second Life or World of Warcraft is an ultimate expression of a front-stage persona. In the multi-user domains (MUD) such as Second Life, people create a virtual self and act in manners not possible in the real world. (Such a notion was illustrated in James Cameron's 2009 blockbuster film *Avatar*). "By role playing, MUDers may adopt characters that express parts of self that they have found necessary to suppress or efface in the offline world, given forces of the 'generalized other's' disapproval. Online, however, these users can invest MUD characters with traits that the offline society regards with contempt or disapproval" (Robinson 2010: 98).

Before we discuss how people use their front-stage personas to interact and form friendships with others in Second Life and World of Warcraft, let's take a quick look at the film *Avatar* as many people who have not participated in the virtual world of MUDers may have seen the film and will better understand what we are about to discuss. At more than $2.78 billion, *Avatar* (2009) is the highest-grossing film of all time. To date, only one other film has grossed more than $2 billion (*Titanic*, 1997 release date); both of these films were directed by James Cameron. The science fiction epic film *Avatar* takes place in the year 2154 on the planet Pandora, where Earthlings are mining a precious mineral called unobtanium (meaning "unobtainable precious metal"). The expansion of the mining industry threatens the existence of indigenous species, including a local tribe of Na'vi (a sentient humanoid species). A team of human researchers interacts with the natives of Pandora through the use of avatars. The use of 3D special effects provides movie viewers with a sense of escape not easily duplicated in traditional 2D film formats. In the film, a number of humans transform their human essence into the avatar bodies of Na'vi. These avatars interact with "real" characters and learn the language and culture of the local beings. The main character, Jake Sully (played by Sam Worthington), is a paraplegic marine who is sent on a mission to help the humans controlled the Na'vi, but he becomes torn between following his orders and protecting the world he feels is his real home (IMDb 2016). Sully loves his avatar body because he can run, jump and feel useful; all of the things he cannot do in his real body. *Avatar's* popularity reflects our growing socialization and human embrace of virtual worlds.

Jake Sully very much prefers his life in avatar form as it provides a positive sense of self and is more congruent with what he prefers to be his presentation of self. In his avatar form, Sully utilizes a front stage persona while his consciousness is outside of the avatar and back in his human body represents his backstage persona. Millions of people around the world enjoy a fantasy-escape world wherein their avatar personas can live out a life much different from their real life. The most popular adult virtual worlds are "Second Life" and "World of Warcraft." "NeoPets" and "FreeRealms" are the two most popular virtual worlds for kids (Virtual Reality Society 2016b).

"Second Life" (also known as "2nd Life") is an internet-based virtual world that was set up by developer Linden Lab in 2003. On its tenth anniversary, Second Life (SL) had one million regular users (Stokel-Walker 2013). At its peak, SL had approximately 1.1 million users and had dropped to about 900,000 active users in 2015 (Weinberger 2015). "Today, the rising tide of virtual reality—with companies like Facebook, HTC, and Sony betting big on immersive 3D technology—means that Second Life's time may have come around" (Weinberger 2015). For now, SL users find the experience quite enjoyable and rewarding.

While SL might be thought of as a Massively Multiplayer Online Role Playing Game (MMORPG), Linden Lab insists that their virtual world in not a game, it is a place for users to reside (SL users are known as "residents"). These residents establish a virtual reality persona and interact with other participants as "avatars." An avatar (often abbreviated to "av," "avi," or "ava") appears in human form with a wide range of physical attributes. An avatar may be customized to a variety of forms. It may reflect the image of the user in the real world or may be made up. (The first-time user begins by choosing an avatar from a range of human forms as well as vampire variations, but the avatar can then be customized after you become a registered user. Some people pick an animal as their virtual self.) SL resident Fee Berry, a 55-year-old graying and overweight mother of three who lives (in the real world) in Middlesex, England, chose an avatar she named Caliandris Pendragon with characteristics of being cool and calm. Berry describes how playing a role in SL is liberating, allows her to forget about her children, her responsibilities and the fact that she does not like the way she physically looks in the real world. Her SL persona is a 25-year-old vampish babe with full lips, long jet black hair, and heavy eyeliner (Stokel-Walker 2013). While Berry's SL character Pendragon is quite a bit different than who she is in the real world, it is believed that more than 50 percent of the women in SL are really men (Stokel-Walker 2013).

Second Life residents have an actual virtual community where they build virtual properties, ranging from homes, bars, universities, hospitals and racing tracks. SL has its own economy and currency (Linden dollars—L$). The economy of SL is more than $500 million in GDP every year (Weinberger 2015). Residents create goods and services, buy and sell items, and attempt to make a living. For example, SL resident Caliandris Pendragon one year earned ($7,600) for her consultancy work, as well as creating music and textures for avatars and locations in-world (Stokel-Walker 2013). The SL residents socialize with one another within their communities and form friendships and romantic partnerships. The virtual friendships they form are what help to keep the community strong. SL residents shop, enjoy holidays, attend sporting events and star as athletes, attend fashion shows, and have their own film festivals. The virtual fashion shows in Second Life included avatar models that display the latest clothing styles available for avatars (Virtual Reality Society 2016a). Participants of the film festival created a film totally within the world of Second Life and were given the opportunity to present their films at the "48 Hour Film Project" at the 2016 Cannes Film Festival.

Caliandris Pendragon formed a relationship with SL resident Oclee Hornet. The two of them own a two-story red brick home together in SL which they spend $295 a month for the freehold to the land. They were so happy in their "2nd Life," they decided to meet in the real world (in what could be called, the First Life). They hit it off in the real world too and were contemplating living together (Stokel-Walker 2013).

While Virtual Reality Society (2016b) claims that "Second Life" is the most popular virtual reality world for adults, and the statistics on the number of actual users vary quite a bit but generally center on just under one million, Statista (2016c) indicates there are approximately 5.8 million users on "War of Warcraft" in 2015. Luckily for us, our focus is on the virtual world itself and its role as a gathering place for people to find entertainment and forge friendships so we are not as concerned about which site is most popular.

World of Warcraft (WoW) is a popular virtual reality world wherein participants create a virtual self via an avatar and participate in virtual interactions with others. According to its website, World of Warcraft (2016) "is an online game where players from around the world assume the roles of heroic fantasy characters and explore a virtual world full of mystery, magic, and endless adventure." Recall that Linden Labs states that SL is not an example of MMORPG; WoW, however, is. Most multiplayer games can accommodate anywhere from two up to several dozen simultaneous players in a game. Massively multiplayer games, however, can have thousands of players in the same game world at the same time, interacting with each other. They are as advertised—massive. In order to participate in a MMORPG, users must be connected to the Internet while they play as they are sharing a virtual world with other players. In World of Warcraft, each player's character has a specific set of skills and abilities that define that character's role. For example, mages are powerful spellcasters who use magic to inflict damage on their enemies from afar but are very vulnerable to attacks (World of Warcraft 2016). Players control their character avatars while going on quests in a virtual world filled with monsters and numerous other avatars. As the characters become more experienced and successful, they complete quests and acquire a variety of talents and skills. Group quests allow for further character development and the achievement of different levels of skills.

The nature and design of WoW encourages groups of friends to play together on teams. These friends may play together in the same geographic place (e.g., someone's living room or basement) or they may be completely remote with players in their own homes or dorms rooms spread across a town, state, country, or across the world. As one would suspect, WoW users are over-represented by younger folks. In 2013, 29 percent of WoW users were aged 16–20; 37 percent were 20–25; and 18 percent were 25–30 (Statista 2016d). More than half of all WoW users spend between 10–25 hours per week playing while another 28 percent spend more than 30 hours per week at the site. Anyone that spend this much time in a virtual world shows signs of disconnect from the real world. But, like any activity people spend a great deal of time with, WoW users find the experience to be enjoyable overall. Participating in WoW helps to reaffirm real friendships in the virtual world and helps to create friendships restricted to the virtual world. Research conducted by Dmitri Williams and associates (2006) on the social life of WoW users indicates that WoW is an important way for players who were friends with each other prior to playing WoW to maintain and reinforce their relationships. For most others, it was an entrée to bridging new social relationships and continued playing helped to forge bonds between them. The researchers also stated, however, that "only a handful of players felt that these relationships mattered more than 'real'-life ones" (Williams, Ducheneaut, Xiong, Yee and Nickell 2006:358).

Implications for the Future of Friendships

Throughout the course of these chapters on friendship, we have demonstrated how the long-held tradition of face-to-face friendships have stood the test of time. However, as a result of the development of communications technology and the rise of the internet, the meaning of friendship has expanded to the cyber and virtual worlds. In these worlds it is possible to forge and maintain friendships without ever having met face-to-face. Still, these friendships are based on the basic characteristics of friendships found throughout history, trust, loyalty, dependability, and so on. In many ways, the world has changed dramatically since the time of Aristotle and we can only venture to guess about the nature of friendships in the future. It is a safe bet, we believe, to suggest that friendships will always be a key component of humanity. Face-to-face friendships will always exist, at least for as long as we possess physical bodies, but, if technology continues to expand at its current pace, we may all eventually reside in a matrix-type of world. On the other hand, in our book *Beyond Sustainability* we warn of an impending sixth mass extinction that will be preceded by a collapse of the power grid. And when the grid goes down the world changes dramatically. It returns to a time prior to electricity (and of course, the internet or any sort of electronic communication) and with people interacting with one another only via face-to-face interactions. Just like in Aristotle's time. So, let that be a lesson to all, be sure to maintain a number (as high as 150!) of close-knit, face-to-face associations as they are the most constant form of friendship.

We would like to reiterate the point that face-to-face friendships have existed throughout history and are highly likely to remain important throughout the remainder of humanity. There is growing evidence that board and card games have become appealing to millennials because they crave face-to-face intimacy in the age of social media (Li 2016). There are an increasing number of locations opening up across the country that offer off-line board and card games. A number of friends and family members still enjoy playing board and card games, and not just at family holiday gatherings, and new games are being created. For example, the off-line "Exploding Kittens" card game sold over 2.5 million copies in a year's time (Li 2016). Games and puzzles were the fastest-growing toy category in 2015, climbing 11 percent to $1.6 billion according to the NPD Group. True, this figure is greatly overshadowed by the video game industry which took in $23.5 billion in sales in 2015, but card and board games is such one small aspect of face-to-face relationships.

The authors, like most other people, enjoy their electronic communications but we still enjoy the company of good friends and close family members. And besides, we have yet to find a virtual beer that equals the taste of a real beer. So, enjoy your friendships and face-to-face associations even while you maintain a virtual cord to the world of electronics. Having good friends, no matter what type, will help you in your pursuit of happiness.

Summary

In this chapter we discussed how people are spending an increasing amount of time in the cyberworld where, among other things, they are forging friendships in virtual worlds of reality. Some people spend so much time online that they have developed a very real problem of internet use disorder. Recognized as an infliction for over a decade now, internet addiction is characterized by an excessive preoccupation, urge, or need to be online to the point where being offline for a length of time causes impairment or distress. Among the symptoms of internet use disorder are measurable amounts of depression and social isolation. We also discussed some of the most popular social network sites including Facebook, Twitter, Tinder, and Snapchat.

The question of whether or not electronic friendships are real friendships was addressed in the context of sociability and social encounters. The question of whether or not there is a limit to how many friends any one person can maintain was also addressed. Data indicates that most humans can handle about 150 close friends and family and that smarter people usually have fewer friends. Virtual reality itself and the distinction between the cyber self and the virtual self was examined. We learned that virtual reality and augmented reality applications represent a growing characteristic of contemporary society. And finally, we look into the concept of residing within a virtual world wherein friendships are restricted to the online domain and yet, sometimes friends from the virtual world (i.e., "Second Life" and "World of Warcraft") enter the realm of the real world.

PART II

Happiness

As we discovered in Part I of this book, among the many positive aspects of having friends is their ability to provide us happiness. In Part II, we will examine the concept of "happiness" from both a philosophical and sociological perspective. We will also describe some of the many sources of happiness. However, before we examine happiness we will take a look at its counterpart, unhappiness. It is important to look at unhappiness for a number of reasons but especially for the very basic realization that often the biggest obstacle in many people's pursuit of happiness is the fact that they are unhappy. This may seem like an unprofound point to make until one realizes that millions of people try all sorts of things to become happy but they fail to realize that they may never be happy until they unburden themselves of the weight of unhappiness that holds them down and impedes their full potential for happiness.

5

Conquering Unhappiness

The American Declaration of Independence contains a famous passage that declares three unalienable rights—"life, liberty and the pursuit of happiness." Other nations profess a tripartite number of rights centered on ideals of liberty, equality and fraternity (France) and unity, justice and liberty (Germany), but only the United States articulated our right to pursue happiness. But what exactly does the right to *pursue* happiness encompass? Can we do whatever we please in order to attain happiness? No, not exactly. Will the government assure us of attaining happiness? No, not at all. As it turns out, the right to pursue happiness gives us a starting point, an opportunity to try and attain happiness. If our pursuit of happiness involves law-abiding methods and we have the means (financial or otherwise) to attain happiness that is good for us. Many people do attain at least some variations of happiness if not pure happiness (to be discussed in chapters 6 and 7); conversely, many people are not very happy. In fact, some people are so frustrated with their failed attempts to achieve happiness that they have flat-out given up. And, in most cases, even the happy people in the world have had to overcome obstacles in their lives in order to overcome unhappiness. Thus, we propose that in order to achieve happiness we must first conquer unhappiness.

How Many People Are Unhappy?

Are you unhappy? If you answered "yes" to that question you are certainly not alone. A large number of research studies have explored the topic of unhappiness and yet, while there are standard happiness indexes in existence, indexes on unhappiness are hard to come by. As a result, in an attempt to determine the number of unhappy people we often have to look at the number of people on the low end of happiness indexes and those who report that they are unhappy. For example, a 2016 Harris poll found that fewer than 1 in 3 Americans (31 percent) are "very happy" but more than 4 in 5 (81 percent) are "happy" (The Harris Poll 2016). (The Poll used a series of questions to determine Americans' levels of contentment and life satisfaction which is determined to be equal to overall happiness.) Women continue to be happier than men (33 percent of women and 29 percent of men report being "very happy"). Past Harris polls have also found that happiness levels increase with age over the long term with Americans over the age of 50 more likely to be "very happy" (36 percent of those ages 50–64, and 41 percent of adults ages 65+) than young people (31 percent of ages 18–24, 30 percent of ages 25–29, and 28 percent of ages 30–39) (Gregoire 2013).

By reversing the focus of Harris polls we could say that 19 percent of Americans are unhappy and that men and younger folks are more likely to be unhappy than women and older Americans. We would like to point out that even people who fall into the categories of "very happy" or "happy" are at times unhappy. Thus, the number of unhappy people at any given time is difficult to determine and this realization leads us to focus on the many causes of unhappiness rather than the number of people who are unhappy.

In our own research, we did not employ an unhappiness index; instead we simply asked survey participants if, "Overall, do you consider yourself an unhappy person?" As the data in Table 5.1 reveals, a much higher percentage (23 percent) of males reported being unhappy than compared to female respondents (7 percent). The causes of their unhappiness are discussed in the following pages.

Table 5.1: Overall, Do You Consider Yourself an Unhappy Person? by Gender, Number and by Percent

Males (N=74)			Females (N=107)		
Yes or No	*Number*	*Percent*	*Yes or No*	*Number*	*Percent*
Yes	17	23	Yes	7	7
No	57	77	No	92	86
			* Sometimes	8	7

(* *Note: While the "Sometimes" option was not given, 8 respondents wrote it in by hand.*)

The Many Causes of Unhappiness

The title of this chapter was inspired by the work of philosopher Bertrand Russell (1872–1970) and his 1930 publication of *The Conquest of Happiness*, a book that predates the contemporary fascination with self-help publications by decades. (For an interesting look at how Russell came to write this bestselling work, as well as his colorful friendship with its publisher Horace Liveright, see David E. White's article "Russell in the Jazz Age" in the 2016 book *Bertrand Russell, Public Intellectual*, edited by Tim Madigan and

Peter Stone.) Russell's use of the word "conquest" in the book's title reinforces his primary contention that happiness, except in rare cases, is *not* something that simply presents itself to people but rather is something that must be achieved (conquered). Following this line of thinking, we have proposed that in order to be happy one must first conquer unhappiness. It is only fitting then to first examine what Russell had to say about the sources of unhappiness before we turn our attention to some of the many other causes.

Bertrand Russell and Unhappiness

The world is filled with avoidable and unavoidable misfortunes, psychological entanglements, a struggle to attain financial security, and a number of other variables that contribute to unhappiness. In *Conquest*, Russell spends more time discussing the causes of unhappiness than he does the causes of happiness. Russell argues that the multitudes of men and women who suffer from unhappiness without enjoying it (this idea will be expanded upon later in this chapter) could find happiness if they heeded the advice offered in *Conquest*. Russell's advice centers on the premise that happiness has as much to do with eliminating the causes of unhappiness as it does with engaging in activities that bring us happiness. Such a perspective seems quite simplistic and yet it is relatively profound, in that many people seem oblivious to the idea that happiness can be attained if one removes the causes of unhappiness. In other words, one can be happy only if one is not unhappy.

Russell acknowledges that there are many causes of unhappiness, some of which have roots in the social system and others as the result of one's individual psychology. The social system, according to Russell, creates war, economic exploitation, unequal access to a quality education among all members of society and tactics of fear designed to make people feel uneasy about their place in society. Elaborating on war, for example, Russell states that the social system cannot avoid war when "men are so unhappy that mutual extermination seems to them less dreadful than continued endurance of the light of day" (p. 15).

Addressing the issue of one's individual psychology, Russell (1930) states this type of unhappiness is caused largely by "mistaken views of the world, mistaken ethics, mistaken habits of life, leading to destruction of that natural zest and appetite for possible things upon which all happiness, whether of men or animals, ultimately depends. These are matters which lie within the power of the individual, and I propose to suggest the change by which his happiness, given average good fortune, may be achieved" (p. 16).

The relevance of Russell's view on "what makes people unhappy" is evident in abundance in contemporary society as social systems, including democracies, create inequality in all the same forms described by Russell;

that is to say, war appears to be a constant, as do economic inequality and education inequality, and a wide variety of scare tactics are used by a variety of social institutions (e.g., politics, government, insurance companies) in an attempt to keep people in support of the status quo. (Scare tactics are also used by some as a way to stimulate a challenge to the status quo as well.) Individuals who are particularly upset with the existing social system and who seek change seem to be particularly unhappy with nearly every social institution and are generally very unpleasant to be around. Such individuals are filled with anxiety; become excessively preoccupied by things beyond their control; have a lack of interest in anything but their self-imposed struggle; are generally incapable of enjoying simple things in life, like play and leisure and pride in their sense of workmanship; and, lack a sense of well-roundedness.

In Chapter 2 of *Conquest*, Russell describes Byronic unhappiness. The origin of the concept of "Byronic" unhappiness dates back to the characteristics of English Romantic poet Lord Byron (1788–1824), or more specifically to his poetic themes, especially romanticism, melancholy, and melodramatic energy (*Dictionary.com* 2016b). Essentially, the Byronic individual has a self-absorbed, brooding personality. The Byronic personality may also include descriptions that include a proud, moody, cynical, defiant and lonely person.

Russell (1930) depicted Byronic individuals as the truly unhappy and yet as those who are also "proud of their unhappiness, which they attribute to the nature of the universe and consider to be the only rational attitude for an enlightened man" (p. 25). Russell counters that there is no superior rationality in being unhappy and that the wise person should allow himself to be happy as circumstances permit. Unless you are a Byronic person, chances are, you will try to avoid being around those who are "happy with being unhappy" as their negative attitudes may rub off on you.

Psychiatrist Jacqueline Olds studies one of the aspects of the Byronic personality—loneliness—and draws at least one conclusion relevant to Russell's analysis of Byronic unhappiness. In her co-authored book *The Lonely American*, Olds and Schwartz (2009) describe how emotions like loneliness and happiness can be contagious based on one's own mood and the moods of associates. It should be noted, however, that Olds and Schwartz (2009) describe loneliness as a universal thing but yet as something that people are embarrassed to admit to others. Russell's usage of the Byronic personality concept would not correspond with loneliness as he believed that such people are proud of their unhappiness status.

Russell (1930) argues that it is *competition* that most interferes with one's pursuit of enjoyment. Competition (which Aristotle would call *agon*) leads to what Russell calls the "struggle for life" and this struggle is enough to lead many members of the masses to believe that "life is too grim, too tenacious" and too tough to bear (p. 55). In the contemporary era we can see that competition is all-prevalent. We are in competition with others over minor things like finding a parking spot or securing a seat on a subway or picking which line will go faster at the grocery store. We are in competition for major things too, such as finding a great career, finding a spouse, and securing a job promotion. Major institutions have elements that are in constant competition too. In sports, individual athletes and teams compete with one another for championships; phone, cable, and car companies fight each other to gain consumer dollars; restaurants compete with one another; dentists, doctors, pharmacies and on and on all compete with another for the right to take money from customers in order to survive. And because competition results in more losers than winners, those who are not best fit for the environment risk dissolution. Competition is indeed a source of unhappiness for many.

In Chapter 4 of *The Conquest of Happiness*, Russell discusses *boredom* as a source of unhappiness. Russell suggests that boredom is exclusively a human emotion. Animals may become listless, pace up and down, and yawn, but in a state of nature what they experience is not analogous to boredom. According to Russell, the opposite of boredom is excitement. Thus, if we are not excited by our environment or circumstances, we are bored by it. Russell (1930) states, "The desire for excitement is very deep-seated in human beings, especially in males. I suppose that in the hunting stage it was more easily gratified than it has been since" (p. 57). From the contemporary perspective we know that suggesting males seek excitement more so than females is a sexist conclusion as nearly everyone, regardless of their gender identification, prefers excitement over boredom.

The dichotomy between boredom and excitement is quite fascinating in the contemporary era as people seek activities that bring them rewards in the form of excitement. In fact, the current era is highlighted by a culture with the need of instant gratification. Paul Roberts (2014) describes America's current age highlighted by the need for instant gratification as the "impulse society." Technology has fueled this impulse age. For example, there are plenty of electronic devices that help to keep people stimulated and seemingly gratified. However, when these e-devices are taken away or forbidden for any length of time many people become very listless, bored or even agitated. Any college professor can tell you that students do not like being told that they cannot use their smartphones in class. Many movie patrons find it necessary to check their phones while at the movie theatre. Couples who are dining at a restaurant often find the need for outside stimuli. Many people walk about conducting their daily activities with their heads held low staring at a bright screen (and are known as "screen sniffers"). In short, too many people seem bored even though there is a form of stimuli right in front of them—other people! Are people who are preoccupied by e-devices truly happy? Or are they missing out on the sources of happiness that surround them? On the other hand, it is the use of electronic devices that alleviates boredom and brings happiness for many people. The time will come, however, when people will not use (or will not be able to use) electronic devices as a means to overcome unhappiness.

Fatigue was the next cause of unhappiness described by Russell (Chapter 5). As is the general case throughout *The Conquest of Happiness*, Russell does not provide a definition of the concepts he uses and this includes the term "fatigue." This may be due in part to the philosophical nature of his writing and/or a belief that the parameters of certain concepts are, more or less, understood by professionals and laypersons alike. The contemporary definition of fatigue includes such descriptions as physical and/or mental exhaustion that can be triggered by stress, medication, overwork, or mental and physical illness or disease (*Medical-Dictionary.com* 2016) and a condition characterized by a lessened capacity for work and reduce efficiency of accomplishment, usually accompanied by a feeling of weariness and tiredness (*MedicineNet.com* 2016). Based on these two definitions, it is easy to comprehend how fatigue can lead to negative consequences.

Russell (1930) himself said that fatigue can become a "grave evil" and, of course, a cause of unhappiness (p. 68). Laborers and peasant women Russell found were old by the time they reached thirty years of age. As with contemporary views of fatigue, Russell also linked stress and anxiety due to fatigue. As a bit of sound advice, Russell proclaimed that a great many worries could be diminished by realizing the unimportance of the matter which is causing the anxiety. Thus, a key to happiness is not giving a damn about what others think of you or what others think is important. This is similar to a sign one of the authors once read at a mechanic's garage—"An emergency on your part does not make it an emergency on my part." Brilliant! Just because someone else, like a college administrator, thinks something is important—like yet another assessment report—does not mean it is an emergency on the part of faculty! Russell describes how he once had a considerable amount of anxiety due to public speaking. In fact, he often dreaded giving a talk in front of others to the point where he became exhausted from the nervous strain. However, Russell (1930) gradually taught himself "to feel that it did not matter whether he [I] spoke well or ill, the universe would remain much the same in either case" (p. 73). Once Russell learned to downplay the importance of giving public talks, the nervous strain he experienced diminished almost to the vanishing point.

Space does not permit an elaboration on the potential positive aspects of fatigue but, in brief, Russell believed that fatigue assisted in one's self-assessment of a job well done; that it leads to sound sleep and a good appetite; and, it gives zest to the pleasures that are possible on holidays. Tim Delaney has conducted research on fatigue and its connection to an endorphin rush, as illustrated by such things as the "runner's high" and the ability of athletes, military personnel and gang members to "press on" despite feeling physically exhausted.

The next cause of unhappiness discussed by Russell is envy. Russell (1930) states, "Next to worry probably one of the most potent causes of unhappiness is envy. Envy is, I should say, one of the most universal and deepseated of human passions" (p. 82). Envy combines traits of jealousy and competition. To be envious of another is to want what others have, to be more like them, or to despise others because of what they have. Among the examples provided by Russell was an interesting presentation of envy as the basis of democracy and women who judge other women based on the clothes they wear. As for democracy, since the time of the Greeks, such a system is based on competition and the attempts of those who control the means of production to encourage citizens to purchase consumer products. If our neighbor has a better product than us, we should want to "keep up with the Jones." With regards to women and clothing, Russell (1930) states, "Among average respectable women envy plays an extraordinary large part" (p. 83). Women, Russell believes, are jealous of other women who have nicer clothing and accessories to the point where they will draw the ire of envious via glances and derogatory inferences. While it could be tempting to conclude that Russell is displaying a sexist attitude by suggesting women are so shallow as to be envious of other women because of the clothes they wear, there exists in contemporary society an adage that "women dress for other women, not men" when they go out for an evening on the town (Levy 2011).

In Chapter 7 of *Conquest*, Russell discusses the idea of "the sense of sin." Earlier in his book (Chapter 1), Russell had described a "sinner" as someone who commits an act that leads to disapproval, especially one's own self-disapproval. Further, if the person is religious, a sinful act is interpreted as the disapproval of God. Interestingly, Russell described narcissism (admiring oneself and wishing to be admired) as a habitual sense of sin. He acknowledged that, up to a point, it is normal to want to be admired and to admire one's own accomplishments, but when such self-directed admiration becomes excessive, it becomes a grave evil. Russell describes "the sense of sin" as one of the most important underlying psychological causes of unhappiness as there exists a corresponding feeling of unease and discomfort. A person who offends his or her rational code of conduct experiences unhappiness because there were alternative behaviors that could have been employed. Upon reflection on an act that violates one's own code of conduct, remorse is likely to take residence within one's consciousness via self-reflection. This remorse, beyond making a person unhappy, is likely to make the individual feel inferior. Worse yet, the unhappy person is likely to act out in a number of harmful ways including setting unrealistic and excessive expectations on others' behaviors and by holding grudges against those who now seem superior. Russell (1930) states, "Nothing so much diminishes not only happiness but efficiency as a personality divided against itself" (p. 107).

In contemporary society there are a near limitless number of examples of people feeling unhappy due to their behaviors that violate a personal code of expectations. Shaking the hand of a rival is often an expectation of social or business protocol but shaking the hand of someone you truly despise is hard to take. Consider, for example, the tradition in hockey playoffs wherein members of each team line up to shake hands with one another following the conclusion of a playoff series. During the course of the playoff series a number of situations may have arrived that leads to tensions between rival team members and, yet, hockey protocol dictates such action. One famous example resonates more than others—the Dino Ciccarelli (Detroit Red Wings) and Claude Lemieux (Colorado Avalanche) handshake following the 1996 Stanley Cup series' concluding game. In the series, Lemieux, known as a dirty player, infamously blindsided Red Wings player Kris Draper, sidelining him for months of rehabilitation. After shaking Lemieux's hand, Ciccarelli told the press, "I can't believe I shook this guy's friggin' hand after the game. That pisses me right off." Many of us may have contemplated at one point or another, "Why did I shake that guy's hand?" In sports, it's a sign of poor sportsmanship to refuse to shake hands with an opponent, even if that opponent was a poor sport. In the case of Ciccarelli, he violated his own personal code of ethics to meet the demands of others and he felt remorseful in doing so.

Russell next discusses persecution mania as a source of unhappiness. In its most extreme form, mania is recognized as insanity. Some people envision that others wish to kill them, or imprison them, or to do some other grave injury (what Russell refers to as "persecution mania"). While it is understandable that mania may be a cause of unhappiness, Russell's analysis reflects the poor understanding of mental health that people had in 1930 and is of little value to us today other than to highlight the tendency of some people to possess a "persecution complex." A persecution complex is a term given to an array of psychologically-complex behaviors centered on an acute irrational fear that other people are plotting one's downfall and that they are responsible for one's failures in life.

The final cause of unhappiness discussed by Russell is the fear of public opinion. Russell (1930) states, "Very few people can be happy unless on the whole their way of life and their outlook on the world is approved by those with whom they have social relations, and more especially by those with whom they live" (p. 126). Hoping to gain the approval of the general public and especially those closest to us is still important to many people today. The field of sociology in particular has produced a great deal of literature that supports the idea that most of us care about the reactions of significant others (e.g., parents, children, best friends, dating partners) toward our behaviors. And yet, while most of us want the approval of others, this is not a universal phenomenon as there remains a sizeable number of people who march to the beat of their own drum. Russell believes that the fear of public opinion, like every other form of fear, is oppressive and stunts growth. Furthermore, it is difficult to achieve any kind of greatness while a fear of this kind remains strong and it is impossible to achieve happiness if we must constantly concern ourselves with the tastes and desires of our neighbors or close relations. Russell (1930) offers this summation, "I think that in general, apart from expert opinion, there is too much respect paid to the opinions of others, both in great matters and in small ones" (p. 136). Still, it would be advisable for employees to heed the directions of their employers; for people to abide by the laws of a particular society; and for spouses to heed their partner's concerns.

While we have now concluded our look at Russell's view of unhappiness, let's continue with a closer examination of the idea that spouses should heed their partner's concerns if they wish to be happy and avoid the unhappiness that often accompanies marriage and other close relationships.

Unhappy with Marriage and Relationships: "Unhappy Wife, Unhappy Life"

A concern with the happiness of one's partner has not always been prevalent throughout history. In fact, in much of the world, throughout most of time, including still today in many cultures, marriage has less to do with love and blissful happiness and more to do with fulfilling arrangements based on more practical issues. This certainly seems to be the case in Aristotle's discussion of marriage in his *Nichomachean Ethics*, for instance. The basic struggle for survival generally took precedence over the pursuit of happiness. Furthermore, the patriarchal nature of nearly every society over the millenniums led to male dominance in nearly all social institutions including marriage. In this regard, the wife was expected to make the husband happy even at the expense of her own happiness. Even during Russell's era, and as told in *Conquest*, there existed an attitude that the wife was supposed to take care of the husband's everyday needs so that he could concentrate on earning a living. The adage of "the husband brings home the bacon and the wife cooks it" was prevalent. (Note: Russell may have been better off concerning himself with the opinion of his wives as he was married four times over the course of his lifetime! He was also a proponent of equal rights for women long before it was considered generally acceptable.)

Today, at least in most Western societies there exists a different outlook on marriage and serious relationships that centers on the premise that it is most important to keep the wife happy and that her opinion is to be heeded. Such a sentiment has led to far different adages (than the one described above) in the contemporary era—"A happy wife equals a happy life" and its corresponding counterpart, "Unhappy wife, unhappy life." Consider, for example, a study conducted by sociologist Deborah Carr and associates (2014) which indicates that a wife's happiness in the marriage has the power to overtake a husband's marital unhappiness and to make his overall life more pleasant. Conversely, Carr's research indicated that women's happiness didn't seem to be affected by husbands' satisfaction with their marriage. Carr and associates explain that if a man is unhappy in the relationship but the wife is happy, she's more likely to provide him with benefits that enhance his overall life—she'll engage in sexual relations, provide emotional support and take on household chores. As with previous research, Carr et al. found that men tended to rate their marriages higher than women did and that this could be the case because women are socialized to think about their relationships and scrutinize them more than men. This notion supports another premise supported by the Carr et al. research that marriage is good for men's health but not necessarily women's.

A great deal of research has been conducted on the link between marriage and steady relationships with happiness or unhappiness. Relationships with significant others can bring love, companionship, an overall sense of well-being, a general happiness; however, because most relationships end in failure, people are left to experience loneliness, emotional distraught, and unhappiness. Any one of us can recollect all the intimate relationships we've had over our lifetimes and realize that nearly all of them ended in failure, generally with hurt feelings and perhaps a broken heart. Even people currently happily married were likely involved in a number of love relationships prior to marriage that ended in disappointment. When people do get married they hope that they have finally found "the one" but, as we know, even marriages that began with high hopes of success risk ending in failure. Divorce is the primary indicator of a failed marriage. We have all heard that nearly half of all marriages will end in divorce and the data seems to support such a notion. The U.S. Department of Health and Human Services, for example, reports that during the 2006–2010 period, the probability of a first marriage lasting at least 10 years was 68 percent for women and 70 percent for men. Looking at 20 years, the probability that first marriages of women and men will survive was 52 percent for women and 56 percent for men (Copen, Daniels, Vespa, and Mosher 2012). U.S. Census Bureau statistics indicate that second marriages have a much higher failure rate (estimates range from 60 to 67 percent) and third marriages an even higher rate (around 75 percent) (AboutDivorce.org

2011). It is also interesting to note the term "un-divorced" which is applied to couples that remain legally married but live separately. The un-divorced may be involved in a trial separation or a full separation but remain married primarily for financial reasons (e.g., neither the husband or wife wanted to pay for the divorce, or they found it monetarily beneficial to remain legally married).

Even in marriages that remain intact, it would be incorrect to assume that all involved are happy. In all likelihood, less than half of those in a relationship are happy. In a study of 3,000 couples, more than six out of ten couples reported that they were unhappy in their relationship; four out of ten admitted they had considered leaving their partner; and, one in ten no longer even trusts their partner (*Daily Mail* 2010). Generally, when the "honeymoon period" ends, couples tend to take each other for granted, which is a leading contributing factor for the number one relationship gripe—the lack of spontaneity (see Table 5.2). This lack of spontaneity is closely tied to the number two relationship gripe, namely a lack of romance. During the courtship/dating period and early on in the relationship couples tend to direct a great deal of attention toward one another in an attempt to make the other happy. When this stops, people tend to become unhappy in their relationship. The top ten relationship gripes are shown in Table 5.2.

Table 5.2: Top 10 Relationship Gripes
1. Lack of spontaneity
2. Lack of romance
3. Terrible sex life
4. No time to give each other attention
5. Lack of time to talk
6. Don't want the same things for the future
7. Don't trust each other
8. Lack of affection
9. No longer fancy each other
10. No honesty

(*Source:* Daily Mail *2010*)

Stress and Depression as Causes of Unhappiness

The idea that one cannot be happy if they are unhappy is connected to the theory that happiness comes from within each of us and, thus, if we are stressed and/or suffer from depression, we cannot be happy. Stress and depression act as harmful toxics to our brains, inhibiting our ability to enjoy life. As Caroline Leaf (2013) explains, the quality of our thinking and our reactions to circumstances and events determine our "brain architecture"— the shape or design of the brain and resultant quality of the health of our minds and bodies. Toxic thinking, then, wears down the brain and thus impedes our pursuit of happiness.

Stress is defined as a state of mental tension or emotional strain or tension resulting from adverse or very demanding circumstances caused by problems in one's life, including work and non-work environments. Synonyms for stress include strain, pressure, nervous tension, worry, and anxiety. Stress causes bodily or mental tension and may be a factor in disease causation. The American Medical Association links stress to more than 60 percent of all human illness and disease (*The Huffington Post* 2013). Stress affects the body in numerous ways including: headaches, dizziness, anxiety, irritability, anger and panic disorders; grinding teeth and tension in the jaw; increased heart rate, strokes, heart disease, hypertension, diabetes; weight gain and obesity; decreased sex drive; muscle tension; and may contribute to alcoholism, suicide, drug addiction, tobacco and other harmful addictive behaviors (*The Huffington Post* 2013). It should be clear that then, that stress can contribute to unhappiness, especially if people do not learn how to control their reactions to stressful events.

Depression is another cause of unhappiness. As defined by the Mayo Clinic (2016), "Depression is a mood disorder that causes a persistent feeling of sadness and loss of interest. Also called major depressive disorder or clinical depression, it affects how you feel, think and behave and can lead to a variety of emotional and physical problems. You may have trouble doing normal day-to-day activities, and sometimes you may feel as if life isn't worth living." The World Health Organization (2016b) estimated that 350 million people of all ages suffer from the mental disorder of depression and adds that "depression is the leading cause of disability worldwide, and is a major contributor to the overall global burden of disease." There are effective treatments for moderate and severe depression including psychological treatments (e.g., behavioral activation, cognitive behavioral therapy) or antidepressant medication (e.g., selective serotonin reuptake inhibitors and tricyclic antidepressants) (WHO 2016b). While there are treatments for depression, it is estimated that 80 percent of individuals affected by this disorder do not receive treatment (Healthline 2012). Individuals that are most likely to suffer from depression are unemployed or recently divorced. In the United States, adults from southern states (Oklahoma, Arkansas, Tennessee, Louisiana, Mississippi, Alabama and West Virginia) have the highest percentage of those meeting the criteria for depression (Healthline 2012). While it is understandable that people who suffer from depression are also unhappy, it might come as a surprise to many that Americans report being among the most unhappy people in the world. Furthermore, whereas 4 out of 5 Americans do not receive treatment, anti-depressant usage increased 400 percent from 1994 to 2013 (Myers 2013).

The bottom line is, happiness does not come naturally for most people; it is something we have to choose to work toward, since otherwise we will be predisposed (but not destined) toward unhappiness. Consciously working toward happiness, and, yes, taking medication when necessary, will help people overcome the causes of stress and depression that contribute to unhappiness.

Work as a Cause of Unhappiness

Work represents a dichotomy when discussing unhappiness. On the one hand, as we just discussed above, individuals most likely to suffer from depression are unemployed (or recently divorced) and as we are about to discover it is the one activity that brings about the greatest unhappiness for people; conversely, as we will describe in chapters 8 and 9 it is work that provides a sense of meaning and gives purpose to the lives of many.

Let's start with a little self-reflection—are you happy with your current job? Based on a variety of poll results, if you answered "no" to that question you are not alone. Just how many people are dissatisfied with their jobs is not completely clear as the data is somewhat inconsistent. Consider the following:

- Beth Stebner (2013), writing for the *Daily News* and citing Gallup Poll results, states that over 70 percent of U.S. workers are unhappy about their job with 20 percent "actively disengaged" and 50 percent "disengaged."
- Alyson Shontell (2010), writing for *Business Insider* and citing Deloitte's Shift Index survey results, states that 80 percent of American workers are dissatisfied with their jobs.
- Susan Adams (2013), writing for *Forbes* and citing Gallup Poll results, states that unhappy employees outnumber happy ones by two to one worldwide; that only 13 percent of workers feel engaged by their jobs; and with 63 percent who are "not engaged" and 24 percent of workers are "actively disengaged."

The statistics cited above paint quite a negative picture for worker satisfaction (using engagement as a criterion) at their places of employment. And while we expected that many people are unhappy with their jobs, these numbers seem high. So, as we encourage our students to do, we went to the original sources and found some conflicting data results. Consider the following:

- In its 2015 report, Deloitte reported that employee satisfaction and commitment with their jobs and workplaces was at 58.1 percent for federal employees and 76.7 percent for private sector employees. The 2015 results represented a modest increase over the past few years (and thus would not account for the discrepancy reported in secondary publications). As a point of interest, the large government agency with the highest percentage of satisfied employees was NASA (76.1 percent), followed by the Intelligence Community (67.1) and the Department of Justice and Department of State tied for third 66.2 percent (Deloitte 2015).

- A 2012 Gallup poll reports that nearly half of U.S. workers employed full- or part-time feel completely satisfied with most aspects of work and that nearly 35 percent were satisfied with all 13 criteria measurements for job satisfaction (Saad 2012). The criteria measurement for job satisfaction that had the lowest response for worker satisfaction was "The amount of on-the-job stress in your job" with just 29 percent of respondents "completely satisfied," 37 percent "somewhat satisfied," and, 33 percent "total dissatisfied." The next three highest percentage of total dissatisfaction among workers was "the amount of money you earn," "the retirement plan your employer offers," and "Your chances for promotion."
- We did find a Gallup poll that stated that 70 percent of U.S. workers were not engaged at work as referenced by Stebner (Gallup 2016). Gallup also reports that younger workers are the least engaged (of all age groups) at work (Adkins 2014).

The data cited above does support the general contention that many workers are not happy with their current jobs. There are a number of specific reasons that people cite for their job dissatisfaction. These reasons include those cited above (stress, low pay, poor retirement plan, and limited chances for promotion) and the following:

- Dissatisfaction with the boss (e.g., the boss is a micro-manager, mean, or unqualified to be the boss)
- Depression (we already reviewed the role of depression with unhappiness)
- Feeling under valued (e.g., the feeling that one's hard work, time and talents are being taken-for-granted)
- Feeling that what one does for work does not really matter (this makes us think of when there is an impending snowstorm coming to a big city and "non-essential" people are told to go home early or not report for work, being labeled "non-essential" cannot be good for one's self-esteem)
- The realization that it is difficult to stay focused on the task at hand (e.g., because the work is tedious or repetitive to the point where there is little to no thinking involved in order to perform the job task)

- Burnout (e.g., exhaustion); other grounds for worker unhappiness including who the boss is, depression, and lack of energy (e.g., the inability to continue to work at peak performance because your mind and/or body needs to be "recharged")
- The job is not challenging enough, leaving the employee feeling under used, under valued and/or bored
- The employee had no idea what they wanted to do with their lives and took the first job they found and now feel stuck (e.g., they once felt aimless in life so they took a job to stop others from hounding them to get a job)
- Taking a job just to make money (let's face it, most people work because they *have* to)
- Taking a job that involved credentials because they felt they needed to do so (e.g., highly educated persons tend to think they must find a career in a profession generally associated with their advanced degree)
- The values of the company are different from those of the employee (e.g., if the employee values the environment but you find yourself working for a gas or oil company)
- Job insecurity (e.g., not knowing if your job will still be there week after week is very stressful)
- Too much interference from administration and/or red tape (e.g., a college professor who has to listen to administrators who think they know your job better than you do and/or having to abide by state politician mandates).
- Relationships with coworkers (if you cannot get along with your coworkers, or in some cases, one coworker in particular, it can be a drag to go to work)
- The flexibility with work hours (this is especially important for single parents who need to leave work to tend to their children's specific needs)
- The amount of vacation time received (the proper amount of vacation time is necessary to avoid burnout as well as to get away from the job for a while)
- Health insurance benefits provided by the employer (it is critical to have a good health care benefits package, one that includes dental too, in order to avoid economic disaster often associated with a major medical procedure).

What can you do if you are unhappy at work? There seems to be just three primary options: change *what* you do (e.g., a new role within the company or a new career); change *how* you do your job (e.g., adopt a new mindset and cultivate new habits and attitudes); or, change *nothing*, and be complicit in your own misery (the worse option but one that may not be avoidable for many people) (Warrell 2014).

To this point, we have discussed a number of specific reasons why people might be unhappy, including the ideas from Russell (e.g., Byronic unhappiness, competition, boredom, fatigue, envy, sense of sin, persecution mania, and fear of public opinion), an unhappy marriage or relationship, stress and depression, and an unhappy work situation. In the following pages we will briefly highlight some other causes of unhappiness.

Many Other Causes of Unhappiness

Undoubtedly, there are many other variables that may cause someone to be unhappy. A highly identified sports fan, for example, will experience unhappiness (along with a number of other emotions) when a favorite athlete or sports team fails to win an important sporting event or championship. The authors have their favorite sports teams and one in particular "lives and dies" with the fortunes of his sports teams—some of which are highly successful but others that are less likely to win a title.

In the following pages we will take a quick look at some of the many other causes of unhappiness. It should be noted that the examples provided below are not meant to be a complete list of sources of unhappiness but they help to illustrate the point that there are many things that can cause of unhappiness. The authors encourage readers to share with them their own ideas on what causes unhappiness in their lives. The items listed below are in no particular order (e.g., from the most severe to the least severe causes of unhappiness) and represent some of the authors' ideas:

- The death of a loved one
- The poor health of a loved one
- The fear of the power grid going down and leading to social chaos
- Lack of true friends, lack of quality friendships
- Lack of meaning in one's day to day life; general feelings of meaninglessness
- Obsession with the past or future
- Being out-of-shape, or feeling poorly about one's physical appearance
- Being unhealthy to the point where desired activities can no longer be pursued
- Suffering from major medical problems
- Suffering from major mental health problems
- Unfavorably comparing oneself to others; jealousy toward others who have more

- Focusing on the negative aspects of one's life
- A lack of tolerance for anything less than perfect and the fear of failure; perfectionism
- Low self-esteem, thinking poorly of oneself leads to unhappiness
- Financial debt, a major source of worry, stress and tension
- A workload that is too heavy and does not allow for time to play or pursue favorite leisure activities
- A lack of time to spend with friends and family members
- Excessive reasoning; over-thinking things
- Negativism; a fixation on the negative—somewhat like Byronic unhappiness
- Assuming the worst of others and social situations
- Worrying too much
- Power freak, the need to control everything and getting frustrated when you realize you cannot control everything
- Holding grudges against others; it sounds like a cliché—and in fact it is—but holding a grudge only hurts you, not the target of your disdain
- Wanting to believe that life is fair when it seldom is
- Wanting everyone to play by your rules
- A glass-half-empty type person
- Loneliness; social isolationism
- Personal insecurity; too afraid to step outside of one's comfort zone
- Hanging out with unhappy people
- Unsure of your purpose in life
- Realizing that you are the actor, not the author of your life; the sheep rather than the shepherd
- Constant need for validation from others (self-worth comes from within not from external forces)
- Procrastination, which leads to an endless spiral of frustration—for you and for others who have to wait on you (no one likes someone who is late all the time for no good reason)
- The realization that your dreams and aspirations have not come true
- Failure to learn new things, something that helps brings joy and personal growth to one's life
- Boredom; if you do not keep busy, you become a dull person and dullness leads to unhappiness (The authors report that they have not been bored in years!)
- Lack of sleep; insomniacs in particular are susceptible to developing depression
- Dependence on others; clinging onto others with no plan of your own leads to low self-esteem, among other things, and unhappiness

- Failure to take time to relax and enjoy life
- Unhappiness with government and politics; a 2013 Gallup poll found that 65 percent of Americans are dissatisfied with the nation's system and efficacy of government (Kopan 2014)
- Failure to take risks in life; when one does not push their perceived limits they fail to grow; excitement is the opposite of boredom
- Impatience, always wanting things/events to occur on time or on a schedule
- Failure to learn from one's mistakes
- You don't love yourself; it is impossible to be happy if you do not love yourself
- Playing the victim card repeatedly instead of taking responsibility for what you can control and moving on
- Failure to allow yourself to be happy; if you are unhappy with your life as it is, chance your life to include things that bring happiness.

In our research on college students we asked respondents to identify some of the things that make them unhappy. Some of these causes of happiness have already been mentioned and others are new (see Table 5.3).

**Table 5.3: Things That Make Me Unhappy
by Gender and by Number**

Males (N=74)		Females (N=107)	
Cause of Unhappiness	*Number*	*Cause of Unhappiness*	*Number*
Economic/financial issues	56	Stress/anxiety	20
Stress, too much work	18	Bad grades	9
Poor school performance	6	Too much school work	9
Poor quality friends/conflict		People in general	5
with friends	4	Rude people	5
People in general	4	Bad weather	4
Family problems	3	Housework	3
Failure	3	Failure	3
Bad weather	3	Being/feeling overwhelmed	3
Being betrayed	3	Not understanding things	
Homework	3	(school)	3
Lack of sleep	3	Loneliness	3
Politics/current affairs	2	Dealing with too many	
Not being able to start my		unfamiliar people	2
career now	2	Fake friends	2
Liars	2	Being talked down to	2
My roommate	1	Being ignored	2
Bad coffee	1	Seeing others upset	2
Death of family member(s)	1	Violence against others	2
Family drama	1	Arguments	2
Political path of the country	1	Fighting	2

(Males)		*(Females)*	
Memories (no elaboration)	1	Lack of money	2
Feeling of not having a purpose	1	Seeing animals or people	
Fake Friends	1	hurt	2
Slow traffic	1	Being separated from	
Being alone	1	friends/family	2
Not exercising	1	Conflict	2
Being judged	1	Overworked	2
Dependency (no elaboration)	1	Negative people	2
Ignorance	1	Negative events	2
Trump supporters	1	Missing someone special	1
My level of intelligence	1	Boys	1
My favorite sports team losing	1	Feeling ignored	1
I don't like where I'm going		Negativity	1
in life	1	Getting a traffic ticket	1
Having my time wasted	1	Losing loved ones	1
Disappointment	1	Unreturned love	1
Negative energy	1	Not sleeping	1
Betrayal	1	Messing things up	1
Ignorance	1	Being hungry	1
Lack of trust in myself	1	People ignorant to world	
Stubborn people that wont'		events	1
listen	1	Being lied to	1
Lack of trust in myself	1	Accidentally messing up	1
Heartbreak	1	Being judged	1
Betrayal	1	Cancer	1
Ignorance	1	People's drama	1
Hypocrites	1	Not having a car	1
People touching my stuff	1	Bad events in our world	1
Fights in my family	1	Dishonesty	1
Politics and poker	1	Fighting with friends	1
Burnt cookies	1	Thinking about the future	1
Seeing people unhappy	1	Prejudice	1
Lack of self fulfillment	1	People who are rude	1
People being critical of one		People who break promises	1
another	1	Prejudice	1
		Being unorganized	1
		Bullying	1
		People being mean for no	
		reason	1
		Running	1
		Rejection	1
		Mean people	1
		Conflict	1
		Changes in daily routines	1
		Losing friends	1
		When my favorite hockey	
		team loses	1
		Hate	1

We have clearly demonstrated that there are many causes of unhappiness. Perhaps you recognized some of these sources of unhappiness in your own life. The primary lesson to learn from this review is that we need to acknowledge the things that cause us unhappiness, address these causes head-on, and learn to eliminate them.

Popular Culture Scenario 5: Mel Brooks' Guide for Overcoming Unhappiness

In 1968 the comedian Mel Brooks wrote and directed a film called *The Producers,* starring Zero Mostel and Gene Wilder. It was the outrageous story of a washed-up Broadway producer named Max Bialystock (played by Mostel) who has had nothing but flops in recent years and is down on his luck. An accountant named Leo Bloom (played by Wilder) comes to do his books and makes the offhand comment that, since Bialystock had actually raised a lot more money than he actually spent on his last production, which closed after the first night, there is a profit in failure. Bloom is only joking, but a delighted Bialystock takes him seriously and lures him into a scheme to raise two million dollars (primarily by Bialystock's seducing little old ladies) and putting on a sure-fire fiasco, after which they can take the unspent profits and go to Rio. They choose a play written by a unrepentant Nazi, entitled *Springtime for Hitler,* which they know is guaranteed to offend everyone (remember, this film came out when World War II was still a living memory). But much to their horror it becomes a huge hit instead, and Max and Leo end up in jail.

The movie was not a huge success at the box office, but Brooks won an Academy Award for Original Best Screenplay, and it was the start of his storied career as a moviemaker, paving the way for such huge successes as *Blazing Saddles, Young Frankenstein, Silent Movie,* and *Spaceballs. The Producers* remained a beloved work for Brooks, and in 1998 he recreated it as a Broadway musical—with no intention of producing a flop. In fact, it became a box office smash, setting records for attendance, and rejuvenating the careers of Nathan Lane, who played Bialystock, and Matthew Broderick, who played Bloom.

Brooks wrote all the songs for the new version of his old work, and one of them, "I Wanna Be a Producer," is directly related to the topic of unhappiness. The nebbish-like Bloom refuses at first to take part in Bialystock's scheme, declaring himself to be an honest man as well as afraid of getting caught. He goes back to his accounting office. However, it is clear that he hates his job. Behind him a chorus of fellow accountants mournfully chants "Unhappy ... unhappy ... very very very very very very very unhappy..." to which Bloom adds: "I spend my life accounting/With figures and such/To what is my life amounting?/It figures, not much" (Brooks

2001). As discussed earlier in the chapter, dissatisfaction with one's job is a leading cause of unhappiness, and Leo is beyond unhappy—he's downright miserable.

But at that point Bloom realizes there's a way out of his doldrums. Secretly, he's always wanted to be a Broadway producer, and he fantasizes about what might happen should he join up with Bialystock. A big production number ensues, in which he imagines himself surrounded by beautiful chorus girls. When his overbearing boss sees him not working, he demands to know what's going on, to which Bloom replies: "Mr. Marks, I've got news for you. I quit! Here's my visor ... my Dixon Ticonderoga number two pencil ... and my big finish!" (Brooks 2001). After the song ends he rushes back to Bialystock's office, and the two begin their search for the world's worst play.

As in the original film version, Bialystock and Bloom's scheme comes crashing down on them when *Springtime for Hitler* becomes a surprise smash. But there's a variation in the Broadway version. Only Bialystock gets caught. Bloom takes the money and runs off with their secretary to Rio. Bialystock is outraged by this betrayal of his trust. But much to his surprise, Bloom returns during Bialystock's trial and sings a humorous but touching song called "'Til Him," which is all about the friendship that has arisen between the two. When Bialystock asks him why he came back and is serenading him, Leo responds "I sang it for you. I sang it because I'm your friend." Max is stunned. "You are? Gee, I've had a lot of relationships, but you couldn't call any of them 'friend.'" And Max then bursts into song as well: "Never met a man I trusted/Always dealt with shysters in the past/Now I'm well adjusted/'Cause I've got a friend at last" (Brooks 2001).

Bialystock and Bloom thus get out of their unhappiness by working together on a project that gives great meaning to their lives—although given its criminal nature the authors of this book don't encourage such behavior. *The Producers* in all its versions (including the 2003 film adaptation of the musical, also starring Lane and Broderick) is a wonderful exploration of the ways in which friendships are formed, and how these can help people break free from unhappiness and bring zest into their lives.

Summary

We chose to write a chapter on unhappiness (rather than simply writing about happiness) because of the simple, and yet often overlooked, reality that in order to be happy one must first conquer unhappiness. In this chapter, we described a number of scenarios that can lead to unhappiness for people. And while it may be difficult, if not impossible, to eliminate *every* source of unhappiness, it is possible to eliminate *enough* causes of unhappiness so that we can pursue happiness.

The next two chapters are designed to inform us how it is possible to find happiness. As a bit of foreshadowing, the authors promote the idea of engaging in as many activities that have the potential to bring you happiness as possible. That way, if one activity you engage in brings you unhappiness (such as a favorite sports team losing a championship game), make sure you counter it with many other activities that can bring you happiness. If you can do that repeatedly, you will have successfully conquered unhappiness.

6

Eudaimonia
A Philosophical Look at Happiness

In our book so far, we have examined various accounts on the nature of friendship, from ancient times to the present-day, as well as looked at why it is important to overcome unhappiness before attending to be happy. In this chapter will look at Aristotle's exploration of the nature of happiness and how this relates to the topic of friendship.

Aristotle Returns

As we saw in our first chapter, one of the most extensive and influential arguments ever made on the importance of friendship can be found in Aristotle's classic work, the *Nichomachean Ethics*. We explored in detail the three-fold nature of friendship—friendship of utility, friendship of pleasure and friendship of the good—that he proposed in this work, as well as how these categories relate to modern views. But it is important to take a step back and ask just *why* Aristotle devoted such more space to this particular issue. It is in fact a component of the much larger project he set out to detail, the importance of happiness to human lives.

Aristotle's overall approach is usually called *teleological,* which means "goal-oriented." In order to understand anything, you have to first ask the question—what is its aim or purpose? What is its essential nature? The essence of a chair, for instance, is to be sat upon. The essence of a hammer is to be used to nail things. But these are nonliving things, so it would be wrong to claim that they have any internal aims. Rather, they are made use of by living things. A living thing possesses something which a nonliving thing does not, namely a *psyche*, or soul.

Thus, one can ask what do non-living seek for their own good? As we read in Chapter 1, Aristotle felt that there are three categories of living things.

The first merely possess what he calls a vegetative soul in that their aim is solely to survive. In order to do so they must take in nutrients, find proper shelter, and engage in some sort of reproductive activity so that their death will not lead to the end of their species. This is the most basic form of life, with the simplest types of activities (mainly just "staying alive").

The second category of living things possess what he calls a sensitive soul. These are creatures which, while engaging in activities to stay alive, also engage in more sensual activities, such as running, playing, raising families, and experiencing pleasure and pain. Their movements are much more complex, and their goals are more complex as well. These creatures constitute the animal kingdom.

And at the very top of the hierarchy of living things are creatures that, while engaging in activities to stay alive and also undergoing sensual activities, have the highest of all natures, in that they have mental activities as well. These are human beings or as he defines them *rational* animals, the possessors of a rational soul.

Thus, for Aristotle the telos or goal of human beings, while sharing some similarities with the vegetative and sensual beings, also in one important way is fundamentally different. The human telos is concerned with the *rational*, that is, with understanding what it is doing.

Telos

Aristotle opens his *Nichomachean Ethics* by asking what is it that human beings seem to seek. This, by the way, is a practical question. He does not imagine scenarios that are fantastic (as is the case in Plato's *Republic*, where the rulers seem to act in ways very unlike any existing set of leaders). Rather, he stays on the foundation of common sense and says that observation holds that there seems to be a limited number of goods that people aim at and hope to achieve for themselves. These include such things as good health; good wealth; and a good reputation. There are not many people who, if asked what they want in life, would answer "to be in ill health and feeling poorly." Likewise, there are not many who would say that their highest goal is to live in dire poverty. And very few would say that they are completely uninterested in what others think about them. In relationship to these higher goals are the more specific professions that one would need to enter into in order to take care of one's health, achieve a proper income, and receive recognition for one's efforts. If, for instance, as was the case with Aristotle's own father, one becomes a medical doctor, then knowledge of proper healthcare will make it more likely that one achieves a good healthy life; the financial compensation connected with the profession will make it more likely that one has a significantly wealthy life; and the community's respect for such members of such a profession will make it likely that one receives good public recognition.

Returning to the discussion of the nature of living things, if one should achieve these goals then the telos of staying alive will certainly be met, since one will have enough food and other requirements to survive without any fear. And the sensual nature of one's soul will be compensated as well, given that receiving recognition is pleasing, and having a good amount of income makes it possible to purchase things that make life more bearable and enjoyable. Surely, then, this seems to be what happiness is all about. As Aristotle phrases it, "It is not unreasonable that men should derive their concept of the good and of happiness from the lives which they lead. The common run of people and the most vulgar identify it with pleasure, and for that reason are satisfied with a life of enjoyment" (Aristotle 1962: 8).

But is this really *reasonable*? Not quite, for as Aristotle goes on to say, our rational self can't help but ask further questions. *Why* do we want to be healthy? *Why* do we desire wealth? And *why* should we care what others think of us? In other words, achieving these things, while perhaps necessary for a good life, is not sufficient to answer the question—what is the ultimate or final goal of human life? They are means to a goal, not the goal itself.

For instance, even if one is completely healthy (whatever that might mean) there is no guarantee that one will be happy. One might become bored with one's life situation, or feel other sorts of dissatisfaction, which would be unpleasant (as we saw in our previous chapter, there are many people who are perfectly healthy but nonetheless quite unhappy in their lives). And there will always be the fear that one's health will decline, due to illness, accident or the ravages of age.

Likewise, one may have a large amount of money, but still not be satisfied. There will always be the fear that the money might be lessened, as can happen in times of great inflation, or may disappear altogether, as can happen during times of economic depression. Or the source of that money—such as one's employment, or an inheritance—may come to an end. But even when this is not the case, if wealth itself is one's goal, then one will never be satisfied with the amount that one has in the bank. There will always be an overwhelming desire for more.

And in regards to recognition, this too, if treated as an end in itself, will prove unsatisfactory. Just how *much* recognition is one looking for? Do you want to be a celebrity, known by everyone in your community? If so, will you be able to lead any sort of private life, outside of the prying eyes of others? And will you be able to maintain this celebrity status? What will happen to your sense of self if that recognition starts to lessen, and people no longer know who you are? Can one ever truly be happy simply by being recognized?

All of these logical questions lead Aristotle to conclude that health, wealth and recognition are not, therefore, ends in themselves but rather aspects of the true final end or goal that all humans seek—namely *eudaimonia*.

Eudaimonia

As previously mentioned, eudaimonia is usually translated into English as "happiness," which is why Aristotle is said to have held the view that happiness is the highest goal for humans. But the problem with this is that the word "happiness" in English is usually identified with feelings and/or emotions, and for Aristotle these relate to what he calls the sensitive soul. If that is the case, then it is not unique to human beings. A dog lying down in the sun or a cat lapping up a bowl of cream can both be said to be enjoying themselves. They are taking great pleasure in such activities, and such pleasures are akin to, if not indeed identical to, what a human being experiences when catching a few rays or downing a tasty drink. While pleasurable, they don't seem to constitute true happiness for humans, since they are fleeting and not based on any particular effort on our parts.

Aristotle's *Nichomachean Ethics* gives a thorough examination of the meaning of the concept of *eudaimonia*. While usually translated from the ancient Greek as "happiness," a better translation would be "self-fulfillment through personal excellence." For Aristotle, the good life consisted of developing one's natural abilities through the use of reason. A virtuous life is one where proper habits are formed that allow one to reach one's full potential.

According to the philosopher Will Buckingham, "The idea of eudaimonia, in focusing not just on what we experience but also on the question of how we lead our lives, draws an explicit connection between happiness and ethics. This connection between happiness and ethics would have been widely accepted in the ancient world. If happiness is, in the eudaimonistic sense, about what might make my life go better for me, then this will require that I come to some kind of decision about what it means for a life as a whole to go well" (Buckingham 2012: 50–51).

Thus, for Aristotle happiness or eudaimonia is something which is desired for its own sake. Clearly, every human being acts with certain aims in view, but what is the reason behind this aims? What is the ultimate motivating factor? It is not merely survival, since if that were the case we'd be no different from plants. Nor it is merely pleasure, since if that were the case we'd be no different from other animals. While these aims have good connected with them, they are not for us good in themselves. What we desire most of all is to cultivate our talents and thus lead fulfilling lives. This is the first principle of ethics: the desire for ultimate good.

The metaphor which Aristotle uses here is that of an archer trying to hit a mark. When we come to understand the true reasons for what we do, then and only then have we "hit our mark," which is to say then and only then do we have true understanding of ourselves (or as Socrates would put it, to "know thyself" is the highest of all goods).

To achieve such knowledge we need maturity. Children and those with mental impairments cannot truly understand themselves. They do not know their own responsibilities, nor can they be held responsible for their actions. They are not autonomous, which is to say they lack the reasoning powers that will guide them to live the best sorts of life. Children, unless they have some sort of mental defect, will naturally develop their reasoning powers, but only if guided properly.

This leads to the important point that, since we are all naturally social beings, in order for us to develop our reasoning powers in the proper way we have to have the right sort of upbringing. We need to be nurtured within a family structure. But we also need education, which goes beyond our own family, so that we can become full members of our society and live a truly political life. But this still requires a level of intellectual maturity. "For that reason," Aristotle writes, "a young man is not equipped to be a student of politics; for he has no experience in the actions which life demands of him, and these actions from the basis and subject matter of discussion. Moreover, since he follows his emotions, his study will be pointless and unprofitable, for the end of this kind of study is not knowledge but action" (Aristotle 1962: 5–6).

The point here is that it takes time and maturity to truly understand what are the best goals one should be seeking that will lead one to real happiness. We must be careful not to let our passions guide us, as is often the case with the young, for this will lead us astray and get us to form bad habits early which, while perhaps making life physically enjoyable in the short run, will ultimately lead us to an unfulfilled and unhappy later life. What we need is a vision of what a good life can be, and thus we need good role models.

Ideally the first sort of good role models should be found within our own family. The love and support that our family members provide for us will ground us properly, and will be the basis for the natural respect that we should show our elders (remember our earlier discussion in Chapter 1 as to why Aristotle felt that one's parents cannot be one's friends).

But there are other role models as well that should guide us to become the best that we can be. And these are found within the society in which we grow up. Who are the leaders—in business, in politics, in entertainment— that inspire us and who we wish to emulate? And more importantly, what sort of people are they? Did they achieve their positions because of their good characters, their virtues, or did they do so by using vicious means? One can judge a society, Aristotle felt, by looking at the nature of those who are held to be its heroes or role models. If they are virtuous people then one is living in a virtuous society; if they are scoundrels, then one is living in a vicious society.

Human Development

For Aristotle, then, in order for anyone to understand what happiness is, it is important to understand how humans should properly develop. Beginning as helpless infants who demand that all their needs be attended to, in a strictly utilitarian way, humans slowly start to develop their emotional connections and become aware and sensitive to the needs of others. They begin to recognize that others have needs similar to their own, and when these are met, there is a more pleasurable existence. In addition, they begin to learn that the more they are able to take care of their own needs rather than rely upon others, the more independent and autonomous they become, which gives them a sense of inner pride. They start to take pleasure in their own abilities, both for what it allows them to achieve and for how these are useful and pleasurable for others as well. Happiness begins to be identified with personal achievement, as this is seen as the highest good attainable through one's own actions. "As far as its name is concerned," Aristotle writes, "most people would probably agree: for both the common run of people and cultivated men call it happiness, and understand by 'being happy' the same as 'living well' and 'doing well'" (Aristotle 1962: 6). Thus, there is, in Aristotle's view, a unifying concept here that identifies happiness with "doing well." But at this point there is still no general agreement as to what "doing well" really means, since people identify this with their given professions. This is why it is important to use one's reason to try to examine different types of human activities and see just how exactly they bring about happiness.

Three Types of Human Activities

Aristotle has a predilection for putting things into three categories (such as the three parts of the human soul and the three types of friendship). So, it's not surprising that in his view there are three different types of human activities: the pursuit of pleasure; the pursuit of virtuous activity; and the pursuit of contemplation. And these can be ranked from the lowest type—that of pleasure—to the highest, namely contemplation. Let's briefly look at these three types of activities, and see how they relate to the concept of eudemonia.

Hedonism: The Pursuit of Pleasure

The Greek word for the pursuit of pleasure is *hedonism*. And it is not surprising that one often identifies happiness with achieving a life of pleasure. It would be odd to think otherwise—not too many people would say that they seek as painful and pleasure-free an existence as possible. And for many this would be a life of amusement, with no responsibilities or concerns. Aristotle perceptively points out that one of the chief ways in which tyrants are able to stay in power is by manipulating those they rule by giving them amusements to keep them passive, not unlike how a bad parent today may keep a child amused by playing video games in order not to have to take proper care of the child. Thus, "most of those who are considered happy find an escape in pastimes of this sort, and this is why people who are well versed in such pastimes find favor at the courts of tyrants; they make themselves pleasant by providing what the tyrants are after, and what they want is amusement. Accordingly, such amusements are regarded as being conducive to happiness, because men who are in positions of power devote their leisure to them" (Aristotle 1962: 286–287). But these amusements are not truly valuable. Aristotle interestingly enough here compares bad men to children—both confuse happiness with a mere life of pleasure. "It is not surprising that as children apparently do not attach value to the same things as do adults, so bad men do not attach value to the same things as do good men" (Aristotle 1962: 287). What is lacking here is genuine virtue, or proper good habits which allow humans to develop or flourish. "Consequently, happiness does not consist in amusement. In fact, it would be strange if our end were amusement, and if we were to labor and suffer hardships all our life merely to amuse ourselves" (Aristotle 1962: 287).

What Aristotle is pointing out here was later called the "Hedonic Paradox." In the words of Will Buckingham: "This paradox is associated with the 19th-century British philosopher Henry Sidgwick (1838–1900), who made the observation that we can't attain happiness by aiming at happiness" (Buckingham 2012: 53). For Sidgwick, as for other English Utilitarian thinkers like Jeremey Bentham and John Stuart Mill (both of whom will be discussed in the next chapter), "happiness" equals "maximizing pleasure." But Sidgwick understood that simply focusing on pleasure itself was inadequate. One needs to examine both the causes of and the effects of pleasure. In Aristotle's view, the truly happy life involves exertion, and a serious commitment to effort. But in developing ourselves in this way we do experience pleasure. The key point here is that it is *earned* pleasure, and is connected with pride that comes from self-achievement. One remembers the analogy of Aristotle's teacher Plato, found in his book the *Republic,* of people in a dark underground cave being amused by shadows cast upon a wall in front of them. They may be experiencing pleasure, but, in reality, they are prisoners who, if they were only made aware of their real situation, would feel ashamed at being so captive, and allowing themselves to mistake happiness with mere amusement. The point is to break your chains—namely the chains of ignorance—and rise out of the darkness into the light of reason.

Honor: The Pursuit of Public Recognition

For Aristotle, then, there is a higher sort of activity than mere pursuit of pleasure. This is a life devoted to honor, based upon virtuous activity. This, he felt, is the sort of activity connected to living in a cultured society, where one's true worth is genuinely appreciated. For instance, if one has musical abilities and cultivates one's talents properly, then one can have the opportunity to achieve recognition from others for one's achievements. "Cultivated and active men, on the other hand, believe the good to be honor, for honor, one might say, is the end of the political life" (Aristotle 1962: 29). This is a more refined existence than that of shallow hedonism. A political life is one where different social activities that contribute to the general welfare should be honored. For instance, there will be a need for medical doctors, who can contribute to the good health of the society. There will be a need for craftsmen who can create items that will make life easier for those around them. There will be a need for artists who can entertain the populace with songs, plays, and creative works. And there will be a need for political leaders, who can make sure that people are governed properly. It is fitting that those who fulfill these roles in the best ways should be rewarded and properly honored, with financial remuneration, the gratitude of the people, and even in some cases with statues erected in their honor or songs written about them so that they will continue to act as role models long after they are gone. The good that they do will thus "live on" after them and continue to inspire others to act in the most virtuous of ways.

However, while the life of virtuous activity is a higher sort of life than that devoted solely to pleasure, it too has its limitations. First of all, it requires a political system or social reality in which the various positions are available for people to aim for. One may have musical talents, for instance, but live in a society where music is not appreciated. Secondly, honor depends upon others, since it is they who bestow praise. But suppose one's talents are not recognized? Or suppose one lives in a society where non-virtuous behaviors—such as lying or using violence to achieve success—are rewarded? One cannot be truly happy in such a world, Aristotle felt, since the removal of or the nonexistence of honor would deprive you of the possibility of proper development.

Contemplation: The Pursuit of Reason

It is the third type of human activity, namely contemplation, which best accords with eudaimonia. This is deeper than either pleasure or honor; rather it is the desire to achieve the good for its own sake. He writes: "We call that which is pursued as an end in itself more final than an end which is pursued for the sake of something else; and what is never chosen as a means to something else we call more final than that which is chosen both as an end in itself and as a means to something else. What is always chosen as an end in itself and never as a means to something else is called final in an unqualified sense. This description seems to apply to happiness above all else" (Aristotle 1962: 14–15). Therefore, he goes on to say, pleasure, honor, and even intellectual development are chosen partly for themselves, since all seem to be good, and we would not pursue them unless they were so. But we also choose them because they lead us to the ultimate good itself—genuine happiness. This is a unique goal, peculiar to humans alone. We wish to have pleasure, honor and rationality because together these three will lead us to eudaimonia, or "self-fulfillment."

For Aristotle, then, it is the proper development of our reason—our rational soul—which is the key to achieving real happiness. Happiness is not a "solid state," something unchanging, but rather an *activity*. Thus, it is not merely accumulating wealth, or having a large amount of possessions, or achieving success and honors. It is the constant use of one's reasoning abilities to understand who you are—what talents you truly possess, what contributions you can make to your society, and what connections you can make to other people close to you to help them develop properly.

Achieving happiness therefore involves both extrinsic and intrinsic factors. The extrinsic are those factors outside of your own control. As mentioned above, if you happen to live in a society that does not appreciate or encourage music, then your possessing musical abilities—which would be an intrinsic factor—would be of no help to you. But should you live in a society that does in fact appreciate and encourage musical development, then you will have the chance to develop your talents in ways that will give you joy. The intrinsic factor also involves how much commitment you put into developing these talents. It is necessary to devote proper time and energy to this. If you do so, then you are acting virtuously. If you do not—if for instance you allow yourself to become lazy and don't practice playing on your chosen instrument—then even if the extrinsic factors exist, you will not achieve success.

This is why for Aristotle the good life involves two main aspects: fortune and skill. There are never any guarantees that one's particular talents will be appreciated or that one will have the chance to fulfill them. For instance, you may be a wonderful architect, but if you can't find a job because in your society there is an overabundance of architects and no job openings, then you will not be able to develop properly. If, on the other hand, such a job opening does occur but you have not kept up with the latest developments or have not gotten the proper credentials, then the good fortune offered to you will be for nothing, since you haven't developed the skills required.

Aristotle gives the vivid example of King Priam of Troy, who witnessed the slaughter of his children at the end of the Trojan War. He was a virtuous man undone by bad fortune. The happiness he had experienced previously was negated by the loss of his kingdom and of his children. Fate has surely dealt him a bad hand. Oedipus, who was cursed by the gods to murder his own father and marry and have children with his own mother, is another example of someone who cannot be happy.

But Aristotle's overall natural law approach is not as grim as these examples might lead one to assume. While realistically pointing out that some situations are so grim that no one could be happy living within them, he feels that these are the extremes, what we might call a "hell on earth." The other extreme would be a utopian system where everyone is always happy all the time because their every need is catered to. The actual world most of us inhabit is neither a hell nor a heaven but rather a place that offers us the possibilities of different experiences.

The Joy of Living

It is important to note at this point that Aristotle feels that true happiness or eudaimonia is a genuine possibility. Virtuous people should feel good about themselves, *because* they are virtuous. "Therefore, a good man should be a self-lover, for he will himself profit by performing noble actions and will benefit his fellow men" (Aristotle 1962: 262). This is the origin of the famous expression "Virtue is its own reward." It is in fact the highest sort of pleasure, because it is directly connected with the good itself, namely being a good soul. "But a wicked man," he adds, "should not love himself, since he will harm both himself and his neighbors in following his base emotions. What a wicked man does is not in harmony with what he ought to do, whereas a good man does what he ought to do. For intelligence always chooses what is best for itself, and a good man will obey his intelligence" (Aristotle 1962: 262).

Happy Medium

Happiness, therefore, is a perfect activity in which a person obeys his intelligence, and unhappiness is an imperfect activity in which a person ignores or goes against his intelligence. This leads to perhaps the most famous notion of Aristotle's ethics, the concept of "the happy medium." Achieving happiness means cultivating a virtue that arrives at a delicate balance between two vices. For Aristotle, the key point is not to go off balance, not to be deficient or excessive in one's activities. A true virtue is a good habit that allows one to "hit one's mark." Some examples of virtues falling within two extremes or vices include the following:

Virtue: Generosity (Two Vices: Miserliness/Being a Spendthrift)
Virtue: Righteous Anger (Two Vices: Spiritedless/Harshness)
Virtue: Wit (Two Vices: Boorishness/Buffoonery)
Virtue: Courage (Two Vices: Cowardliness/Rashness)

When one achieves such a happy medium, then one experiences true happiness, because one is achieving one's personal best, or excellence. To excel is to be one's best. But not only must one have good fortune (remember poor King Priam); one also needs proper guidance and support. And, in addition to one's family members, who else can be of assistance in urging one to develop one's talents in the best ways possible? Well, as we have stressed throughout the book—and as the Beatles would put it—you get by with a little help from your friends.

Friendship and Happiness

Now that we have explored in greater detail Aristotle's overall conception of what happiness or eudaimonia is all about, we can return to the topic of friendship. For he argues strongly that it is not possible to be truly happy without the constant support of friends around you, even if you should have wealth, health and honor. He writes, "It seems strange that we should assign all good things to a happy man without attributing friends to him, who are thought to be the greatest of external goods. Also, if the function of a friend is to do good rather than to be treated well, if the performance of good deeds is the mark of a good man and of excellence, and if it is nobler to do good to a friend than to a stranger, then a man of high moral standards will need people to whom he can do good" (Aristotle 1962: 263).

It is friends—especially friends of the good—who will encourage us to be our best, who will understand our true nature and guide us in the best possible ways. It is friends who share our lives with us. Friends have genuine concern for our well-being, and we share goodwill with them. We relate to them better than to anyone else—even in some ways our own family members—because they are our equals. There is true reciprocity involved in this relationship because we know each other so well.

As we discussed earlier, friends of utility can help us fulfill activities that make life more bearable; and friends of pleasure can make life more pleasant and enjoyable for us. But it is only friends of the good who can help us to truly develop our rational souls, that part of us which Aristotle deemed to be most special (and indeed most godlike). In the words of Jean Vanier: "Through friendship I communicate in the consciousness that my friend has of his own existence. For in the same way that we feel that we are alive and exist through activity and derive pleasure from it, so through friendship, we feel our friend live and exist. And the union is so profound that the goodness of the life of our friend extends to us and gives us pleasure. In friendship there is almost a communion, a merging of two beings and their rightful good" (Vanier 2012: 71–72). Friendship of the good is thus essential to living a fully human life, and to achieving genuine happiness. Eudaimonia in this sense is best described as a human flourishing, or as the authors of this book have described it in their work *Beyond Sustainability: A Thriving Environment*, it is *thrivability*. As we define it, "Thrivability emerges from the persistent intention to create more value than one consumes" (Delaney and Madigan 2014: 6). The good life in this sense means maximizing one's potential to bring out one's best, through cooperating with like-minded friends.

Criticisms of Aristotle's Views on Happiness

Much like the earlier criticisms leveled against Aristotle's views on friendship, there are genuine criticisms that can be made regarding his concept of eudaimonia. First of all, it is elitist. While humans may be the highest living beings on earth, because they possess reason, Aristotle did not feel that all humans are created equally. For him, the Greeks were the most superior of all humans, and non–Greeks were literally barbarians, or uncivilized. Those humans who lack proper reasoning abilities are closer to non-human animals than they are to properly rational humans. He takes this so far as to justify slavery, saying that it is the natural lot of some human beings to serve others in this way.

And his view is most definitely sexist as well. Since he felt that women were naturally inferior to men, Aristotle doubted that they can ever truly achieve eudaimonia in the full sense. Women are less rational then men, and therefore more prone to be guided by their emotions. That is why he argued it would be unnatural to grant them political power or any autonomy at all.

Thus, Aristotle felt that only a small number of people—excluding poor men, those without families, those who were unattractive, and *all* women— had the intellectual capacities and the strength of will to achieve eudaimonia. This narrowly-focused and downright offensive concept of happiness is not one that most people today would feel rightly comfortable espousing. But, taking all of these criticisms into consideration, can Aristotle's overall views on eudaimonia still be defended?

Martha Nussbaum on Eudaimonia

As mentioned at the end of Chapter 1, one of the most important defenders of Aristotle's views in the modern age is, remarkably enough, someone who goes against Aristotle's own claim that women cannot be philosophers, namely Martha Nussbaum.

One of today's most prominent philosophers, Nussbaum is author of such books as *The Fragility of Goodness* (1986), *Love's Knowledge* (1990), *The Quality of Life* (co-written with Amartya Sen in 1993), *Sex and Social Justice* (1998), *Upheavals of Thought: The Intelligence of Emotions* (2001), and *Frontiers of Justice; Disability, Nationality, Species Membership* (2006). Her writings demonstrate a thorough understanding of the classical Greek world, as well as expertise in contemporary literature and legal studies. Ironically enough, she has been influenced most by the writings of Aristotle—the scholar who argued that women are by nature intellectually inferior to men, and thus unfit to master the rigors of philosophical analysis. She has given demonstrative proof of the unsoundness of that empirical claim.

Nussbaum was for many years a professor of philosophy, classics, and comparative literature at Brown University. Since 1995 she has been a professor of law and ethics at the University of Chicago, teaching in the law faculty there. She is a well-known public intellectual. A frequent contributor to *The New Republic* and other journals of influence, she has championed such social causes as equal rights for homosexuals and the elimination of world poverty. She is especially active in movements to increase the participation of women in philosophical endeavors.

Nussbaum has been strongly involved with the United Nations, acting as a research advisor for economic development. She has also chaired the Committee on International Cooperation and the Committee on the Status of Women for the American Philosophical Association, and was one of its three co-presidents in 1999–2000. Nussbaum lectures throughout the world, and remains a strong advocate for the development of women in all cultures. To bring all citizens of a nation to the same level, she argues, more resources must be devoted to those who encounter obstacles from traditional hierarchies and prejudices. She calls this "the Capabilities Approach"—is a person capable of performing certain actions or not? There are functions which are central to human life, and by fulfilling these functions we become more human. Thus, the need to cultivate certain skills, as well as provide for basic needs, is a political reality, which exerts a moral claim on all members of society. Clearly, Nussbaum remains a modern-day Aristotelian, who takes seriously Aristotle's concept of eudaimonia as "human flourishing." For her, the Capabilities framework is an attempt to argue for a universal set of guidelines that are not incompatible with cross-cultural norms. She is herself an example of a person who is a virtuous role model for others, especially for women who wish to cultivate the pursuit of reason.

Why Aristotle Still Matters

Thus, while bearing in mind the limitations inherent in Aristotle's defense of eudaimonia, there are still important ways in which it can be defended. It is a down-to-earth, common sense approach to the topic. He bases his views not on pure speculation but rather on observation, and argues that his findings can be tested.

Aristotle's emphasis on human excellence or flourishing is also an important contribution to our understanding of happiness, and differentiates it from more hedonic-based ideas. He rightly points out that pleasure as an end in itself is self-defeating.

And as we have stressed throughout this book, one of Aristotle's main contributions to the study of happiness is his emphasis on the need for good companions in one's personal development, most especially the need for friends.

No thinker is perfect. All of them present theories based in part on their own prejudices or biases. With Aristotle, though, you have the important point that he wished his theories to be both practical and testable. His writings on happiness have stood the test of time because many who have achieved happiness find them to be on the mark.

Popular Culture Scenario 6: Aristotle Is Watching You

As we discussed in chapters 3 and 4, we are living in a cyber age. Most of our information comes to us from the internet and through the use of smartphones and computer technology. And for those born in the new millennium this interaction with computers begins at birth.

To capitalize upon this, Mattel has developed a voice-controlled device to help parents monitor their baby's movements and assist in the child's intellectual development. And they have named it "Aristotle."

According to *USA Today* columnist Ed Baig, "The voice-controlled Aristotle hub bundle consists of a Bluetooth and Wi-Fi Direct speaker with multicolored LED lights, and Wi-Fi camera with object recognition.

The company is employing 256-bit encryption through the cloud and complying with COPPA, the Children's Online Privacy Protection Act, which aims to protect the privacy of children younger than 13" (Baig 2017).

But this technology is not limited to infants. "Aristotle is meant to work with both parents and kids. So, the system might detect when a child is low on diapers and let mom or dad order a fresh supply by voice, fulfilled by such retailers as Babies R Us, Target and Amazon" (Baig 2017).

"Aristotle" will thus be a digital assistant and a sort of postmodern "nanny." One assumes that children will form an attachment to this companion, which will not only make sure their diapers are changed and their stomachs are filled, but also see that they receive intellectual stimulation that will help them to develop as rational beings. "So with toddlers, Aristotle might flash different-colored lights with the child trying to name the correct color. It might engage kids with sing-a-longs or reading them bedtime stories. And when your kids get into their tween years, Aristotle promises social networking integration or more sophisticated lessons, perhaps quizzing them on U.S. presidents or helping them learn a foreign language" (Baig 2017).

This leaves us with a rather interesting question. Should "Aristotle" really take off and be such a lifelong companion, encouraging us from infancy throughout the rest of our lives to constantly develop our rational souls, just what would be the nature of our relationship? Can one be a friend of the good with a robot?

Russell Returns: The Causes of Happiness

In Chapter 5 we examined the 20th century philosopher Bertrand Russell's look at causes of unhappiness. So it only seems fitting to end Chapter 6 by returning to Russell's 1930 work *The Conquest of Happiness* and explore his views on what actually makes life enjoyable for those who have overcome the causes of unhappiness. In other words, what are the causes of happiness?

In Part Two of *The Conquest of Happiness*, Russell ponders whether or not happiness is possible and then describes a number of causes of happiness. He expresses concern as to whether happiness in the modern world is a possibility. He concludes that via his own introspection, foreign travel and conversations with his gardener that happiness is indeed possible. It is worth noting that Russell acknowledges, once again, that the ideas presented in *Conquest* (1930) are not scientific. He states "I am at the moment not concerned to prove any thesis, but merely to describe" (pp. 143–144.) Despite its unscientific approach to the study of happiness he seems to employ an elitist attitude nonetheless when he declares that there are two forms of happiness that can be distinguished as: plain and fancy, or animal and spiritual, or of the heart and of the head. Upon further elaboration, Russell (1930) states, "Perhaps the simplest way to describe the difference between the two sorts of happiness is to say that one sort is open to any human being, and the other only to those who can read and write" (p. 144). The second category of happiness is only available to the more highly educated sections of the community and the happiest of these folks are the men of science. One can see the similarity here with Aristotle's argument that it is only a life of contemplation (a life of reason) that can bring about true happiness. But then, Aristotle and Russell were both philosophers, so it stands to reason they'd say that!

It would appear too, that if half of the sources of happiness come from pursuits of high education achievement that the adage of "ignorance is bliss" would be inaccurate.

Perhaps the best bit of advice Russell offers in Chapter 6 of his book is this summation to the secret of happiness: "Let your interests be as wide as possible, and let your reactions to the things and persons that interest you be as far as possible friendly rather than hostile" (p. 157). Such sentiments would certainly appear to be true today; after all, the more interests one has the more opportunities there are for happiness.

In chapters 11–17 of Russell's *Conquest*, the philosopher describes a number of specific topics that he believes helps to provide happiness. Starting our review with Chapter 11, Russell describes zest as a potential contributor to happiness.

Zest

"Zest" refers to a hearty pleasure or appreciation for life. In Chapter 11 of *Conquest*, Russell equates zest to a thirst for happiness. Among the examples provided by Russell is the idea that while many people eat their daily meals as a matter of utility that must be completed, others approach the preparation and/or consumption of a meal with a great deal of gusto.

Russell indicates that the more things a person is interested in, the more opportunities for happiness will present themselves. If one potential source of happiness fails to bear fruit there are other things one can fall back on. Russell describes how a person who likes chess sufficiently enough to look forward to a game at the end of the day is fortunate. The authors, like billions of other people around the world, look forward to sporting events, especially football. One of them, Tim Delaney, is a season ticket holder of a major college and NFL franchise, and looks forward all week to the weekend's game. The tailgating experience is also something to look forward to as he happily serves as the grill master as he grills up favorite foods (which the other author, Tim Madigan, enjoys consuming!). Other participants in our tailgate will bring food dishes as well. The festive atmosphere and the zest that his fellow tailgaters bring to the day's events further maximizes the potential for happiness.

Russell notes that zest for life varies by gender. "In women, less nowadays than formerly, but still to a very large extent, zest has been greatly diminished by a mistaken conception of respectability" (Russell 1930:173). Russell's description of women and zestly pursuits is less of a sexist attitude on his part than an observation of the differences in expected behavior between men and women during his time. Today, women are less likely to be condemned from pursuing their interests with a zest for life but still, a double-standard exists. Consider that women who wish to have sex with as many men as possible are likely to be frowned upon more severely than it is for men who seek to have sex with as many women as possible. Having sex, of course, is another fine example of having a zest for life!

Affection

As Russell (1930) explains, "One of the chief causes of lack of zest is the feeling that one is unloved, whereas conversely the feeling of being loved promotes zest more than anything else does" (p. 176). Russell adds, those who face life with a feeling of security are much happier than those who face it with a feeling of insecurity. "It is affection received, not affection given, that causes this sense of security, though it arises most of all from affection which is reciprocal" (Russell 1930:178). Thus, in Chapter 12 of *Conquest*, he turns to the role which affection plays in human happiness.

Obstacles, psychological and social, to the blossoming of reciprocal affection are a grave evil, he felt, from which the world has always suffered and still suffers. Affection comes in many forms. Remember Aristotle's discussion of the desire for public recognition. Russell likewise uses the example of persons whose trade is to secure public admiration, such as actors, preachers, speakers, and politicians, who come to depend more and more upon applause from an audience. When they received their due amount of public approbation their life is full of zest; when they do not, they become displeased and unhappy. Perhaps the best form of affection is that given and received from parents, or children, and intimate others, especially sexual partners.

The Family

As sociologists oft promote, the family serves as a primary agent of socialization and plays a hugely significant role in personal security, affection and happiness. The family structured has changed a great deal since the time of Russell—a period wherein the traditional definition of the family originated and centered on the idea of a breadwinner father with his stay-at-home wife and their dependent children all living under a single dwelling until the kids are grown, move out of the home, and start their own families. Sociologists have conducted a great deal of research to explain the growing number of alternative family types including, couples who cohabitate without marriage; couples who chose not to have children; same-sex couples; dual-income couples; and so on. The traditional family is often romanticized in American culture and a number of people promote the idea of a return to traditional roles.

However, after learning what Russell had to say about the family of his era in Chapter 13 of *Conquest* we would have to wonder why anyone would want to return to such an institution. Russell (1930) states, "Affection of parents for children and of children for parents is capable of being one of the greatest sources of happiness, but in fact at the present day the relations of parents and children are, in nine cases out of ten, a source of unhappiness to both parties, and in ninety-nine cases out of a hundred a source of unhappiness to at least one of the two parties. This failure of the family to provide the fundamental satisfactions which in principle it is capable of yielding is one of the most deep-seated causes of discontent which is prevalent in our age" (p.187). While Russell does not provide any statistical data or sources for his statistics, it is clear that his opinion of the family is not romanticized!

According to Russell, family unhappiness comes from a variety of causes including psychological, economic, social, educational, and political. The conquest of happiness within the institution of the family comes as a result of respect for one another and for parents to maintain a life with meaning separate from their children. In other words, for parents, their children's lives should not dominate their every activity. Children too, need meaning in their lives away from that provided by the family. Interesting, the single person, Russell suggests, can have a happy life provided they have a good education and have no difficulty in making a comfortable living.

Russell (1930) does state, however, that for him personally, "I have found the happiness of parenthood greater than any other that I have experienced" (p. 198).

Work

Although the act of working may be an example of unhappiness for some people, having employment is not only a sign of being a productive member of society, it can bring a great sense of happiness unto others. Russell (1930), in Chapter 14 of *Conquest,* states, "provided work is not excessive in amount, even the dullest work is to most people less painful than idleness" (p. 209). And certainly, anyone who has been unemployed, or is currently unemployed, despite efforts to find employment can attest to the unhappiness than unemployment brings.

Work, therefore, is desirable and provides us with many opportunities for happiness, including the following:

- It provides us with an escape from boredom
- It makes holidays more enjoyable
- Provided that the work is not so hard as to impair one's vigor, it allows for more zest for life during one's free time.
- Paid work allows people the opportunity to earn money to pay bills and pursue leisure pursuits
- It affords individuals with a chance to demonstrate their skill, and that too brings about happiness.

Impersonal Interests

Russell explains in Chapter 15 of *Conquest* that impersonal interests are those minor interests which help to fill in one's leisure time and afford relaxations from the tenseness of more serious preoccupations—such as family, work and financial stability. Reading a book, watching games, going to the theatre, and playing golf are among the examples impersonal interests that Russell provides. And certainly today, people still find enjoyment from these same activities. Some find it enjoyable to regularly go to the movie theater while others like to keep up with the Kardashians or follow along with pointless reality TV shows as it brings them happiness.

Russell (1930) explains that "All impersonal interests, apart from their importance as relaxation, have various other uses. To begin with, they help a man to retain his sense of proportion. It is very easy to become so absorbed in our own pursuits, our own circle, our own type of work, that we forget how small a part this is of the total of human activity and how many things in the world are entirely unaffected by what we do" (p. 224). Then again, when we heed Russell's advice here, it may make you feel unhappy to realize your life is essentially unimportant in the grand scheme of things!

So, let's revisit the main point of impersonal interests—they help to keep us preoccupied and they are a source of happiness. Russell (1930) summarizes this chapter by stating, "the man who pursues happiness wisely will aim at the possession of a number of subsidiary interests in addition to those central ones upon which his life is built" (p. 230).

Effort and Resignation

The key to Russell's view of happiness resides in the realization that happiness is not, except in very rare cases, something that simply happens; rather, it is something that must be achieved (conquered) through effort.

Resignation, however, has also its part to play in the conquest of happiness, and it is a part no less essential than that played by effort. Russell discusses this in detail in Chapter 16 of *Conquest*. He argues that a wise person will learn to resign from the pursuit of certain desired forms of happiness so as not to interfere with attainable forms of happiness. In other words, sometimes we have to resign ourselves to the reality that not everything we desire in life will happen.

Russell (1930) states, "Nothing is more fatiguing nor, in the long run, more exasperating than the daily effort to believe things … [will magically] become more incredible. To be done with this effort is an indispensable condition of secure and lasting happiness" (p. 241).

So, good things do not come to those who wait; instead, they come to people who actively seek happiness and conquer the obstacles that come between one's pursuit of happiness and happiness itself. One can see the similarity here with Aristotle's idea that eudaimonia involved genuine effort. Happiness will also come when one learns to stop pursuing the unattainable. Again like Aristotle, Russell is stating here that we must use our rational minds to determine what are realistic goals for ourselves.

The Happy Man

In the final chapter of *The Conquest of Happiness* (Chapter 17), like Aristotle and his idea of intrinsic and extrinsic values, Russell explains that happiness depends partly upon external circumstances and partly upon oneself. Some people are born with certain advantages and yet we all, potentially, have the opportunity to pursue happiness.

The happy person is one who has affections, wide interests, pursues happiness with a zest, is free from suffering, is a citizen of the universe, and does not give a damn about what others think of you or what others think is important.

Happiness and Human Effort

After reading Russell's *The Conquest of Happiness* and reflecting upon its meaning and relevance to contemporary society, we can conclude that happiness is not, except in very rare cases, something that drops into the mouth, like a ripe fruit, by the mere operation of fortunate circumstances. For in a world so full of avoidable and unavoidable misfortunes, of illness and psychological tangles, of struggle and poverty and ill will, the man or woman who is to be happy must find ways of coping with the multitude of causes of unhappiness by which each individual is assailed. Individuals must then pursue activities that will bring them happiness while also resigning to the fact that not everything one wants in life is achievable.

And here we see again Aristotle's point that eudaimonia or happiness is based upon our own efforts—it is something to be achieved, rather than something merely innate. And it is the fulfillment of our abilities which brings about the sense of self-satisfaction which Russell calls zest, and the authors of this book call thrivability.

Summary

In this a chapter, we returned to an examination of Aristotle's philosophy. To truly understand what he meant by friendship, as detailed at the beginning section of the book, it is necessary to put this in its proper context. Friendship is a subset of eudaimonia (usually translated as happiness) and connects to the understanding of the nature of the human soul.

Human beings, in Aristotle's view, are the only living things which possess rationality. Happiness is the ultimate goal, or telos, that human beings at aim. Achieving things such as good health, good wealth or public recognition are important to humans but are not the ultimate goal we seek. Rather, they are means to that end.

The ultimate goal of happiness is a fulfillment of our talents. This relates to the three types of human activities: hedonism, honor, and contemplation. The last is the most important since it directly relates to our rational self.

In order to be happy we need two things: good fortune and skill. We need to develop our talents so that when good fortune arrives we will know how to make the most of it. But in order to develop our skills we need the support of others, most particularly good friends. They will encourage us to make good use of our reasoning skills and avoid vices (deficiencies or excesses of behavior) that lead us astray. The key to a good life is therefore to achieve a "happy medium" between extremes.

While there is no guarantee that good fortune will smile upon us, Aristotle felt that nature generally allows the possibility for human beings to develop their talents in ways that will allow them to be happy.

Aristotle's writings on ethics are too narrowly focused and can rightly be accused of being elitist, racist and sexist. But they are still relevant to the present day, especially in their focus on human development (what the authors call thrivability) and on their emphasis on the importance of friends in one's life. Philosopher Martha Nussbaum, in her writings on human capabilities, has shown that Aristotle's concept of eudaimonia is very much alive and well in the present day.

The 20th century philosopher Bertrand Russell has spelled out in detail many causes of happiness, including affection, family, work, impersonal interests, and effort and resignation. Like Aristotle and his idea of intrinsic and extrinsic values, Russell explains that happiness depends partly upon external circumstances and partly upon oneself. When combined, these give one a zest for life and a sense of genuine self-fulfillment.

7

The Pursuit and Attainment of Happiness

A Sociological Look at Happiness

In Chapter 5, we noted that the "Declaration of Independence" guaranteed Americans the right to pursue happiness. Specifically, the original phrase written by Thomas Jefferson that addresses happiness reads, "We hold these truths to be sacred & undeniable; that all men are created equal & independent, that from the equal creation they derive rights inherent & unalienable, among which are the preservation of life, & liberty, & the pursuit of happiness." The Committee of Five (Jefferson, VA; John Adams, MA; Benjamin Franklin, PA; Roger Sherman, CT; and Robert R. Livingston, NY), appointed by Congress on June 11, 1776, to draft the Declaration of Independence edited Jefferson's draft to read: "We hold these Truths to be self-evident, that all Men are created equal, that they are endowed by their Creator with certain unalienable Rights, that among these are Life, Liberty and the Pursuit of Happiness." The profoundness of this statement cannot be underestimated. As Slauter (2011) explains, "In America's revolutionary history, no document is more iconic than the Declaration of Independence." This declaration of independence from the rule of Britain was approved by Congress on July 4, 1776.

The iconic phrase granting Americans the rights of life, liberty and the pursuit of happiness, has been dissected quite a bit over the nearly two and a half centuries since its initial introduction into social and political discourse by sociologists, philosophers, political scientists, historians, and lawyers, among others. For example, much has been made about the fact that the phrase clearly states that all *men* are created equal instead of saying all people are created equally. Beyond the obvious exclusion of many basic rights given to *women* at this time (e.g., women were not allowed to vote until the passage of the 19th Amendment to the Constitution in 1920; and once a woman married, she forfeited her legal existence—she couldn't sign a contract, make a will, or sue in a court of law [Gurko 1974]),—rights were not given to *all* men either as many black males (in addition to black females) were still slaves at this time and free black men were forbidden from voting (until the 15th Amendment to the Constitution was ratified in 1870). The presumption that there exists a "Creator," let alone that all people share the same vision of such an entity, is also a matter of conjecture and opinion and, thus, problematic to say the least.

Addressing the issue of social inequality framed by the early composers of the "Declaration of Independence" and the U.S. Constitution is not within the scope of this chapter; instead, we are interested in their notion of the unalienable right to pursue happiness. It is well recognized that, while the right to pursue happiness has no binding effect in judicial courts, the concept of the "pursuit of happiness" has been embedded in a number of state constitutions and judicial interpretations of the U.S. Constitution. Furthermore, it is now common for all Americans, no matter how diverse they may be, to demand the right to pursue happiness.

It is much more than a matter of semantics that the Declaration of Independence gives us the right to *pursue* happiness and not the right to *be* happy. Reflecting on the elusiveness of attaining happiness, Benjamin Franklin receives credit for having said, "The Constitution only gives people the right to pursue happiness. You have to catch it yourself" (*Think Exist* 2016). While this quote seems reasonable, especially from such a wise man, it is highly unlikely that Franklin made such a statement. Alexander Marriott, for example, points out that this is obviously a spurious statement as the U.S. Constitution never uses the phrase "the pursuit of happiness" and there is no attribution of the quote documented in any of Franklin's papers (Marriott 2011). In this, the era of social media and fake memes that attribute quotes to famous people, it's no wonder that many quotes that may seem plausibly to have been made by famous people such as Franklin are not actually true. Blaine McCormick, an associate professor and chair of the management department at Baylor University, debunks a number of famous and infamous sayings attributed to America's "founding fathers." For example, there is a popular t-shirt that reads, "Beer is proof that God loves us and wants us to be happy" citing Benjamin Franklin as the source of such a saying. McCormick states that Franklin did not make such a proclamation of beer; however, he did say something remarkably close in 1779, when he wrote to his French friend, Abbe Morellet, and remarked, "We hear of the conversion of water into wine at the marriage in Cana as of a miracle. But this conversion is, through the goodness of God, made every day before our eyes. Behold the rain which descends from heaven upon our vineyards; there it enters the roots of the vines, to be changed into wine; constant proof that God loves us, and loves to see us happy." As McCormick summarizes, the attribution of beer as proof of a God who loves us and wants us to be happy is close to his actual comments on wine and the role of nature—which Franklin credits to God—in converting water into wine, but that is much harder to put onto a t-shirt (Eckert 2015).

We might wonder why the founders of the United States felt that it was important enough to mention the "pursuit of happiness" in their Declaration of Independence from England in the second paragraph, which followed a first paragraph that consists of one long sentence stating the intentions of the colonists to dissolve political associations with the existing power structure. It would seem clear that the framers of the Declaration believed that the colonists were not reaching their full human potential under the rule of England because, in short, they were unhappy with the arrangement. Declaring independence from an imperialist regime certainly implies a level of unhappiness with the status quo. By using the phrase "pursuit of happiness" the architects of the Declaration were leaving the door open for people to figure out for themselves what makes them happiest, whether it involves material or nonmaterial, spiritual or otherwise, or whatever it might take someone to be happy so long as this pursuit for happiness was free from tyrannical rule (Delaney and Madigan 2014).

Having established that Americans have the right to pursue happiness we can now focus on the primary areas of concern in this chapter—sources of happiness and categories of happiness. We begin first however by examining the *meaning* and *value* of happiness.

The Meaning and Value of Happiness

On the surface, the concept of "happiness" would seem to be relatively straightforward as nearly all of us possess a general understanding of its meaning. This understanding of happiness is strengthened by our own experiences with happiness, as everyone is likely to have had, at the very least, moments of happiness, while others tend to be quite happy nearly all the time. Nonetheless, there is some ambiguity surrounding the term "happiness" because of its subjective nature. That is to say, happiness has different meanings for different people and diverse forms of stimuli can trigger the emotional state of happiness in some but not in others. For example, passionate sports fans can find great happiness when their favorite player or team is victorious but for people who do not find enjoyment in following the sporting accomplishments of others they will not find such happiness.

As the above paragraph implies, the notion of happiness begins with the realization that it involves a mental or emotional state of well-being and positive and/or pleasant reactions to stimuli ranging from general contentment to intense joy. Other emotions that can be associated with happiness include inner peace, absence of want, blissfulness, being true to oneself, confidence, freedom, and viewing one's life favorably. The idea of an individual evaluating their life favorably is a central aspect of J.C. Ott's definition of happiness. Ott (2010) defines happiness as the degree to which an individual judges the overall quality of his or her life, on the whole, favorably or unfavorably. From this perspective, the more favorably one views their own life, the happier they are. In her popular book *The How of Happiness*, Sonja Lyubomirsky (2008) states that happiness can be measured in terms of experiences of joy, contentment, positive well-being, "combined with a sense that one's life is good, meaningful, and worthwhile" (p. 32). Diener (1984) defines happiness as the "experience of positive affect coupled with high life satisfaction." Brockmann and Delhey (2010), like the authors of this book, use a multi-disciplinary approach to the study of happiness and state, "Happiness has a long philosophical tradition, a biological core, a close match with economics, psychological standing, sociological significance, and political implications" (p. 1).

In Chapter 5, we acknowledged that many people are unhappy and that there are a wide variety of causes of unhappiness; however, nearly everyone who is unhappy—except, perhaps those who enjoy Byronic unhappiness—would rather be truly happy than unhappy. Such a statement seems quite obvious and of the domain of common sense; after all, we like to be happy and we feel better when we are happy. Still, there are many specific and sound reasons why we pursue happiness. Listed below are a sampling of studies that demonstrate that happiness improves aspects of our lives (Note: the term "positive emotions" is often used to describe "happiness"):

- Happiness improves our attitudes toward education, academic aspirations, academic achievement, life satisfaction, altruism, self-esteem, and parental relations—Proctor, Linley and Maltby (2010), who conducted research on 410 adolescents (ages 16–18) who were divided into three life satisfaction groups—very high (top 10 percent), average (middle 25 percent) and very low (lowest 10 percent)—found that "very happy" adolescents had significantly higher mean scores about their attitudes toward education, academic aspirations, academic achievement, life satisfaction, altruism, self-esteem and parental relations. The "very happy" adolescents also felt that it was very important to protect the environment, placed a greater importance on recycling, and reported to recycle more often than those who reported to be "very unhappy" (Proctor et al. 2012).

- Happiness is good for our health—Happy people are less likely to get sick, and they live longer. Happiness protects the heart (e.g., lowers heart rate and blood pressure; reduces heart rate variability); happiness strengthens your immune system (e.g., one study showed that happy adult volunteers who were exposed to the common cold were less likely to get sick than were unhappy adult volunteers); happiness combats stress (happiness seems to temper psychological and biological changes in our hormones and blood pressure caused by stress); happy people have fewer aches and pains (e.g., one study suggests that positive emotion mitigates pain in short-term aches and pains); happiness combats disease and disability (positive emotion is associated with improvements in more severe, long-term conditions as well); and, happiness lengthens our lives (supported by a number of studies) (Greater Good Science Center 2016a). Flynn and MacLeod (2015) reviewed a number of studies on the connection between happiness and health and found that happiness has also been associated with better dietary habits and the maintenance of normal body weight (Chang and Nayga 2010; Piqueras et al. 2011), better oral health practices (Dumitrescu et al. 2010), and being more physically active (Piqueras et al. 2011).
- Happiness is good for our relationships—Happy people are more likely to get married and have fulfilling marriages, and they have more friends (2016). In a study conducted by Lyubomirsky, King, and Diener (2005), who examined cross-sectional, longitudinal, and experimental data, they found that happy individuals are more likely than their less happy peers to have fulfilling marriages and relationships, high incomes, superior work performance, community involvement, robust health, and a long life.
- Happy people make more money and are more productive at work—The Lyubomirsky, King and Diener research cited above showed a correlation between happiness and financial productivity and productivity at work. Additional research, such as that conducted by Zelenski, Murphy, and Jenkins (2008), as well as other publications in the *Journal of Happiness Studies*, have shown the same positive correlation.
- Happy people are more generous—A variety of studies have shown that people report happiness when looking back at times when they were kind to others or spend money on others without expecting anything in return (altruism) (Greater Good Science Center 2016a). In contrast, however, there is research that indicates happy people are more selfish as they find possessing things rewarding (Vedantam 2010).

- Happy people use positive emotions to bounce back from negative emotional experiences—Research conducted by Tugade and Fredrickson (2004) indicates that resilient people use positive emotions to rebound from, and find positive meaning in, stressful encounters and that positive emotions contributed, in part, to participants' abilities to achieve efficient emotion regulation.
- Happy people are more creative and are better able to see the big picture—Barbara Fredrickson (2011) argues that positive emotions (e.g., feelings of gratitude, feelings of serenity and tranquility, and feelings of love and closeness for the people we care for) don't just make us feel good, they transform our minds, our bodies, and our ability to bounce back from hard times. In her own research, Fredrickson concluded that positive emotions literally change the boundaries of our minds and our hearts and change our outlook on our environment. Using an analogy of the warmth of sunlight that opens flowers, Fredrickson puts forth the notion that the warmth of positivity opens our minds and hearts and that it changes our visual perspective at a really basic level, along with our ability to see our common humanity with others.

The above sampling of research that connects happiness and positive emotion to a wide variety of topic areas helps to underscore the importance of the study of happiness as happiness is not simply a giddy feeling we have but rather something that affects us in a number of social realms. As we saw in the previous chapter, this accords with Aristotle's concept of *eudaimonia*, which while usually translated as "happiness" should more appropriately be translated as "self-fulfillment." The study of happiness has led to the development of academic journals that are designed for such purposes as seeking to broaden our understanding of happiness and how it may relate to development from economic, political, psychological, and/or sociological perspectives (the *International Journal of Happiness and Development*) and to create an "interdisciplinary forum on subjective well-being" which addresses such topics as life-satisfaction and enjoyment (including mood levels), job satisfaction, and the perceived meaning of life (*The Journal of Happiness Studies*). A number of academic conferences are held annually with a friendship and happiness theme wherein scholars from multiple disciplines, including sociology and philosophy, share their ideas on the meaning and value of friendship and happiness. Non-academics, of course, have also found the value of pursuing the meaning of happiness (e.g., via self-help books and blogs) because, as we have previously stated, nearly all of us would prefer to be happy rather than unhappy and we are willing to listen to advice on how to achieve this happiness goal.

Explaining How Happiness Is Attained

Perhaps one of the most profound aspects in the study of happiness is explaining how happiness is attained. To that end, many theories have been brought forth. In the following pages we will provide a brief review of a number of theories on how happiness is achieved and conclude with our own thoughts. We begin with "The 40 Percent Solution" notion put forth by Sonja Lyubomirsky.

The 40 Percent Solution

In her book *The How of Happiness* (2008), Lyubomirsky puts forth the opinion that happiness is 50 percent determined by our genes, 10 percent by our life circumstances, and 40 percent by our daily activities. (Note: A number of people who have reviewed this conception refer to this categorization of happiness as the "Happiness Pie.") In the Foreword to her book, Lyubomirsky states that "The 40 Percent Solution" was one of the original book title ideas "because it is effectively the tool that underlies the promise of becoming happier" (p. 6). The "promise of becoming happier" is designed to inspire people who are currently unhappy that they too can find happiness later in life. Lyubomirsky shares with readers that she grew up in both Russia and the United States and that she knew many unhappy people in her life that became genuinely happier as they grew by changing their daily activities.

Lyubomirsky (2008) believes that genetics is responsible for fifty percent of our happiness and that genetics determines a "set point" in an individual's level of happiness. Lyubomirsky compares this "happiness set point" to one's predisposition to being skinny as some people easily maintain their weight without much effort while other people have to work very hard to keep from gaining weight. In turn, those with low happiness set points will have to work harder to achieve and maintain happiness while those with high set points will find it easier to be happy under similar circumstances.

Our life circumstances play just a ten percent role in our happiness according to Lyubomirsky. Life circumstances include such socioeconomic variables as one's wealth, or lack thereof; good health or poor health; being attractive or plain-looking; married or divorced; and so on. Relying on her psychological training that includes over-inflating the value of genetics, Lyubomirsky argues that if we could use a magic wand and reverse the life circumstances of people (e.g., poor individuals become wealthy, unhealthy people become healthy, etc.), differences in happiness levels would be increased by only ten percent. Unfortunately, Lyubomirsky has no way of proving such a notion without actually changing the life circumstances of a large enough sample size to support such a notion.

Intentional activities accounts for 40 percent of our happiness according to Lyubomirsky. Intentional activities are "happiness strategies" that people can utilize in their attempt to alter genetic set points. From the vantage point of the authors of this book, intentional activities represent our pursuits for happiness; these are the activities that make us happy. (Note: We will share a number of such activities later in this chapter.) For Lyubomirsky, there are a dozen activities that she describes as "evidence-based happiness-increasing strategies." They include:

- Expressing gratitude
- Cultivating optimism
- Avoiding overthinking and social comparison
- Practicing acts of kindness
- Nurturing social relationships
- Developing strategies for coping
- Learning to forgive
- Increasing flow experiences
- Savoring life's joys
- Committing to your goals
- Practicing religion and spirituality
- Taking care of your body (via meditation, physical activity and acting like a happy person)

The sociological perspective strongly questions the overwhelming weight that Lyubomirsky bestows upon the role of genetics (nature) in determining happiness and gives far greater credence to an individual's daily activities and life circumstances (nurturing and the social environment).

Hedonism

Supporting the notion of engaging in intentional pleasurable activities as a significant influence on explaining how happiness is achieved is the principle of "hedonism." Hedonism involves the pursuit of activities that bring us joy while avoiding activities that cause us pain. Happiness, then, is a matter of experiencing pleasure and avoiding painful situations. A happy person is someone who smiles a lot, is ebullient, enjoys intensity in pleasurable activities and whose pains are few and far between (Seligman and Royzman 2003). A variation of hedonism is "desire theory." Desire theories hold that happiness is a matter of getting what you want with the content of the "want" left up to the person who does the wanting (Griffin 1986; Seligman and Royzman 2003).

Among the more famous early proponents of hedonistic principles are Jeremy Bentham and John Stuart Mill, who developed the ethical system known as Utilitarianism. In his *An Introduction to the Principles of Morals and Legislation* (1781), Bentham, an English philosopher, states (in Chapter 1: Of Principle of Utility), "Nature has placed mankind under the governance of two sovereign masters, *pain* and *pleasure*. It is for them alone to point out what we ought to do, as well as to determine what we shall do.... The *principle of utility* recognizes this subjection, and assumes it" (pp.1–2) to be the foundation of behavior. As we can see with this quote, Bentham links hedonism with utility. Bentham, along with Mill, promoted the idea of utilitarianism— the greatest good for the greatest number of people—as a moral construct. Bentham and Mill also connected "the good" with pleasure. Seeking pleasure, which is viewed as good and morally ethical, becomes then, a sound manner in which one should lead their life. Additionally, seeking to live a good and moral life, from the hedonistic and utilitarian perspective, stimulates one's desire and motivation to achieve happiness.

The Savanna Theory of Happiness

We referenced the savanna theory of happiness in Chapter 4. If you recall, evolutionary psychologists Norman Li and Satoshi Kanazawa (2016) found that people who live in more densely populated areas tend to report less satisfaction with their lives overall than people who live in less dense areas, like a savanna. The savanna theory of happiness combines the life circumstances aspects of an individual (something that Lyubomirsky believes accounts for just 10 percent of our happiness) with ancestral consequences as an explanation for one's life satisfaction (happiness). In their attempt to explain why some people are happier than others, the researchers examined two variables—population density and frequency of socialization with friends. As they predicted (and as we stated above and in Chapter 4), population density is negatively, and frequency of socialization with friends is positively, associated with life satisfaction.

Li and Kanazawa (2016) propose that hunter-gatherer lifestyles of our ancient ancestors have shaped the foundation for what makes us happy today. In such simpler societies people interacted with a smaller number of people and such interactions generally brought about happiness; except for more intelligent people who found greater happiness with fewer interactions. The researchers believe that in the past, people who lived in less-densely populated areas like savannas were happy; similarly, people who live in rural areas today are happier than those who live in the suburbs, and those who live in the suburbs are happier than those who live in large cities. Why is high population density life a less happy environment than life in less-populated areas you might ask? The researchers point out the large number of social problems often cited by sociologists as an inhibitor of overall life satisfaction. Such social problems would include traffic, pollution, crime, small living spaces, and so on.

The savanna theory of happiness is an intriguing attempt to explain happiness but certainly has its limitations. For example, the link between ancestral happiness and modern happiness that Li and Kanazawa attempt to make is not strong. The researchers seem to ignore that fact that many people who live in highly-populated areas such as New York City love their lives and the diversity of activity options such a living style provides; and they seem to ignore the fact that many people in low-density population areas are bored by such a lifestyle. In addition, while sociologists regularly point out the many social problems that exist in large cities, they also point out the many social problems that exist in less-populated area. Nonetheless, Li and Kanazawa's study included analysis of a large national survey of 15,000 respondents (adults aged 18 to 28) which gives empirical data to support their theory.

Anticipation as a Motivator for Happiness

What type of person are you? Are you the type of person who enjoys the "thrill of the chase" or, the type of person that prefers the "joy of conquest?" Another variation of the "thrill of the chase" cliché is, "life's a journey, not a destination." With each cliché we have polar opposite viewpoints as, on the one hand, the conquest, or reaching the destination, means that you accomplished your goal and that should bring people joy and happiness. On the other hand, many people find the anticipation of a climatic finish as a joyful reward (happiness) in itself. Consider, for example, the man or woman who pursues the affection of another and yet the desired other is all but unattainable. The object of desire may be married or otherwise involved in a serious relationship, or the other person may be "out of the league" of the pursuer. So, why even attempt to gain the affection of another if there is so much work involved or the chase involves a great deal of costs (e.g., the pursuer may already be in a serious relationship; the time spent on the chase comes at the expense of other role expectations)? The thrill of the chase can involve seeking other rewards much like following clues for a treasure map. During the pursuit of the treasure the treasure hunters may envision all sorts of riches and their anticipation grows and grows during the chase period. Whether or not they will be pleased or disappointed at the conclusion of the chase explains why some people prefer the chase (the anticipation of riches was more pleasurable than the found valueless treasure) or why some people prefer the conquest (e.g., the pursuit of the treasure came with many costs but the treasure was priceless). Thus, the chase itself may bring happiness, the conquest of a successful pursuit may bring happiness, or both the chase and the conquest together may bring happiness.

Kumar, Killingsworth, and Gilovich (2014) are among the researchers that have examined the role of anticipation as a motivator for happiness. Specifically, Kumar and associates examined the role of anticipatory consumption of experiential and material purchases. Experiential purchases refer to money spent on *doing* things while material purchases involve spending money on *having* things. They found that experiential purchases tend to provide more enduring happiness than material purchases. The authors state that their conclusions are far more profound than simply the hedonic consequences of finding happiness in joyful activities, as people find happiness *before* consumption, an aspect not typically applied to hedonistic forms of happiness. In their research, Kumar and associates (2014) argue that waiting for experiences tends to be more positive than waiting for possessions and conclude that consumers derive value from anticipation, and that value tends to be greater for experiential than for material purchases.

Kumar and associates also wanted to explain why anticipation plays a more satisfying role with experiential purchases compared to material purchases and they offer a number of possible explanations. For one, they reasoned that when people are thinking of a future material purchase, such as a new pair of shoes or a sweater, they have relatively concrete images of how they will look while wearing the purchase and, thus, the anticipation factor is limited to mostly known entities. However, when it comes to experiential purchases, such as a vacation, there are more unknown variables to anticipate. Sure, people going on a vacation are likely to know the specific place they are heading to and how they will get there and so on, but they also realize the trip could introduce all sorts of unknown stimuli and experiences. Thus, the more abstract thoughts about experiences seem more significant and hence more gratifying.

Another possible explanation put forth by Kumar and associates is the idea that the possession of material goods brings about a competitive mindset much like the idea of "keeping up with the Joneses"—the idea that if a neighbor, friend, rival, or relative buys a new car, you too will want a new car and while you can find joy in the anticipation of purchasing a new car it may come with the realization that you will never be able to afford a new car as nice as the Jones' car. In this regard, the ending conclusion has diminished the anticipation factor. On the other hand, it is far more difficult to compare the happiness that an experience may have brought to individuals. Wealthy friends may have gone on an exotic vacation spending tens of thousands of dollars but that does not mean they had more fun than you did while going camping or taking a much more modest vacation. If a modest vacation experience brings joy and happiness it has a higher value than a vacation that was miserable and costs tens of thousands of dollars. Even if the expensive vacation was filled with happiness, how is one to say which experience was truly happier? Thus, the experience, and the prior anticipation of the experience, are what have the value.

Kumar et al. used the example of waiting in line in their third proposed explanation of why an experiential purchase may be more rewarding than a material purchase. Kumar and associates suggest that waiting in line for an experiential purchase is more likely to lead to friendly conversations with fellow consumers which in turn would make them feel more connected and make the experience of waiting more pleasurable. Writing for *NPR*, Maanvi Singh (2014) reviews the research of Kumar, Killingsworth and Gilovich and agrees that waiting in line for experiential purchases, such as concert tickets or a taco from the latest rave food truck, is a far happier experience than waiting in line for the latest material gadget, such as the newest smartphone. Waiting in long lines for material purchases seems more like an irritant and may lead to a fist-fight with people who try to jump the line. In such instances it is clear that material purchasers waiting in line care far more about the conquest than they do the chase.

Another fascinating aspect of anticipatory experiential purchases involves the idea that extending the period of anticipation of experiences leads to higher levels of happiness (because we have longer to enjoy the idea of the future experience). Happiness associated with material purchases on the other hand tends to foster more of a "give it to me now" mindset (Kumar et al. 2014).

Good Governance Fosters Happiness

Good governance as an explanation for how happiness is achieved might seem like an odd theory to discuss, especially in the United States as Americans seem more divided than ever before due to polarizing political beliefs and perceived government foul-ups at every turn. And yet, research conducted by J.C. Ott (2010) found that good governance fosters a higher level and more equality of happiness. Because happiness is often a vague term, Ott used data collected from the World Database of Happiness which utilizes a series of "Happiness Measures" questions which are used to determine the level of happiness. Ott uses the World Bank's definition of governance (the traditions and institutions by which authority in a country is exercised) and a number of specific aspects that lead to "good" governance. These sociological variables include: voice and accountability (e.g., the freedoms that a country's citizens have to express themselves; and a free media); political stability and absence of violence (e.g., perceptions of the likelihood that the government will be destabilized or overthrown by unconstitutional means; and the level of domestic violence and terrorism); government effectiveness (e.g., quality of public services and civil services); regulatory quality (e.g., the ability of the government to formulate and implement sound policies and regulations that permits and promotes private sector development); rule of law (e.g., the extent to which agents have confidence in and abide by the rules of society); and control of corruption (e.g., the extent to which public power is exercised for private gain, including both petty and grand forms of corruption, as well as capture of the state by elites and private interests). Ott refers to the average score of the first two variables as "democratic quality" and the average score of the last four variables as the "technical quality" of government.

If we use these same variables as Ott to examine the United States in 2017 we can see why some people are so unhappy with government. For one, there is an attack on the free media from many sources including the current U.S. president (Donald Trump); and yet, people have the freedom to voice their concerns via a number of avenues including social media. There appears to be governmental stability, at least in terms of few worries about the government being overthrown unconstitutionally. And yet, there are a number of social problems that the U.S. government has not successfully addressed including protecting the environment and the human right to clean air and clean water; increased levels of terrorism on American soil, from both domestic and foreign sources; racial and class inequality in the criminal and judicial systems; millions of Americans living in poverty and without proper health care coverage; and, the continued dependency on burning fossil fuels as a primary source. There is little wonder why so many people have grave concerns over the manner in which our government operates.

Still, it is the government that can assure our relative freedoms and provide relief in times of disasters (natural or man-made) and it is the overall quality of government that Ott links to national happiness. After examining government and happiness in 130 nations, Ott concludes that there is a positive relation between the quality of government, the technical quality in particular, and average happiness in nations. "There is a bell-shaped relation with inequality in happiness. The relations are up to a point based on causality. These findings suggest that improvement of the technical quality of governance will usually lead to a higher average happiness. Starting at a low level this improvement will also lead to more inequality in happiness firstly and to less inequality later. The relation between the size of government and average happiness depends on the quality of governments; big government adds to happiness only when its quality is good" (Ott 2010).

Ott (2010) adds, "It seems plausible therefore that government can promote happiness, and reduce inequality eventually, by improving their quality and their technical quality in particular. This conclusion is interesting because the improvement of technical quality is usually not a controversial issue. Most people will agree that improving the technical quality is perfectly all right, even if they have different priorities otherwise."

We will examine happiness around the world later in this chapter when we discuss the concept of "Gross National Happiness."

The Delaney and Madigan Theory of Happiness

Delaney and Madigan emphasize the role of engaging in pleasurable intentional activities as a fundamental aspect in individuals' attempt to attain happiness. We also recognize that life circumstances play a significant, albeit a lesser, role than engaging in pleasurable intentional activities, as a fundamental feature in reaching happiness. Genetics, on the other hand, plays a minor role in our pursuit of happiness as genes and DNA do not dictate the courses of action we choose to engage in. Genetics plays a limited role in who we are as individuals but generally plays a small role in how we choose to react to life's challenges.

There is no question that the intentional activities we choose to participate in may have a hedonistic quality to them, as the primary reason we engage in unobligated forms of behaviors—in contrast to obligated forms of behavior (e.g., work and household chores)—centers on having pleasurable experiences. In many instances, people engage in what Thorstein Veblen described as *conspicuous consumption* and *conspicuous leisure*. Both of these activities are a form of hedonistic happiness. According to Veblen (1899), conspicuous leisure refers to a lifestyle where the pursuit of leisure and the appearance of privilege are used in order to gain approval or envy. It is a self-esteem enhancement technique. Those who engage in conspicuous leisure are attempting to present evidence, in a public forum, of their ability to survive without having to work. There is a great deal of evidence of conspicuous leisure presented in social media wherein people are constantly making posts of leisure activities that bring them happiness. Demonstrating to others our leisure activities has in itself become a method for happiness for many; it may also convey a "keeping up with the Joneses" attitude as well. The ability to pursue experiences that one finds rewarding and pleasurable reflects our commitment toward attaining personal happiness. Nixon and Frey (1996) describe conspicuous consumption as "a public display of material goods, lifestyles, and behavior in a way that ostentatiously conveys privileged status to others for the purpose of gaining their approval or envy" (p. 211). From this perspective, individuals gain happiness by purchasing material goods or by spending time and money on non-work activities (at the expense of engaging in activities that may lead to further work production). Diener's (1984) definition of happiness as the experience of positive affect coupled with high life satisfaction is consistent with Veblen's ideas of conspicuous leisure and consumption.

Anticipation is a great motivator for happiness as it stimulates our desire to engage in certain activities over others. Not only can the anticipation of certain behaviors bring us happiness but of course so too will the completion of tasks bring us happiness. Ott (2010) is correct when he points out that good governance can provide happiness. When government officials actually have the best interests of their citizens in mind and successfully execute their roles as civic leaders, the people can benefit; which in turn can lead to happiness among the citizenry.

Delaney and Madigan believe strongly that individuals must eliminate the sources of unhappiness in their life if they wish to become truly happy. We discussed many of the causes of unhappiness in Chapter 5 and put forth the notion that individuals cannot be truly happy unless they eliminate or minimize the causes of unhappiness in their life. We pointed out in Chapter 5 that while this seems like a relatively straightforward notion, many people, including others who propose theories on happiness, tend to ignore the fact that unhappiness must be conquered if happiness is to be attained. We cannot eliminate all forms of unhappiness but, rather, we have to find a way to downplay the negative impact of sources of unhappiness in our lives.

There are other important aspects of happiness that are also important including the idea that most people are capable of enjoying moments of happiness even when their life circumstances are primarily unhappy. For example, a person living in a war-torn area is unlikely to experience constant moments of happiness but will find a few opportunities to be happy. People who are fighting cancer with chemo treatments are also likely to have their level of happiness compromised but even they will find some moments of happiness. In less extreme situations, generally unhappy people may still find moments of happiness from a wide variety of sources—and if they open themselves to more pleasurable intentional activities they can increase happiness levels from momentarily to regularity. Thus, whether the life circumstances of someone is extremely or mildly detrimental to an individual's life there is still a chance for moments of happiness.

We acknowledge that there are short-term and long-term variations of happiness too. Long-term happiness would involve situations wherein people are engaged in pleasurable intentional activities that bring about good health, love and security (financial and otherwise). Short-term happiness comes in many forms too including the simple things in life that bring us joy like someone holding the door open for us, an unexpected smile or nod of approval from a stranger, random acts of kindness (both as the provider and receiver of such an act), or having a one-night stand.

In addition, as we hope we have shown throughout this book, happiness involved to a very large extent the cultivation of the right sorts of friends who will help you develop into the best sort of person you can be.

We conclude this brief look at our theory of happiness by emphasizing that individuals should find as many avenues of pleasurable intentional activities to pursue as possible; but, advise that individuals limit the number of such pursuits during a short timeframe.

Pleasurable Intentional Activities That Make Us Happy

As previously stated, Delaney and Madigan emphasize the active engagement in pleasurable intentional activities as the core aspect of an individual's attempt to attain happiness. Increasing the number of pleasurable intentional activity pursuits generally results in a higher probability of something emotionally-positive and joyful occurring. As with Etkin and Mogilner (2016) however, we caution that the pursuit of too many activities at one time may be too daunting a task and result in stress and feelings of being overwhelmed. Etkin and Mogilner found that happiness is the result of a proper balance between the number and variety of activities individuals engage in. Variety within a day can promote happiness whereas variety within an hour is more likely to decrease happiness. "This reversal stems from people's sense of stimulation and productivity during that time. Whereas longer time periods with more varied activities makes the time feel more stimulating (which increases happiness), filling shorter time periods with more varied activities makes time feel less productive (which decreases happiness). These effects are robust across actual and perceived variety, actual and perceived time duration, and multiple types of activities (work and leisure, self-selected and imposed, social and solo)" (Etkin and Mogilner 2016).

There exists a wide variety of pleasurable intentional activities of which we may chose to participate in. Sean Moran (a friend and colleague of the authors of this book), a philosopher from the Waterford Institute of Technology (Ireland), organizes conferences on happiness and in his detailed "Call for Papers" he included many possible sources of happiness including the following:

- creativity
- music
- the arts
- work
- exercise
- sport
- craft skills
- philanthropy/volunteering
- culture
- entertainment (real and virtual)
- travel
- relationships
- sex
- self-efficacy
- self-esteem
- self-actualization
- wealth and achievement

- contentment
- family
- spirituality

- the sublime
- terror

In our own research of college students we asked survey participants to identify some of the activities that make them happy. As the data in Table 7.1 reveals, being with friends and family were the two most common responses for both males and females. We were not surprised by this result as the theme of this book is to establish and demonstrate the link between friendship relationships and happiness. Other commonly reported pleasurable intentional activities engaged in by our survey participants were being with a significant other, watching sports, listening to music, playing sports and working out, and eating good food. It is also clear that survey participants have found a wide variety of sources of happiness. Some activities are passive, such as reading, watching TV or movies, and listening to music; while other activities, such as playing sports, dancing and cheerleading, are far more active. (Note: We will take a closer look at how music can make us happy in this chapter's popular culture box at the end of the chapter.)

Table 7.1: Pleasurable Intentional Activities That Contribute to Happiness by Gender and by Number

Males (N= 74)		Females (N=107)	
Happiness Activities	Number	Happiness Activities	Number
Hanging out with friends	44	Hanging out with friends	80
Being with family	34	Being with family	65
Watching sports	26	Being with significant other	25
Being with my significant other	18	Playing with pets	23
Listening to music	10	Eating good food	19
Playing sports	9	Watching sports	15
Having high quality friends	8	Sleeping	13
Working out/physical activity	8	Listening to music	13
Eating/preparing great food	6	Watching TV/Netflix	13
Smoking pot	5	Playing sports	10
Being outdoors	4	Doing school work	10
Beautiful women	4	Going to classes	10
My school	4	Reading books	6
Earning good grades	4	Working at my job	6
Having good health	4	Dancing	5
Eating/preparing good food	4	Achieving personal goals	5
Playing with pets	4	Leading a healthy lifestyle	4
		Being physically active	4

(Males)	
Sleeping	3
Watching television	3
Watching old movies	3
Playing video games	3
Having money	3
Drinking alcohol	3
Seeing family members happy	2
Making videos/films	2
Life	2
Learning	2
Making a positive impact	2
Traveling	2
Personal achievements	2
Going to the theatre	2
Film/photography	2
Being alive	1
Summer time	1
Being able to laugh	1
Philosophy	1
Comedy	1
Freedom	1
Simplifying Things	1
Self-reliance	1
Having fun	1
Reading	1
Winning at anything	1
Being organized	1
Earning a degree	1
Math	1
Writing	1
God	1
Holidays	1
Committing deviance	1
Success	1
Receiving praise	1
Being financially stable	1
Time for hobbies	1
Work	1
Fly fishing	1
My faith	1
Firefighting	1
Eating cookies	1

(Females)	
Going out on the town	3
Being in love	3
Having money	3
Enjoying good weather	3
Going to the movies	3
Volunteering	2
Watching sunsets	2
Relaxing	2
Enjoying nice weather	2
Talking/good conversations	2
Planning for my future	2
Enjoying nature	2
Cooking	2
Meeting new people	2
Art/drawing	2
Enjoying my life blessings	2
Helping others	2
Shopping	1
Doing things I am passionate about	1
Writing	1
Going on vacation	1
Laughing	1
Participating in my religion	1
Playing video games	1
Laughing	1
Putting on make-up	1
Online shopping	1
Cuddling	1
Eating ice cream	1
Cleaning	1
Celebrating Christmas	1
Drinking good tea	1
Cheerleading	1
Going to new places	1
Looking at the stars	1
Losing weight	1
Playing cards/games	1
Having a daily routine	1
Drinking good coffee	1
Doing something nice for someone	1

As we noted earlier, individuals can participate in more than one activity at any time, or in a short period of time, but they must watch against trying to combine too many activities at one time. Like Etkin and Mogilner (2016), we note that trying to participate in too many activities in a short period of time can result in stress for participants. In addition, there is another warning we would like to give with regard to multi-tasking and that is, while it is possible to engage in some activities, such as listening to music while also social networking, it is much more difficult to try and study for an exam while gaming, listening to music, watching a ballgame, drinking alcohol and hanging out with friends all at the same time. Thus, while it is wonderful to have many avenues of pleasurable intentional activities to pursue, it would be advisable to limit the number of such pursuits during a short timeframe. It would also be prudent to prioritize chosen courses of actions whether they have happiness as a goal or are guided by some other form motivation. .

Categories of Happiness

We have just learned about some of the many pleasurable intentional activities available to people to pursue in their attempt to attain happiness. Undoubtedly, the reader has thought of some other sources of happiness as well. In the following pages, the authors have compiled sixteen categories of happiness (the first 10 which first appeared in our 2014 book, *Beyond Sustainability: A Thriving Environment*; and the last 6 which are new categories that we have added for this publication). It is important to note that there are so many different categories of happiness because so many people today struggle with several challenges and are hard pressed to be happy. Furthermore, happiness is not something that comes easily for a lot of people. (Note: We discussed many possible causes of unhappiness in Chapter 5.) Perhaps if more people were made aware of these different categories of happiness it would significantly affect their lives in a positive way. Some people may feel as though they are either happy or they are not. However, when one realizes that happiness comes in many forms, it may be easier to acknowledge the experience of happiness more often; and this is a beneficial development for everyone.

We do not proclaim this to be an exhaustive list of categories of happiness and we welcome feedback from all readers on their views of happiness. The discussion of our categories of happiness are in no particular order of importance and do not represent any form of happiness that we consider to be most important. Our discussion on categories of happiness begins with religious and spiritual happiness.

Religious and Spiritual Happiness

Religion is a system of beliefs and rituals that binds people together in a social group while attempting to answer the dilemmas and questions of human existence by making the world more meaningful to adherents. *Religious happiness* refers to the joyous emotional feelings that believers gain by maintaining faith in their convictions. Many forms of organized religion promise an afterlife (i.e., Heaven) wherein the righteous will benefit from their good deeds on Earth via salvation and a blissful existence throughout eternity. The idea of eternal salvation in a perfect afterlife is more than enough to make billions of people happy while they reside in the here and now.

Spirituality has many interpretations but is generally viewed as believing in a power operating in the universe that is greater than oneself. While spirituality has religious undertones, the referenced higher power is not necessarily the same higher power that religious people believe in. Spirituality involves a sensitivity or attachment to a set of ideal values; a quest for special (ultimate/sacred) meaning and personal growth; a deep concern with a sense of spirit; a lack of concern with material or worldly things; and/or, inner peace. Finding peace in the world is a goal for spiritualists. *Spiritual happiness* is characterized by such traits as serenity, kindness, humility, and joy for self and others.

Physical and Touching Happiness

Physical happiness is associated with exercise, a healthy diet, touching and intimacy and is the result of the release of endorphins. An arduous exercise routine, such as a long and fast run, releases endorphins within the human body. Endorphins provide individuals with an adrenaline rush. Endorphins are morphine-like substances in the brain that block pain, heighten pleasure, and have been associated with some additions (Delaney 2013). Endorphins are neurotransmitters produced in the brain which function to transmit electrical signals within the nervous system that may lead to feelings of euphoria, modulate appetite, release sex hormones, and enhance our immune responses. Endorphin release varies among individuals and this explains why two people experiencing the same stimuli (e.g., physical exercise or physical threat) may release different levels of endorphins and consequently lead to different reactions among participants. The "runners high" that some people experience and others do not is explained, in part, by the varying release of endorphins among runners (Delaney 2013).

Physical touching can also bring about happiness as a result of the release of oxytocin, a bonding hormone which strengthen the relationships between people and produces such feelings as trust, contentment and sexual pleasure, as well as reduces stress, anxiety, and fear. Hugging someone (or cuddling) stimulates the production of oxytocin which makes you feel closer to the person and relaxes you. Simply laying down next to someone slows down the heart rate and reduces cortisol levels (the stress hormone) (DeAngelis 2008; Coulon et al. 2013; and Grewen et al. 2005). It is also interesting to note that this same sort of hormonal reaction happens when we interact with animals, such as petting them or playing with them (Coulon et al. 2013). If we look back at Table 7.1 we can see that many respondents included having pets as a source of happiness and this physical touching aspect helps to explain why that is the case.

Intellectual Happiness and Happiness of the Mind

A number of people find happiness through intellectual pursuits. They too can experience an endorphin rush via the sense of learning something new, supporting existing claims of knowledge, or discounting claims of knowledge. Attaining new knowledge is an ultimate form of intellectual happiness that we call the "researcher's high." Academic authors may accomplish "writer's high" when they accomplish a great deal of work in any given time period. Ask any prolific or first time author to explain how they feel when they finish writing a book or see the book in publication and they may explain to you how this writer's high feels. (The authors of this text will tell you that the writer's high is very real!) Teachers and professors may experience the "teacher's high" when they realize students have grasped the material at hand. Conversely, students can achieve intellectual happiness when they learn new material, write an excellent paper, or do extremely well on an exam. Receiving an "A" is not a criterion for intellectual happiness for students as the real happiness comes from learning. Students may feel elated when they receive graded material back from their teachers/professors and learn that their hard work paid off via a high grade and/or praise on the quality of their work.

Limbasiya (2015) argues that intellectual happiness is only possible because of the mind's ability to interpret stimuli and the corresponding ability to convert stimuli into intellect. The mind, according to Limbasiya, allows for the development of intellect by assisting individuals to properly understand life and the many forms of stimuli; and thus, the mind represents the forces within us that make intellect possible. Achieving *mind happiness* reflects our ability to understand the importance of gaining intelligence and knowing what to do with such information.

John Stuart Mill believes that intellectual happiness lasts longer than physical pleasures. As he famously put it, "better to be Socrates dissatisfied than a fool satisfied" (Mill 1863/1979: 54). Thus, while the runner's high represents a great blast of endorphin release within the body, that sense of accomplishment will dissipate rather quickly; the intellectual achievement lasts, potentially, indefinitely. From this perspective, intellectual pleasures such as reading a good book; seeing an intriguing, thought-provoking movie; or having a deep conversation with someone can stay with you longer than a physical touch.

While some people may question the legitimacy of intellectual happiness, intellectual people may wonder how people can be happy pursuing trivial interests, such as finding happiness due to a sports outcome or by watching television. As we have seen previously, for Aristotle this is the highest type of happiness possible, since it corresponds to the highest part of our soul, the rational. Still, intellectual people often find their happiness compromised when they try to reason with people who lack the same level of intelligence as they possess when discussing specific topics in such areas as social policy, politics, economics, the environment, and so on.

Going with the Flow Happiness

Psychologist Mihaly Csikszentmihalyi (1990, 1996) believes that there exists a link between happiness and those heavily involved in an activity to the point where they lose track of everything else, even the time of day. This "going with the flow" activity can contribute to the previously mentioned "writer's high," "researcher's high," the "runner's high" and so much more. Anyone who works can attest to the fact that the work day seems to go by so much faster when they are busy. This is because when we are busy, we get caught up with the task at hand, we become consumed by accomplishing all the deeds, chores, and activities associated with the work day. Before we know it, the work day is over, and we are happy.

Going with the flow happiness does not rely on one being happy at the conclusion of some activity, however. Rather, the process of achievement presents itself as a feeling of happiness to the participant. In this regard, life's a journey, not a destination, is applicable; and yet, expanded upon because the journey is so all-encompassing that the participant enjoys a "high" while doing it. The "flow" represents an optimal experience and consequently, offers the opportunity for happiness (Csikszentmihalyi 1990).

Cultural Happiness

Culture refers to the shared knowledge, values, norms, and behavioral patterns of a given society that are passed on from one generation to the next, forming a way of life for its members (Delaney 2012a). Celebrating one's culture is like celebrating one's place in society. This helps to explain why so many people take pride in their cultural heritage and ancestral origin. Across the globe, societies have special days to celebrate their culture. In heterogeneous societies like the United States, many ethnic people celebrate specific days of the year of the year that acknowledge their cultural heritage (Americans celebrate Independence Day on July 4th; Irish Americans celebrate St. Patrick's Day on March 17th; and Mexican Americans celebrate Cinco de Mayo on May 5th).

Many people like to feel as though their lives have meaning and this meaning can be achieved by contributing, in a positive manner, to the general well-being of society, in contrast to being a drain on society. Putting in a good honest day's work, helping out others through volunteerism, cleaning local neighborhoods of trash and graffiti, and so on, are ways that people can feel like they are contributing to society. Once they feel as though they have made a positive contribution to society, such people have achieved *cultural happiness*.

BIRG and CORF Happiness

The authors have conducted a great deal of research in many areas of sports, including the concepts of BIRG and CORF (Delaney and Madigan 2015; Delaney 2001). BIRG is short for "basking in reflected glory," a phenomenon that involves people connecting themselves with successful others, often using the expression "we" (as in "we won the game!") as a way to enhance their own positive sense of self. The BIRGing behavior leads to happiness as we have identified ourselves with those considered "winners" or "successful."

CORFing refers to "cutting off reflective failure," a technique utilized by folks who want to distance themselves from perceived losers often by using the term "they" (as in "they lost the game"). Cutting ourselves off from perceived failures serves a defense mechanism. People may CORF so that they don't feel unhappy and that, in turn, may trigger happiness.

While the concepts of BIRG and CORF are most noticeable within the institution of sport, they are also applicable in most spheres of life including politics, popular culture and even with our friends and family members who either achieve or fail miserably at something (especially when such results are publicly known by others). BIRGing and CORFing are quite common reactions to various instances of behavior because humans tend to live vicariously through the lives of others. As the old ABC TV show *Wide World of Sports* so memorably put it, we have all experienced the thrill of victory and the agony of defeat in vicarious ways.

Ignorance Is Bliss

Have you ever noticed that some people go through life seemingly oblivious to the problems of the world that surround them? Some people have no idea of major world events or even the decisions made by local politicians, lawmakers and business people. They avoid the news and ignore public debates of cultural importance. And yet, many of these oblivious people are very happy because of the fact that they employ an ignorance is bliss approach to life and have managed to remain happy because they do not concern themselves with the problems of others or the major social problems of society. While remaining ignorant to major world events or significant local events may keep people seemingly happy, they run the risk of such problems suddenly becoming all too real in their immediate lives. Thus, while some people choose to ignore all the ways in which the environment has been compromised, they may be forced to deal with this reality when it's too late to do anything about saving the environment.

Economic Happiness

While we have all heard the cliché that "money can't buy you happiness" most of us also realize that money can buy us experiences and material goods that help provide us with pleasurable intentional activities that do provide happiness. Just think of the many things you would like to do, like visiting exotic places or owning a big, comfortable home, and yet due to the lack of economic prosperity, you cannot do such things. People with the economic means however, are not restricted in their activities and therefore have far more opportunities to attain happiness.

Economic riches and success does not guarantee happiness; nonetheless, economic success affords us the opportunity to secure the essentials of life—food, clothing, and shelter—and it provides us with the means to pursue our interests that lead to happiness. So, while there are people who enjoy economic success and are not happy and there are happy people who do not enjoy economic success, most people benefit from economic security if for no other reason than the realization that the bills and expenses are covered. This economic realization makes many people happy.

Love and Happiness

Perhaps nothing is more identified with happiness than love. There is the love for an intimate other, love for friends and family, love for a pet, love for country, love for religious beliefs, and love for idealistic principles among the many categories of love.

Many philosophers, sociologists and a slew of other theorists from nearly every academic discipline, along with countless laypersons have attempted to define love. Love is generally considered an emotional state that involves deep affection, fondness, tenderness, warmth, intimacy, admiration, and passion for another person. However, as we already stated, love can be extended beyond intimate persons. Philosopher Irving Singer, author of the monumental three-part work *The Nature of Love* (1984–1987), attempts to provide a naturalistic outlook toward the concept of love. Singer argues that there are three broad categories of love: the love of things, the love of persons, and the love of ideals. All of these give meaning to our lives, and we are at our best when we can somehow combine these in a pluralistic approach, a kind of equilibrium (or what the Ancient Greeks would call a harmony of the soul).

There is one thing that everyone who studies love can agree on and that is, when two people are in love with each other it contributes to their happiness.

Environmental Happiness

In our *Beyond Sustainability* book, *environmental happiness* was the last category of happiness we discussed. We emphasized this particular form of happiness because of our desire to inspire people to do all that they can do to try and save the compromised the environment. In trying to understand why *environmental happiness* is so crucial the phrase, "a breath of fresh air" comes to mind. Metaphorically, it has come to mean a pleasant change in direction or and new way of looking at a problem that allows one to come up with a better solution. But of course there is the literal meaning as well. Without fresh air we cannot survive, nor can most of the other living things in our ecosystem. Due to human activities and naturally-caused actions that can end our existence in a relatively short period of time, the reality of fresh air remains constantly at issue.

Saving the environment should be the number one goal of everyone, especially our political and corporate leaders. Unfortunately, many of these same people value economic profits over the future of our planet. The evidence of our compromised environment is overwhelming and cannot be denied by any rational person. As Delaney and Madigan explain in *Beyond Sustainability*, we are currently in the 6th mass extinction period. A mass extinction occurs when the vast majority of species (including humans) on the planet are wiped out forever. Mass extinction periods can take millions of years but due to human behavior this mass extinction is happening at an accelerated rate and could be completed within a few hundred years or hundreds of thousands of years from now (depending on circumstances).

Clearly, it is in everyone's best interest to help save the environment and whenever one does their part to help the environment sustain itself, or ideally help the environment thrive, they will be happy.

Relaxation Happiness

Perhaps one of the more obvious forms of happiness that Delaney and Madigan did not mention in their *Beyond Sustainability* book is relaxation happiness. The *Oxford English Dictionary* defines *relaxation* is the state of being free from tension and anxiety and allows for the restoration of equilibrium following a disturbance. Relaxation also involves a relief from bodily or mental work, effort and application of required deeds. Relaxing provides relief to the physical and mental aspects of our body; it is a diversion from the normal daily sources of stress. *Relaxation happiness* then refers to times when we are doing nothing in particular, we are free from commitments, and we are slacking off and enjoying life. There is little wonder why people would prefer to relax than find themselves in highly stressful situations, especially those of which they have little, or no control over.

Gift of Time Happiness

What is more precious than time, especially when one considers that each of us has a limited time to live? Without dwelling on this fact to the point where we become unhappy with the inevitability of our own pending deaths should come the desire to enjoy every moment we have. And that is why the authors believe that the gift of time is one of the best sources of happiness. The gift of time may come in the form of an *extended lifetime*—something we should truly be happy about, especially if we have good or relatively good health—or it may come in the form of some sort of *situational unexpected free time*. If you've ever received an unexpected day off from work or from school, or had a meeting cancelled, or had some other type of appointment cancelled (especially one that you really didn't want to tend to), you understand the gift of situational free time and its corresponding variation of happiness. In the second scenario of free time we react as if we have "bonus" time, time to do something that makes us happy because we didn't expect to have that extra time in the first place. As for the extended life variation of the gift of time, that is something we enjoy day-by-day as this too represents a true unexpected gift. Recovering from a disease or an accident in which you were given little chance of survival but eventually overcoming such obstacles is a real gift of time. If you have ever had a doctor tell you that you have incurable cancer but then you recovery, you will surely understand how precious every "extra" day really is.

Research conducted by Hershfield, Mogilner and Barnea (2016) reveals that Americans who want more time in their lives are happier than those who want more money. Across studies, the researchers asked thousands of Americans whether they would prefer more money or more time. "Although the majority of people chose more money, choosing more time was associated with greater happiness—even controlling for existing levels of available time and money" (Hershfield et al. 2016). Research suggest that more money is associated with greater daily happiness up to an approximate annual income of USD\$75,000 and with life satisfaction beyond that (Kahneman and Deaton 2010). Research also suggests that even after controlling for material affluence, having more time is associated with greater feelings of happiness and life satisfaction (Kasser and Sheldon 2009).

Undoubtedly, many of you feel the same way as the authors—we love the *gift of time happiness.*

Work Happiness

In Chapter 5 we discussed work as a cause of unhappiness and reviewed statistics about the number of people who are unhappy with their jobs. Some of the reasons that people are unhappy with their jobs include the related stress, burnout, low pay, job insecurity, too much interference from supervisors/administrators, poor retirement plan, and limited chances for promotion.

It is unfortunate that so many people find their work to be a source of unhappiness especially in light of the fact that we spend a large portion of our awake time working. There are, however, many people who enjoy their jobs as they find great meaning in their work and their identities are positively correlated with their job. The following are among the reasons people like to work:

- They like their co-workers
- They have freedom, autonomy and flexibility
- The work environment is a positive one and workers feel appreciated
- There are new things to learn
- They like the challenges that their job provides
- They feel engaged, which fuels their desire to continue working
- They are building their portfolios
- They are good at their work and receive outside recognition
- They like being a part of a succession of past and future workers in their field
- They are highly motivated to achieve goals and will not be stopped
- They are passionate people and inspire others to work hard
- They care about their job and see the value of it
- They like the financial benefits (e.g., salary, health and dental benefits, and retirement benefits)
- They would be bored if they weren't working

Some people love working so much that they become workaholics. Workaholics work compulsively, generally enjoy their work, feel compelled to work, and constantly think about work. Working compulsively comes at the expense of other pursuits but the workaholic seems fine with that. There are researchers, however, including Andreassen et al. (2016) that argue an underlying psychiatric disorder is associated with workaholism—defined as "being overly concerned about work, driven by an uncontrollable work motivation, and to investing so much time and effort to work that it impairs other important life areas." Andreassen and associates found that just 7.8 percent of people in their studies qualified as workaholics. While we acknowledge that workaholism is an addictive form of behavior, we see it as a potentially positive thing as workaholics counterbalance the work slackers that exist in society. Further, if the workaholic is single (or has a relationship with a significant other who keeps busy as well) and maintains a relatively balanced life, it is fine to be so driven as to want to be an overly productive member of society.

The authors of this book are workaholics. We have full-time teaching jobs as professors which involve teaching, holding office hours, advising students, engaging in service activities on campus and in the community, and of course writing. We generally work 6–7 days per week and while we each have our own separate diversionary pursuits, thoughts of work are almost always at the forefront. As tenured professors we could just do our jobs, go home, and be done with it. Instead, we do our jobs, retreat to our respective homes, and work. We do manage to find time for leisure but even those pursuits are often connected to work. Thus, as we travel to various places around the world, whether together, alone, or with others, and we are asked by a flight attendant, "Is this work or pleasure?" We generally answer, "Both!" Although being a workaholic is a form of addiction, it is an addiction that can lead to happiness.

Personal Happiness

We are using *personal happiness* here to refer to a number of related variations of happiness including self-happiness, being single happiness, and being proven right happiness. *Self-happiness* refers to any activity that a person participates in that brings them joy and fulfillment. Being satisfied with oneself—whether this involves personal achievements, personal appearance, or being in a happy relationship—is a rewarding type of happiness as we can reflect upon our own personal achievements. Self-happiness can be achieved by modifying thoughts and habits that get rid of sources of happiness and heighten feelings of happiness; using affirmations or mantras; filtering your inner circle so that you are surrounding by positive people or people who appreciate you; allowing yourself to feel gratitude when things are going well; and helping others. Helping others, or engaging in selfless or altruistic behaviors, are very good sources of attaining self happiness. Someone who has achieved self-happiness also has a positive sense of self. Truly loving yourself is also a way to attain self happiness.

While being involved in a personal relationship with a significant other (e.g., being in love) is generally a good way to attain happiness, some people find true happiness in being single, especially if they have an active social life or a fulfilling job. Being single is often viewed as a gift to those who were in destructive or dysfunctional relationships. Being single means not having to explain your daily activities or whereabouts to another. Single people often snicker when they hear their married friends talk about "needing permission" or "running it past" their spouses before they can do something. Single people can just do what they want, when they want, without going through a quasi-interrogation or some sort of guilt trip for wanting to do something on their own or with friends instead of with a spouse/significant other.

An interesting variation of personal happiness involves the idea of being proven right. Some people, especially experts in a specific field, will often find themselves offering (or being asked) advice on a topic of which they have knowledge. When this is the case, they do not generally like being told they are wrong. There are certain things that each of us know to be true and when we are challenged by others who clearly have less knowledge on the topic, it is very rewarding when the activity/event plays out and you are proven right. There is a certain rush to being proven right and a corresponding degree of happiness.

Humor Happiness

Perhaps one of the most straightforward sources of happiness is humor. Humor comes in many forms and can be enjoyed with friends, family, significant others or by oneself. As described by *Dictionary.com* (2016c), humor is a comic, absurd, or incongruous quality that causes amusement; with such sources as talk in general, comical books, skits, plays, and so on. Many of us truly appreciate humor and enjoy watching television shows and movies that fit the comedy genre. We may also enjoy listening to comedy albums and comics who perform standup routines. Some of us even find humor in daily events that might otherwise be frustrating but we choose to find the humor in such inconveniences. Humor can alter or mental disposition or temperament and provide a temporary mood or frame of mind that brings us joy, and of course, happiness.

The Free Dictionary.com (2016c) describes humor as the quality that makes something laughable or amusing; acts that were intended to induce laughter or amusement; the ability to perceived, enjoy, or express what is amusing, comical, incongruous, or absurd; and often a temporary state of mind or mood. While some people find the humor in a wide variety of activities, others may fail to see the humor in a given situation.

Regardless of the source of humor, if something occurs that makes one feel better or brings joy into their lives, *humor happiness* is something that should be embraced and enjoyed; whether it is enjoyed periodically or on a regular basis. Finding the humor in certain events is certainly a way to "take the edge off" stressful and sad situations and the authors recommend that you find some source(s) of happiness as life is too precious to be wasted being stressful all the time. So, if you are a good joke teller, keep telling jokes; if you are a bad joke teller, be sure to laugh at the jokes of others.

Experiences of Awe Happiness

Among the more intense forms of happiness is experiencing awe. Being in *awe* of something involves an overwhelming feeling of reverence, admiration, and respect for something that is grand, extremely powerful, or beyond words. Dacher Keltner, who heads the University of California, Berkeley's Social Interaction Lab, is a pioneer in the study of emotions, and who helped Facebook create those new "like" button emojis, describes awe as "the feeling of being in the presence of something vast or beyond human scale, that transcends our current understanding of things" (Scott 2016). (Note: Keltner is also the founding director of the Greater Good Science Center, an organization we have cited in this chapter.) Awe is the response to things we view that seem so vast or overwhelming that it alters the way we understand the world. "This sense of vastness can by physical (e.g., a panoramic view from a mountaintop) or psychological (e.g., a brilliant idea). People may experience awe when they are in the presence of a beautiful natural landscape or work of art, when they watch a moving speech or performance, when they witness an act of great altruism, or when they have a spiritual or religious experience" (Greater Good Science Center 2016b).

Many people may experience awe as that spine-tingling feeling you get gazing at the Milky Way, the Grand Canyon, Niagara Falls, ocean waves, or some other vastness of nature. In fact, 75 percent of awe is believed to be inspired by the natural world (Scott 2016). One can only imagine the feeling of awe astronauts in space experience when they get to look out at the vastness of space but also look at the planet earth as a distant object. Feelings of awe generally make us "stop and think" about the world we can observe and it allows deep thinkers to ponder what exists beyond our sight. Paul Piff of the University of California, Irvine believes that awe makes us act more generously, ethically and fairly, and generally makes us nicer, and of course, happier people (Scott 2016). Experiencing awe alters our bodies with positive emotion that reduces levels of cytokines, a marker of inflammation that's linked to depression, according to research from Jennifer Stellar at the University of Toronto (Scott 2016). While awe-inspiring events generally come from the natural world, human activities such as a newborn's hand curling around a parent's finger, outstanding sports performances, and acts of altruism and people of great beauty, can all create moments of awe.

Research suggests that people experience 2.5 incidences of awe per week. If that seems like a low number, congratulations, you are enjoying life's awe-inspiring moments more than others. However, if that seems like a high number to you, perhaps you could heed the following advice on how to find awe in your everyday life:

- Put down your electronic devices and gaze at the clouds or stars.
- Visit local, state or national parks.
- Take an Awe Walk in your neighborhood, noticing things as if for the first time (similar to the adage of taking time out to "smell the roses").
- Describe to a friend or write about a time you once felt awe.
- Visit a museum or planetarium.
- Get up early to watch the sunrise.
- Play amazing music (Scott 2016).

Experiencing awe is like experiencing nirvana; it is an ultimate form of happiness that should free your soul, or your essence, from suffering and desire and bring you to a state of perfect happiness and peace. And wouldn't such happiness be truly awe-inspiring?

We have just concluded our look at 16 categories of happiness. Perhaps you can think of a category that we missed. For the most part, happiness is a subjective reality. Nonetheless, a number of researchers have attempted to create indexes of quizzes that are designed to measure one's level of happiness. In our following discussion, we will review an index that is meant to be an objective analysis of happiness at the national level.

Gross National Happiness

In 1972, Bhutan's former king Kigme Singye Wangchuck coined the term "gross national happiness" (Nelson 2011; Leigh 2006). From this concept, the "Gross National Happiness" (GNH) index was created. The GNH index has four pillars:

- The promotion of equitable and sustainable socio-economic development

- The preservation and promotion of cultural values
- The conservation of the natural environment
- The establishment of good governance

Wangchuck developed the GNH while transforming Bhutan, a landlocked mountain monarchy, into a more modern society. He wanted to promote equitable and sustainable socio-economic development but preserve and promote Bhutan's traditional Buddhist spiritual and cultural values. It was Wangchuck's hope that people would find happiness when socio-economic development was combined with the preservation of cultural values and the conservation of the natural environment under the guidance of good governance. (Note: Think of Ott's work on good governance discussed earlier in this chapter.)

The GNH scale has its detractors. For one, critics point out that Bhutan is a far cry from paradise. It is a society that has faced criticism for expelling residents it claims are illegal Nepali immigrants, but whom some human rights groups assert were citizens opposed to the monarchy (Nelson 2011). Bhutan also has a culture that accepts domestic violence.

Despite the criticisms of Bhutan's cultural norms and values and the perceived vagueness of the concept of happiness, there is a "World Database of Happiness" that offers an ongoing register of scientific research on the subjective enjoyment of life; a happiness bibliography; measures of happiness; happiness measurements in different nations; correlational findings on happiness; and happiness measurements in publics (World Database of Happiness 2011).

With a database on happiness, GNH Index, and the intriguing Happy Planet Index (HPI) in place, we can rank over 150 nations across the globe. For example, the HPI calculates scores for each nation based on the life expectancy of its citizens, the well-being (happiness) of its citizens, and the ecological footprint of that nation. These nations are then given a color code—green for nations that score positively in these three areas, amber for those in the middle, and red for those who rate as having a bad performance on the HPI index. The United States, by the way, received a "red" grade because of its extremely low rating on environmental issues (it has a very high ecological footprint). The nations score the highest (green) grades were Vietnam, Argentina, Chile and Mexico (to see the HPI site, visit http://www.happyplanetindex.org/data/).

The World Would Be a Happier Place If People Would Just ...

We conclude this chapter with a sampling of the results of our survey question that asked respondents to finish this sentence, "The world would be a much happier place if people would just...." (See Table 7.2 for our survey results.)

Table 7.2: The World Would Be a Much Happier Place If People Would Just ... by Gender

Males:

* Drive faster
* Get along
* Realize that they don't need a significant other to be happy
* Connect and interact in non-electronic ways
* Overthrow the bourgeoisie
* Be nice to each other
* Be honest and more friendly with each other
* Do more research and be more aware
* Learn to accept others
* Not be so sensitive
* Relax
* People would stop committing crimes and violence
* Would have better attitudes
* Stop complaining and do something about improving their lives
* Coexist
* Follow the rule, "If you don't have anything nice to say, don't say anything at all"
* Mind their own business
* Honestly, nothing can make the world happier
* Simplify everyday life
* End violence, prejudice and injustice
* Education
* Love/respect each other
* Smile
* Sweep their own front porch
* Think. Take a step back. Breathe
* Say hi to strangers
* Stop being so sensitive
* Realize we are smaller than a grain of sand in the grand scheme of the universe
* Everybody dies but not everyone lives
* Treat people the way they want to be treated
* Have a profound respect for human life from conception to death
* Exercise!
* Bake more cookies and spread the treats around (this is the same respondent that said cookies make him happy but burnt cookies make him unhappy!)
* Not get offended so easily
* Stop being greedy
* Calm down
* Everyone was open minded and did not see physical differences as "different" and "abnormal"

* If everyone just accepted the way everyone dresses, functions, and interacts than people would just socialize rather than judge
* The world would be much happier without judgment
* Keep it real with each other instead of talking behind their back
* Let people finish their sentences and thoughts
* Love each other and the planet we live on
* Mind their own business!
* Stop whining about everything

Females:

* Try to understand others and have more compassion for each other
* Listen to each other/and get rid of prejudgments
* Be nice/kind to one another
* Get along, not be so selfish and care for one another
* Would just chill out
* Accept cultural and personal differences among people
* Stop being nosey/mind own business
* Accept each other as they are
* Be nice to one another
* Be more honest with one another
* Read more
* Exercise more
* Eat more vegetables
* Care about people outside their own social circles
* Stop judging others
* Forget about things we cannot control
* Think before they speak
* Weren't so stubborn
* Realize that everybody has their own issues and you must not judge others
* Be kinder to others
* Be more considerate of others
* Get along with one another
* Love one another
* Enjoy the little things and live care free
* Stop agreeing with Donald Trump!
* Be more open-minded
* Act their age
* Put down their phones and have an actual conversation with someone
* Calm down
* Confront their problems in a healthy and constructive manner
* Stop hate crimes
* Take the easy way out
* Be honest
* Realize what a wonderful gift life is and just look up from their phones and experience the world with the people around them
* Listen, we have two ears so we can listen more than we talk. Be open to new ideas and get old ones like racism and homophobia out of people's heads

* Be upfront with each other and understand that everyone is fighting a fight you know nothing about so just be kind
* Be more positive
* Stop taking offense at everything they hear, or finding ways to make something that wasn't supposed to be hurtful, hurtful
* Not vote for Donald Trump (Author's Note: This survey was taken in October 2016)
* Help not spread global warming
* Stop hating each other
* Mind their own business
* Look at the positive sides of things and not dwell on the bad

As we can see from the results of Table 7.2, college students have a wide variety of ideas on what would make the world happier. What do you think would make the world a happier place?

Popular Culture Scenario 7 examines a formula for making music that will bring happiness to others.

Popular Culture Scenario 7: The Formula for Making Music That Brings Happiness to Others

Earlier in this chapter we provided survey results of pleasurable intentional activities that contribute to happiness and not surprisingly, music was one of the activities cited by survey respondents. We would suggest that if we had specifically asked respondents if they find music pleasurable and/or as a source of happiness that nearly all respondents would agree that music has that capability. Recall also that in Chapter 4 we described special-interest friendships and noted that music has the ability to draw people together simply by sound, a sound that is appealing to the listener.

But what is it about music that has this capability of making us happy? Listeners of music are likely to cite a number of reasons including such simplistic responses as, "I like the sound," "I like the message," "Because it reminds of past happy moments, such as a special place or person," "I can relate to the lyrics," and "I like to dance and music helps me to feel free." The idea that music with a certain beat allows people to experience happiness, whether it involves dancing or not, is something many people may acknowledge but is also something immortalized by the TV show, *American Bandstand* (1952–1989). During a popular segment in the show, "Rate-A-Record," audience members on the show were asked to rank new single releases on a scale of 0–100. The common response (and perhaps one prompted by the show's producers) was, "It's got a good beat and it's easy to dance to."

According to Jacob Jolij, a cognitive neuroscientist at the University of Groningen in Holland, who studied pop songs from the past fifty years, the "feel good" experience associated with listening to music is the beat and this beat is primarily responsible for triggering happiness. Jolij found that while positive lyrics were important, it is a high tempo of 150 beats per minute that subconsciously makes people feel energized and thus, happy (Woollaston 2015). Jolij adds, putting the song into a third major key—the third note or chord in a musical scale—also produced a happy sounding song (Woollaston 2015). Jolij states, "A feel good song is very personal. Music is intimately linked with memory and emotion, and these associations strongly determine whether a song will put you in a good mood or not. However, there are some key criteria for composers to consider when creating feel good songs—namely, lyrical theme, musical key, and tempo" (Woollaston 2015). Holiday songs certainly make people happy and are pleasant to our ears; however, a high tempo of 150 beats per minute also subconsciously triggers a sense of energy (Woollaston 2015). With these criteria in mind, we can look at Jolij's formula as: FGI = ?L postivie / (BPM − 150) + (K − [1/3 + ?, 1/3 ,1/3 − ?]) + 1. "FGI" refers to a feel good song, "L" stands for positive lyrics, "BPM" represents beats per minute, and "K" as the third musical key to produce the ultimate feel good song that will make people happy.

Using his formula, Jolij produced a top ten of the most feel good songs from the past fifty years. Jolij's list is topped by Queen's "Don't Stop Me Now," a song that was released in 1978. The complete Top Ten list is described below:

1. Don't Stop Me Now—Queen
2. Dancing Queen—ABBA
3. Good Vibrations—Beach Boys
4. Uptown Girl—Billy Joel
5. Eye of the Tiger—Survivor
6. I'm a Believer—The Monkees
7. Girls Just Wanna Have Fun—Cyndi Lauper
8. Livin' on a Prayer—Bon Jovi
9. I Will Survive—Gloria Gaynor
10. Walking on Sunshine—Katrina & The Waves

Jolij also broke down the top feel good songs from each of the past 6 decades with Pharrell Williams' "Happy" as the top song of the 2010s.

While everyone's own taste in music varies quite a bit, an aspiring songwriter hoping to hit the charts with a best seller should consider heeding the formula put forth by Jolij. Such a musical achievement will not only make the songwriter happy, but it will likely make millions of others happy too.

Summary

In this chapter we examined the aspects related to the pursuit and attainment of happiness from a sociological and multi-disciplinary approach. The pursuit of happiness is ingrained in all Americans and perceived as a right as a citizen. The pursuit of happiness originates with the "Declaration of Independence" and has existed as a mainstay value of American society and of most societies around the world.

Happiness, while having different meanings for different people, is the emotional state of well-being and positive reactions experienced due to triggering stimuli. Happiness may involve such other emotions as inner peace, absence of want, blissfulness, confidence, being true to oneself, freedom, and viewing one's life favorably. The value of happiness is plentiful and general manifests itself in the form of improved physical and mental health; improved attitudes toward education, academic aspirations, academic achievement, life satisfaction, altruism, self-esteem, and parental relations (for youth); happiness is good for our personal relationships; happy people make more money and are more productive at work; happy people are more generous; happy people use positive emotions to bounce back from negative emotional experiences; and, happy people are more creative and better able to see the big picture.

A number of theoretical explanations were brought forth in order to explain how happiness is attained. The authors put forth their own theory which emphasizes the role of engaging in pleasurable intentional activities; recognizing that life circumstances impacts one's happiness, albeit in a lesser role than engaging in pleasurable intentional activities; acknowledges the potential hedonistic component of happiness; recognizing anticipation as a motivator for happiness; stressing that happiness can only be achieved when the sources of unhappiness are diminished; and acknowledging that there are short-term and long-term variations of happiness.

A large variety of pleasurable intentional activities that make us happy were discussed including responses from our survey participants. Sixteen different categories of happiness were presented. Although the authors do not proclaim their list as an exhaustive list of categories of happiness, they do cover a wide range of sources of happiness. The Gross National Happiness (GNH) index and the four pillars of the index were discussed. And the chapter concluded with survey respondents offering up their ideas as to what it would take to make the world happier and a Popular Culture Scenario that offered up a formula for the elements of the happiest songs.

Conclusion:
The Connection Between Friendship and Happiness

In parts I and II we reviewed a number of key aspects of friendship and happiness respectively. We have learned a great deal about both of these fundamental components and we have also discovered the relationship between the two. In this portion of the book, the conclusion, we provide a brief review of each of the preceding chapters and highlight the relationship between friendship and happiness. In particular, we will return to Aristotle's threefold categorization of friendship and see that, while it definitely needs refinement, it still has great relevance to the present-day.

Parting Thoughts

It is safe to say that we are all better off if we have a number of close friends and if we can find activities that bring us happiness. Having friends is one of the most fundamental aspects of finding and achieving happiness. Having friends has always been important throughout human history and will remain so in the future. While we have traditionally relied on face-to-face encounters with others as the means of attaining friendships, in the contemporary era it is possible to make friends electronically in the cyberworld. Whether they are face-to-face, cyber or virtual, all of our friends have the ability to bring us happiness.

In Chapter 1 we looked at the life and teachings of the Ancient Greek philosopher Aristotle and how his views regarding the nature of friendship continue to influence modern-day discussions of the topic. In particular, we examined his threefold categorization of friendship—utility, pleasure and the good.

We also examined Aristotle's claim that we are by nature social beings, and that in order to develop in the best possible ways we need connections with many other humans. This begins with the family, which in Aristotle's view is an unequal relationship. Parents cannot be friends, in his view, since the relationship with them is not on equal terms, nor is it a chosen one. The same holds for siblings and other family members.

Friends are thus those people with whom we choose to form intimate bonds (as opposed to "familiar strangers" whom we choose not to form such bonds with), based on a sense of equality and reciprocity.

Friends of utility, for Aristotle, are those for whom such reciprocity is based on specific situations. We rely upon each other for mutual aid. But such relationships are fragile, and in Aristotle's terms "imperfect." They are likely to end when our life situations change and we are no longer of use to each other.

Aristotle's second category of friendship, friends of pleasure, are based upon human emotions, especially the joy that people feel in being in each other's company. Such friendships are thus of a higher nature, and tend to be more important to one's development. But these two are fragile since once the pleasure ceases to be reciprocated, the basis for the friendship ends.

Thus, both friends of utility and friends of pleasure are "imperfect" in their nature, and are contrasted with the "perfect" or strongest type of friendship, friends of the good. "Perfection" does not imply that such friendships will never end or have no flaws, but it does mean that their foundation is the most solid, since the basis for them is the concern each has for the other's continued well-being. Friends of the good encourage virtuous behavior, and are reliable and trustworthy to the highest degree. Such friendships take time to develop, and because of the commitment necessary one can only have a limited number of friends of the good.

For our natural development as humans, it is important to cultivate friendships of the good, since these allow us to develop in the highest of ways, and life would be inadequate without such friendships.

We ended with a brief look at criticisms that Aristotle's views are elitist, sexist, and inadequate in relationship to modern times but we argued that nonetheless his threefold concept is still relevant in trying to understand the nature of friendship in the present day.

In Chapter 2, we discussed how forming friendships is preceded by group formation. Group formation has been a characteristic of humanity throughout our time on this planet and was primarily the result of our need to do so for our own safety and basic survival. Even as humans continued to evolve physically and intellectually over hundreds of thousands of years the need for companionship and a strong communal bond with others would remain intact. As we evolved, group formation became more selective and as a result of evaluating experiences, or expected experiences and the benefits provided by each alternative. The people we grade the highest are sought out as friends because we wish to spend our time with them. From a sociological perspective, the socialization process is the key aspect of group and friendship formation. Socialization is a lifelong process of social development and learning that occurs as individuals interact with one another and learn about society's expectations of proper behavior so that they can fully participate and properly function within cultural standards. Individuals also attain a social identity as they learn various values and norms while interacting with others. Individual social identities (individualism) help to establish differences and leads to attraction by some and rejection/repulsion by others.

As we learned in Chapter 1, Aristotle argued there were three types of friends. In Chapter 2 we too describe three primary categories of friends; albeit different categories—casual, close and best friends—as well as a number of other categories including, old friend, older friend, new friend, wild friend, scary friend, the confidant, and the dormant friend (all subcategories of close friends); frenemies; friends with benefits; friends of friends, or secondhand friends; ex-friend; bromance friends; work friends; single-modifier friends; and, special-interest friends. We concluded this chapter by examining the end of a friendship. Most of us have experienced this and there are a number of reasons why people "fall out of friendship" including, one of the friends moves away, the friends grew apart, issues of dishonesty and distrust, betrayal, and the lack of shared interests that once formed the bond between them.

Cyber socialization and its role as a transitional step toward electronic friendships was the focus of Chapter 3. Cyber socialization emerged for a number of reasons but especially because of the development of communications technology and the rise of the Internet along with the changing cultural norms and values that encourage impersonal forms of communication. Following the time of U.S. independence from Great Britain, communication among members of American society was assisted via the Postal Service and for a short period of time the telegraph system. By the end of the 19th century and the start of the 20th century, Americans were beginning to use the technological advancement of the telephone to communicate with one another. Continued technological growth led to communication via computers, including sending electronic messages (e.g., emails) to one another. As telephone technology continued to develop we started to communicate with one another via wireless and hand-held smart phone devices small enough to fit in our pockets that allowed people in both urban and remote areas to communicate with one another by either talking on the phone or by sending electronic messages (texts). Technology and communications evolved to the point wherein the Internet was established. The "Net" allows users to gain immediate access to a communications system that allows for long-distance social interactions through a series of networking sites that further allows for (among other things) the maintenance of existing friendships—those originally formed via face-to-face contact—and for the creation of new friendships—electronic friendships—wherein those involved in the relationship have not necessarily ever met and do not have face-to-face interactions.

Electronic socialization also includes changing some of the basic norms and values of social interactions and the maintenance of relationships. For example, language itself has been modified via such symbolic modifications that encourage the use of emoticons rather than the use of words as a means of communicating with one another. Emoticons are text gestures that take on meaning for the sender and the receiver. They are tiny pictures used to add a little flavor to text messages and tweets. Emoticons developed from emoji. Many people, in particularly friends, who communicate with one another electronically, rely heavily on the use of emoticons especially as a way to express sentiment in an otherwise emotionless form of interaction.

Cyber socialization represents a critical aspect in the development of electronic friendships, the focus of Chapter 4. The cyber socialization process, among other things, indoctrinated us into accepting the fact that an increasing number of social interactions once done in person could, and would, now take place in the cyberworld. Following our acceptance for the need of a cyberworld we have become further drawn into virtual worlds where an escalating number of social interactions take place. It will not come as a surprise to anyone that the amount of time people spend using the electronic media and communicating with one another in cyberspace rather than in face-to-face interactions has increased dramatically over the course of the past few decades. The amount of time spent in the cyberworld generally comes at the cost of less time spent with personal relationships in the real world. Some people are so consumed with spending time on the internet that they have developed compulsive internet use disorder—characterized by such behavior as people having an inability to stop themselves from using computers, developing an increased tolerance that allows users to seek even longer sessions online, and suffering from withdrawal symptoms like anger and craving when prevented from logging on. The authors often notice that many college students display this disorder but also recognize that compulsive internet use disorder extends far beyond college campuses.

People spend a great amount of time online and in particular on social network sites. Social networking sites are popular for many reasons but in particularly because they provide users an opportunity to control their presentation of self via the posts they make and the photos they share. Facebook is by far the most popular social network site. Research has shown that the positive experience enjoyed by users on Facebook affects the nucleus accumbens, a small but critical structure located deep in the center of the brain and responsible for the reward system of the brain. The nucleus accumbens is the part of the brain that's associated with motivation, pleasure, and addiction—sometimes called the brain's "pleasure center." The positive feedback users receive from friends in the form of "likes" and positive comments to posts can stimulate the nucleus accumbens. While many younger people maintain an account with Facebook, they tend to find other sites like Instagram, Snapchat, YouTube, Yik Yak and Tumblr far more enjoyable.

Social network sites provide us with a realm for focused encounters of interactions with others. For example, the relationship status feature on Facebook provides a big advantage for people seeking certain types of friends, such as a single person looking for another single person, or someone in an open relationship looking for hookups with others who share that same feature. In the conventional world, we do not know the relationship status of people we first encounter. Social network sites allow users an opportunity to maintain current relationships while also providing an opportunity to establish new friendships and relationships. These new relationships are known as electronic relationships and they are just as real as face-to-face relationships minus the physical closeness. Electronic relationships are as real as the participants make them. With electronic relationships, communication, even if limited to electronic communication, seems to be the key variable when describing e-relationships as true friendship or romance relationships. And isn't good communication the key to all relationships? Furthermore, we all seem to value friendships and whether we secure them electronically or in-person, the desire for friendship itself remains constant.

Our socialization into the cyberworld and compliance with spending an increasing amount of time in electronic relationships leads to the next step in the transformation process of friendships; one that involves further heading away from face-to-face interactions to friendships that can only exist in virtual realities. Virtual reality, among other things, allows people to create personas (the virtual self) that are real only in virtual worlds. Thus, virtual relationships become a distinctive sub-category of electronic friendships previously discussed.

In chapters 5–7 (Part II), we examined the concepts of unhappiness and happiness. A key aspect of our own theory on happiness (explained in Chapter 7) incorporates the idea that in order to achieve happiness, we must overcome unhappiness. The topic of unhappiness was discussed in Chapter 5.

Inspired in part by the work of philosopher Bertrand Russell and his classic book *The Conquest of Happiness*, Chapter 5 provides a review of the sources of unhappiness articulated by the English philosopher which included: the realization that some people are simply unhappy people due to their individual psychology; Byronic unhappiness; competition (the struggle for life); boredom; fatigue; envy; the sense of sin (one's one self-disapproval); persecution mania; and, the fear of public opinion. We also describe a large number of other possible sources of unhappiness including: someone who is suffering through an unhappy marriage or relationship; stress and depression; work/ employment; the death of a loved one, or the poor health of a loved one; one's own poor health; a fear of the grid going down, leading to social chaos; a highly identified sports fan who suffers because of the defeat of a favorite team; lack of true friends, lack of quality friendships; lack of meaning in one's day to day life; general feelings of meaningless; focusing on the negative aspects of one's life; a lack of tolerance for anything less than perfect and the fear of failure; low self-esteem; financial debt; lack of time to spend with loved ones; being a power freak and yet in control of one's own life; holding grudges against others; wanting to believe that life is fair when it seldom is; wanting everyone to play by your rules; a glass-half-empty type of person; loneliness; personal insecurity; constant need for validation; the realization that your dreams and aspirations have not come true; failure to learn new things; boredom; failure to take time to relax and enjoy life; unhappy with politics and government; failure to risks in life; impatience; playing the victim; and failure to allow yourself to be happy.

In Chapter 6 we returned to an examination of Aristotle's philosophy. To truly understand what he meant by friendship, as detailed at the beginning section of the book, it is necessary to put this discussion in its proper context. Friendship is a subset of eudaimonia (usually translated as happiness) and connects to the understanding of the nature of the human soul.

Human beings, in Aristotle's view, are the only living things which possess rationality. Happiness is the ultimate goal, or telos, that human beings aim at, but it is a unique type of happiness. Achieving things such as good health, good wealth or public recognition are important to humans but are not the ultimate goal we seek. Rather, they are means to that end.

The ultimate goal of happiness is a fulfillment of our talents. This relates to the three types of human activities: hedonism, honor, and contemplation. The last is the most important since it directly relates to our rational self, which he felt is something that only humans possess.

In order to be genuinely happy we need two things: good fortune and skill. We need to develop our talents so that when good fortune arrives we will know how to make the most of it. But in order to develop our skills we need the support of others, most particularly good friends. They will encourage us to make good use of our reasoning skills and avoid vices (deficiencies or excesses of behavior) that lead us astray. The key to a good life is therefore to achieve a "happy medium" between extremes.

While there is no guarantee that good fortune will smile upon us, Aristotle felt that nature generally allows the possibility for human beings to develop their talents in ways that will allow them to be happy.

Bertrand Russell has spelled out in detail many causes of happiness, including affection, family, work, impersonal interests, and effort and resignation. Like Aristotle and his idea of intrinsic and extrinsic values, Russell explains that happiness depends partly upon external circumstances and partly upon oneself.

In Chapter 7, we learned about the manner in which people pursue and attain happiness. While the notion of happiness is a little vague—as its subjective meaning varies from one person to another—it is generally understood to involve a mental or emotional state of well-being and positive and/or pleasant reactions to stimuli ranging from general contentment to intense joy. A number of studies were cited that demonstrate that happiness improves many aspects of our lives, including: our attitudes toward education, academic aspirations, academic achievement, life satisfaction, altruism, self-esteem, and parental relations; our physical and mental health; for our relationships; happy people make more money and are more productive at work; happy people are more generous; happy people use positive emotions to bounce back from negative emotional experiences; and, happy people are more creative and are better able to see the "big picture."

A number of theoretical explanations on how happiness is attained were put forth in this chapter including the authors' own theory of happiness. The authors emphasize the role of engaging in pleasurable intentional activities as a fundamental aspect in individuals' attempt to attain happiness. We also recognize that life circumstances plays a significant, albeit a lesser role than engaging in pleasurable intentional activities, as a fundamental feature in reaching happiness. Genetics, on the other hand, play a minor role in our pursuit of happiness. Anticipation is a great motivator for happiness as it stimulates our desire to engage in certain activities over others. We believe strongly that individuals must eliminate the sources of unhappiness in their life if they wish to become truly happy. There are important aspects of happiness that are also important including the idea that most people are capable of enjoying moments of happiness even when their life circumstances are primarily unhappy; the acknowledgment that there are short-term and long-term variations of happiness; and, emphasizing that individuals should find as many avenues of pleasurable intentional activities to pursue as possible; but, advise that individuals limit the number of such pursuits during a short timeframe.

In this chapter, we also described a wide variety of pleasurable intentional activities that people engage in during their pursuit of happiness. Among these activities are: spending time with friends, creativity, seeking knowledge, music, sports, work, exercise, arts and crafts, entertainment, sex, travel, family, spirituality, the sublime, thrill-seeking, watching movies, sleeping in, volunteering, and doing something nice for others. We also discussed sixteen different categories of happiness. The idea behind categorizing happiness is that it allows for people to realize that while they may feel unhappy about certain aspects of their lives, there are still many other areas wherein they may find happiness and come to realize that life is not so gloomy after all. The categorization of happiness also allows people who are already relatively happy to realize that there are many things in their lives that bring them happiness.

As Aristotle argued long ago and as modern science continues to prove, there is a solid link between friendship and happiness. We provided many examples of this link throughout the book. A sampling of the research on friends and happiness includes: one person's happiness triggers a chain reaction that benefits not only their friends, but their friends' friends, and their friends' friends' friends, with the effect lasting for up to a year; quality real-life friends are correlated with subjective well-being (SWB) even after controlling for income, demographic variables and personality differences. Happiness in life is real possibility, but it can only happen with a little help (or in the case of friends of the good with a lot of help) from your friends.

We conclude this chapter with a Popular Culture Scenario that sends a clear message on the value of friendship and happiness. In Popular Culture Scenario 8 we can see that when people have friends they truly do have a happy and wonderful life.

Popular Culture Scenario 8: It's a Wonderful Life When You Have Friends (and Happiness)

A holiday film staple at the end of every calendar year and just prior to Christmas is the 1946 film, *It's a Wonderful Life*. Directed by Frank Capra, *It's a Wonderful Life* stars James Stewart as George Bailey and Donna Reed as his wife Mary. The storyline of this classic film centers on the life of George Bailey who was raised in Bedford Falls, a small community highlighted by the simpler activities of life. Throughout his life, George longed to travel to places and locales of places he had only seen in magazines. His dreams would never be realized and this reality often haunted him as he considered himself a failure in life.

For the townspeople of Bedford Falls, a fictional place meant to be a "small town USA" so that it could be relatable to many people who live in, or yearn for, a simpler life, George Bailey was anything but a failure. (Note: A few American towns have claimed to be the inspiration for Bedford Falls, including Seneca Falls, New York, a village known as the "birthplace of the U.S. women's rights movement." The film acknowledges that Bedford Falls is a short plane ride from New York City.) George took on the responsibility—or burden as he would come to see it as—of running his late father's unpretentious building and loan company. The Bailey

Bros. Building & Loan Association provided low-interest loans for the townspeople, many of whom could barely afford their own homes and small businesses.

As with any good film that withstands the test of time, Bedford Falls was also home to an antagonist, Mr. Potter (played by Lionel Barrymore), much akin to other Christmas villains like Ebenezer Scrooge and the Grinch. Mr. Potter lacked the altruism that characterized George Bailey. He was a rich and greedy man who was intent of owning much or all of Bedford Falls so that he could benefit financially. On one particular Christmas Eve, George's Uncle Billy loses the building and loan's substantial cash receipts that he was supposed to deposit at the bank. Potter finds the misplaced money and hides it from Uncle Billy. The scheming Mr. Potter alerts the bank examiner of the building and loan's shortage. George Bailey realizes that he will not only be held responsible for the shortage and mostly likely sent to jail, he also realizes that this incident could lead to Mr. Potter taking over the Bailey business and, as a result, take ownership over the rest of the town.

George is so distraught at the thought of these consequences that he begins to think that his wife and children, as well as all the town folks, would be better off if he was dead or never born at all. Such a notion leads George to ponder suicide. As he is about to jump off a bridge that rises above a river that flows through the town, an angel named Clarence (Henry Travers) is sent down from Heaven to help save George. Via spiritual intervention, Clarence is able to show George just what would've happened to Bedford Falls and all the townsfolk if he had indeed never been born. As one would imagine with this type of film (and by the title of the film), the life of all of George's friends, family members, and others in the community were far worse off without him. By the conclusion of this heavenly intercession, Clarence is able to convince George not to take his own life.

Filled with renewed vigor, George happily runs through town saying hello to everyone and all the businesses that his loan company has helped. He now realizes that he has more friends than he can count. He also has a very loving and supporting wife who, while George was going through his mental meltdown, alerted the townsfolk of the financial crisis facing the building and loan company. Realizing that without George's financial help and friendship throughout the years they would all be much worse off, people from the town quickly gather all their cash and run it over to the Bailey house, thus saving him from possible incarceration, saving the building and loan company, and keeping Mr. Potter from taking over the town. With the Bailey family gathered around the Christmas tree and the cash continuing to pour onto a table in front of them, George's brother Harry arrives. (Note: George had saved Harry's life when they were children.) Harry proposes a toast to his brother by saying, "To my big brother, George, the richest man in town!" The implication of such a toast is obvious: if you have friends, you have riches.

The film's final scenes conclude with George opening up a gift from

Clarence. It's a book, Mark Twain's *The Adventures of Tom Sawyer*, with an inscription inside that reads:

Dear George:

Remember no man is a failure who has friends.
Thanks for the wings!

Love,
Clarence

Just then, a bell on the Bailey Christmas tree rings and the Bailey's young daughter Zuzu proclaims, "Look, Daddy. Teacher says, every time a bell rings an angel gets his wings." George, and the viewing audience, are left to believe, that the bell must have been for Clarence. Acknowledging Zuzu and looking upwards (presumably toward Heaven), George replies, "That's right. That's right. Attaboy, Clarence."

Aside from the religious aspects of this film, the true meaning of *It's a Wonderful Life* rests with the realization that as long as we have friends, we are successful in life. And when we have friends, we are happy.

Bibliography

AboutDivorce.org. 2011. "Divorce Rate—USA." Retrieved circa August, 2012 (www.about divorce.org/us_divorce_rates.html).

Adams, Susan. 2013. "Unhappy Employees Outnumber Happy Ones by Two to One Worldwide." *Forbes*, October 10. Retrieved August 21, 2016 (http://www.forbes.com/sites/susanadams/2013/10/10/unhappy-employees-outnumber-happy-ones-by-two-to-one-worldwide/#18ab653d2f29).

Adkins, Amy. 2014. "Majority of U.S. Employees Not Engaged Despite Gains in 2014." *Gallup*, January 28. Retrieved August 21, 2016 (http://www.gallup.com/poll/181289/majority-employees-not-engaged-despite-gains-2014.aspx).

Aelred of Rievaulx. 1977. *Spiritual Friendship.* Kalamazoo, MI: Cisternian Publications.

Akin, Jennifer. 2005. "Mass Media." *Beyond Intractability*. Retrieved June 12, 2016 (http://www.beyondintractability.org/essay/mass-communication).

Allen, Woody. 1980. "The Shallowest Man." *Kenyon Review,* Winter, 1980: Vol. II, No. 1. Retrieved July 12, 2016 (http://www.kenyonreview.org/kr-online-issue/weekend-reads/woody-allen-342846/)

Anderson, Elizabeth. 2015. "Teenagers Spend 17 Hours a Week Online: How Internet Use Has Ballooned in the Last Decade." *The Telegraph*, May 11. Retrieved December 14, 2015 (http://www.telegraph.co.uk/finance/newsbysector/mediatechnologyandtelecoms/digital-media/11597743/Teenagers-spend-27-hours-a-week-online-how-internet-use-has-ballooned-in-the-last-decade.html).

Andreassen, Cecilie Schou, Mark D. Griffiths, Rajita Sinha, Jorn Hetland, and Stale Pallesen. 2016. "The Relationships Between Workaholism and Symptoms of Psychiatric Disorders: A Large-Scale Cross-Sectional Study." *PLOS One*, 11(5). Retrieved November 26, 2016 (https://www.ncbi.nlm.nih.gov/pmc/articles/PMC4871532/).

Aristotle. 1962. *Nicomachean Ethics* (translated by Martin Ostwald). New York: Macmillan Publishing Company.

Barrett, David. 2015. "What is the Law on Revenge Porn?" *The Telegraph*, April 13. Retrieved June 17, 2016 (http://www.telegraph.co.uk/news/uknews/law-and-order/11531954/What-is-the-law-on-revenge-porn.html).

BBC News. 2014. "Many Young People Addicted to Net, Survey Suggests." October 15. Retrieved June 19, 2016 (http://www.bbc.com/news/technology-29627896).

Beck, Julie. 2015. "How Friendships Change in Adulthood." *The Atlantic*, October 22. Retrieved June 7, 2016 (http://www.theatlantic.com/health/archive/2015/10/how-friendships-change-over-time-in-adulthood/411466/).

Bellis, Mary. 2015. "The History of the Electric Telegraph and Telegraphy." Retrieved June 12, 2016 (http://inventors.about.com/od/tstartinventions/a/telegraph.htm).

Beneito-Montagut, Roser. 2015. "Encounters on the Social Web: Everyday Life and Emotions Online." *Sociological Perspectives*, 58(4):537–553.

Bennett, Shea. 2014. "The Year of the Selfie—Statistics, Facts & Figures." *Social Times*, March

19. Retrieved June 14, 2016 (http://www.adweek.com/socialtimes/selfie-statistics-2014/
497309).

_____. 2015. "28% of Time Spent Online Is Social Networking." *Social Times*, January 27,
2016. Retrieved June 19, 2016 (http://www.adweek.com/socialtimes/time-spent-online/
613474).

Bentham, Jeremy. 2007. [1781]. *An Introduction to the Principles of Morals and Legislation.*
Mineola, NY: Dover.

Benzaquen, Adriana S. 2006. *Encounters with Wild Children: Temptation and Disappointment
in the Study of Human Nature.* Montreal: McGill-Queens University Press.

Bierly, Mandi. 2008. "'Boston Legal' Finale: I Now Pronounce You Denny and Alan." *Entertainment Weekly.* December 9. Retrieved October 10, 2016 (http://ew.com/article/2008/
12/09/boston-legal-1/).

Blass, Thomas. 2004. *The Man Who Shocked the World.* New York: Basic Books.

Blau, Peter. 1964. *Exchange and Power in Social Life.* New York: Wiley.

Borgueta, Maya. 2015. "The Psychology of Ghosting: Why People Do It and a Better Way to
Break Up." *Huffington Post*, August 17. Retrieved June 13, 2016 (http://www.huffington
post.com/lantern/the-psychology-of-ghostin_b_7999858.html).

Boston Legal. 2008. Retrieved October 10 (http://www.imdb.com/title/tt0402711/quotes).

Bradley, Carl Marshall, and Philip Blosser, eds. 1989. *Of Friendship: Philosophic Selections on
a Perennial Concern.* Wolfeboro, NH: Longwood Academic.

Brady, Erik, and Rachel George. 2013. "Manti Te'o 'Catfish' Story is a Common One." *USA
Today*, January 18. Retrieved June 18, 2015 (http://www.usatoday.com/story/sports/ncaaf/
2013/01/17/manti-teos-catfish-story-common/1566438/).

Bro Code. 2016. "The Code." Retrieved June 7, 2016 (http://www.brocode.org/page/16/).

Brockmann, Hilke, and Jan Delhey. 2010. "Introduction: The Dynamics of Happiness and
the Dynamics of Happiness Research." *Social Indicators Research*, 97: 1–5.

Brody, Jane. 2016. "The Challenges of Male Friendship." *The New York Times,* June 28: D5.

Brooks, Mel. 2001. *The Producers: The New Mel Brooks Musical Original Broadway Cast
Recording.* New York: Sony Music Entertainment Inc.

Bryan, Bradley. 2009. "Approaching Others: Aristotle on Friendship's Possibility." *Political
Theory*, 37 (6): 754–779.

Bryant, J. Alison, and Jennings Bryant. 2003. "Effects of Entertainment Televisual Media on
Children," pp. 195–218 in *The Faces of Televised Media: Teaching, Violence, Selling to
Children*, 2nd edition, edited by Edward L. Palmer and Brian M. Young. Mahwah, NJ:
Lawrence Erlbaum.

Buckingham, Will. 2012. *Happiness: A Practical Guide.* London: Allen & Unwin.

Cafferty, Jack. 2011. "Technology Replacing Personal Interactions at What Cost?" *CNN*, January 3. Retrieved June 19, 2016 (http://caffertyfile.blogs.cnn.com/2011/01/03/technology-
replacing-personal-interactions-at-what-cost/).

Cannarella, John, and Joshua A. Spechler. 2014. "Epidemiological Modeling of Online Social
Network Dynamics." *arXiv:1401.4208*, v1. Retrieved June 21, 2016 (http://arxiv.org/pdf/
1401.4208v1.pdf).

Carr, Deborah, Vicki A. Freedman, Jennifer C. Cornman, and Norbert Schwarz. 2014. "Happy
Marriage, Happy Life? Marital Quality and Subjective Well-being in Later Life." *Journal
of Marriage and Family*, 76(5): 930–948.

Cartwright, Dorwin, and Alvin Zander, eds. 1968. *Group Dynamics,* 3rd ed. Evanson, IL:
Peterson.

Cash, Hilarie, Cosette D. Rae, Ann H. Steel, and Alexander Winkler. 2012. "Internet Addiction: A Brief Summary of Research and Practice." *Current Psychiatry Reviews*, Nov, 8(4):
293–298.

Castells, Manuel. 2009. *Communication Power.* Oxford: Oxford University Press.

CBS This Morning. 2016. "Virtual Reality Check." Original air date, May 13, 2016.

Chalabi, Mona. 2014. "The 100 Most-Used Emojis." *FiveThirtyEight*, June 5. Retrieved June
14, 2016 (http://fivethirtyeight.com/datalab/the-100-most-used-emojis/).

Chamorro-Premuzic, Tomas. 2014. "The Tinder Effect: Psychology of Dating in the Technosexual Era." *The Guardian*, January 17. Retrieved June 21, 2016 (http://www.theguardian.com/media-network/media-network-blog/2014/jan/17/tinder-dating-psychology-technosexual).

Chang, H.H., and R.M. Nayga, Jr. 2010. "Childhood Obesity and Unhappiness: The Influence of Soft Drinks and Fast Food Consumption." *Journal of Happiness Studies* 11: 261–275.

Chokshi, Niraj. 2016. "If You're a Racist, Say You Have Minority Friends. It Helps." *The Washington Post*, February 16. Retrieved June 6, 2016 (https://www.washingtonpost.com/news/wonk/wp/2016/02/16/if-youre-a-racist-say-you-have-minority-friends-it-helps/).

CNN. 2016. "Excessive Selfie-taking Could Be Sign of Mental Illness, Study Says." October 8, 2016. Retrieved October 9, 2016 (http://raycomgroup.worldnow.com/story/33341644/excessive-selfie-taking-could-be-sign-of-mental-illness-study-says).

Cockerham, William. 1995. *The Global Society*. New York: McGraw-Hill.

Cooley, Charles Horton. 1909. *Social Organization*. New York: Scribner.

Cooper, John M. 1977. "Aristotle on the Forms of Friendship." *The Review of Metaphysics* 30 (4): 619–48.

Copen, Casey E., Kimberly Daniels, Jonathan Vespa, and William Mosher. 2012. "First Marriages in the United States: Data from the 2006–2010 National Survey of Family Growth." U.S. Department of Health and Human Services, *National Health Statistics Reports*, 49 (March 22). Retrieved August 20, 2016 (http://www.cdc.gov/nchs/data/nhsr/nhsr049.pdf).

Coulon, Marjorie, Raymond Nowak, Stephane Andanson, Christine Ravel, Pierre G. Marnet, Alain Boissy, and Xavier Boivin. 2013. "Human-lamb Bonding: Oxytocin, Cortisol and Behavioral Responses of Lambs to Human Contacts and Social Separation." *Psychoneuroendocrinology*, 38(4): 499–508.

Creedon, Jeremiah. 2001. "The 19 Kinds of Friends." *UTNE Reader*, September/October. Retrieved June 5, 2016 (http://www.utne.com/community/the-19-kinds-of-friends.aspx).

Crockett, Zachary. 2016. "The Tragic Data Behind Selfie Fatalities." *Priceonomics*, January 29. Retrieved June 14, 2016 (http://priceonomics.com/the-tragic-data-behind-selfie-fatalities/).

Cronin, Anne M. 2015. "Gendering Friendship: Couple Culture, Heteronormativity and the Production of Gender." *Sociology*, 49(6): 1167–1182.

Csikszentmihalyi, Mihaly. 1990. *Flow: The Psychology of Optimal Experience*. New York: HarperCollins.

_____. 1996. *Creativity: The Psychology of Discovery and Invention*. New York: HarperCollins.

Cuckle, Pat, and June Wilson. 2002. "Social Relationships and Friendships Among Young People with Down's Syndrome in Secondary Schools." *British Journal of Special Education*, 29: 66–71.

CyberBully Hotline. 2013. "Catfishing: A Growing Trend in Cyberbullying." Retrieved June 19, 2015 (http://www.cyberbullyhotline.com/catfishing.html).

Daily Kos. 2012. "75 Ways Socialism Has Improved America." Retrieved June 26, 2016 (http://www.dailykos.com/story/2012/3/29/1078852/-75-Ways-Socialism-Has-Improved-America).

Daily Mail. 2010. "Six Out of 10 Couples 'Unhappy in Their Relationship.'" May 31. Retrieved August 20, 2016 (http://www.dailymail.co.uk/news/article-1282851/Six-10-couples-unhappy-relationship.html).

Dastagir, Alia E. 2016. "Why There's Nothing Fake about Facebook Friendship." *USA Today*, February 7. Retrieved June 23, 2016 (http://www.usatoday.com/story/tech/columnist/2016/02/04/facebook-anniversary-future-friendships/79765832/).

Dave, Paresh. 2016. "Snapchat Allows Users to Bring Back Old Images." *Los Angeles Times*, July 7: C3.

Davidson, Lauren. 2015. "Is Your Daily Social Media Usage Higher than Average?" *The Telegraph*, May 17. Retrieved June 19, 2016 (http://www.telegraph.co.uk/finance/newsbysector/mediatechnologyandtelecoms/ 11610959/Is-your-daily-social-media-usage-higher-than-average.html).

Days of the Year. 2016. "Unfriend Day." Retrieved June 29, 2016 (https://www.daysoftheyear. com/days/unfriend-day/).

DeAngelis, Tori. 2008. "The Two Faces of Oxytocin." American Psychological Association, Monitor on Psychology, 39(2): 30.

Dear Abby. 2015. "Family Offers Little Sympathy after Online Boyfriend's Death." As it appeared in *The Citizen*, November 6: B6.

Dear Amy. 2015. "Sisters Engage in 'Friending' War." As it appeared in *The Post-Standard*, April 30: C-8.

Delaney, Tim. 2001. *Community, Sport and Leisure*, 2nd Edition. Auburn, NY: Legend Books.

_____. 2004. *Classical Social Theory: Investigation and Application*. Upper Saddle River, NJ: Prentice Hall.

_____. 2008. *Shameful Behaviors*. Lanham, MD: University Press of America.

_____. 2012a. *Connecting Sociology to Our Lives*. Boulder, CO: Paradigm.

_____. 2012b. "Georg Simmel's Flirting and Secrecy and Its Complicated." *Journalism and Mass Communication*, 2(5) (May): 637–647.

_____. 2013. *American Street Gangs*, 2nd edition. Upper Saddle River, NJ: Pearson.

_____. 2014. *Classical and Contemporary Social Theory: Investigation and Application*. Upper Saddle River, NJ: Pearson.

Delaney, Tim, and Tim Madigan. 2014. *Beyond Sustainability: A Thriving Environment*. Jefferson, NC: McFarland.

_____. 2015. *The Sociology of Sports: An Introduction*, Second Edition. Jefferson, NC: McFarland.

_____. 2016. *Lessons Learned from Popular Culture*. Albany, NY: SUNY Press.

Delaney, Tim, and Allene Wilcox. 2002. "Sports and the Role of the Media," pp. 199–215 in *Values, Society, and Evolution*, edited by Harry Birx and Tim Delaney. Auburn, NY: Legend Books.

Deloitte. 2015. *The Best Places to Work*. Retrieved August 21, 2016 (https://www2.deloitte. com/content/dam/Deloitte/us/Documents/public-sector/us-fed-best-places-to-work-2015.pdf).

Derrida, Jacques. 1997. *Politics of Friendship* (translated by George Collins). London: Verso.

Dictionarywww. 2014. "Frenemy." Retrieved June 28, 2016 (http://www.dictionary.com/browse/frenemy).

_____. 2016a. "Avatar." Retrieved June 28, 2016 (http://www.dictionary.com/browse/avatar).

_____. 2016b. "Byronic." Retrieved April 24, 2016 (http://www.dictionary.com/browse/byronic).

_____. 2016c. "Humor." Retrieved November 27, 2016 (http://www.dictionary.com/browse/humor).

Diener, Ed. 1984. "Subjective Well-being." *Psychological Bulletin*, 95(3): 542–575.

Digi-Capital. 2016. "Augmented/Virtual Reality to Hit #150 Billion Disrupting Mobile by 2020." Retrieved June 27, 2016 (http://www.digi-capital.com/news/2015/04/augmented virtual-reality-to-hit-150-billion-disrupting-mobile-by-2020/#.V3FWjKKPacE).

D'Innocenzio, Anne. 2016. "Virtual Reality Tools Let You Redecorate from the Sofa." As it appeared in *The Post-Standard*, June 21: A-11.

Dumitrescu, A.L., M. Kawamura, B.C. Dogaru, and C.D. Dogaru. 2010. "Relations of Achievement Motives, Satisfaction with Life, Happiness and Oral Health in Romanian University Students." *Oral Health & Preventive Dentistry*, 8: 15–22.

Dunbar, Robin I.M. 2016. "Do Online Social Media Cut Through the Constraints that Limit the Size of Offline Social Networks." *Royal Society Open Science*, January 20. Retrieved June 23, 2016 (http://rsos.royalsocietypublishing.org/content/3/1/150292).

Ebert, Roger. 2010. "Review: Catfish." RogerEbertwww, September 22. Retrieved June 18, 2016 (http://www.rogerebert.com/reviews/catfish-2010).

eBiz. 2016. "Top 15 Most Popular Social Networking Sites/June 2016." Retrieved June 20, 2016 (http://www.ebizmba.com/articles/social-networking-websites).

Eckert, Eric. 2015. "Baylor Expert Affirms, Debunks Founding Father's Famous—and Infamous—Sayings." Baylor Media Communications, July 1. Retrieved November 21, 2016 (http://www.baylor.edu/mediacommunications/news.php?action=story&story=15 7950).

The Economist. 2016. "Done, Bar the Counting." January 23:73–74.

Elkind, David. 2001. *The Hurried Child: Growing Up Too Fast Too Soon*, 3rd ed. Cambridge, MA: Perseus.

Ellie Bean Design. 2013. "11 Characteristics of a True Friend." Retrieved June 7, 2016 (http://elliebeandesign.com/11-characteristics-of-a-true-friend/).

Etkin, Jordan, and Cassie Mogilner. 2016. "When Variety Among Activities Increase Happiness?" *Journal of Consumer Research*, 43 (4): 210–229.

Facebook. 2016. "Facebook Statistics." Retrieved June 20, 2016 (http://www.statisticbrain.com/facebook-statistics/).

Fackler, Martin. 2008. "Internet Addicts Get Help." *Honolulu Star-Bulletin*, January 13: A4.

Farganis, James. 2000. *Readings in Social Theory*, 3rd edition. Boston: McGraw-Hill.

Farran, D.C., and R. Haskins. 1980. "Reciprocal Influence in the Social Interactions of Mothers and Three-Year-Old Children from Different Socioeconomic Backgrounds." *Child Development*, 51: 780–791.

Farren, Michael. 2016. "Pokemon Go Represents the Best of Capitalism." A Medium Corporation, July 14. Retrieved July 26 (https://medium.com/concentrated-benefits/if-you-play-pok%C3%A9mon-go-team-rocket-wins-b2d04efd2ea0#.k2naoiygl).

Flavel, John, Patricia H. Miller, and Scott A. Miller. 2002. *Cognitive Development*, 4th ed. Upper Saddle River, NJ: Prentice Hall.

Flynn, Deborah M., and Stephanie MacLeod. 2015. "Determinants of Happiness in Undergraduate University Students." *College Student Journal*, 49(3): 452–460.

Fredrickson, Barbara. 2011. "Are You Getting Enough Positivity in Your Diet?" Greater Good Science Center, June 21. Retrieved November 21, 2016 (http://greatergood.berkeley.edu/article/item/are_you_getting_enough_positivity_in_your_diet/).

The Free Dictionary. 2016a. "Virtual." Retrieved June 23, 2016 (http://www.thefreedictionary.com/virtual).

_____. 2016b. "Frenemy." Retrieved June 28, 2016 (http://www.thefreedictionary.com/Frienemy).

_____. 2016c. "Humor." Retrieved November 27, 2016 (http://www.thefreedictionary.com/humor).

Freud, Sigmund. 1989. *The Ego and the Id: The Standard Edition*, with a biographical introduction by Peter Gay and edited by James Strachey. New York: W.W. Norton.

Friedlander, Ruthie. 2014. "21 Types of Best Friends Everyone Has." *Elle*, February 27. Retrieved June 6, 2016 (http://www.elle.com/life-love/news/a15306/twenty-one-types-of-best-friends/).

Gabillet, Annie. 2009. "You Choose: Best Female Version of 'Bros Before Hos.'" PopSugarwww. Retrieved June 7, 2016 (http://www.popsugar.com/love/You-Choose-Best-Female-Version-Bros-Before-Hos-3281647).

Gallagher, Conor. 2012. *If Aristotle's Kid Had an iPod: Ancient Wisdom for Modern Parents.* Charlotte, NC: Saint Benedict Press.

Gallup. 2016. "70% of U.S. Workers Not Engaged at Work." Retrieved August 21, 2016 (http://www.gallup.com/services/178514/state-american-workplace.aspx).

Genzlinger, Neil. 2016. "In the Footsteps of Harry and Sally." *New York Times*, December 24. Retrieved December 25 (http://www.nytimes.com/2016/12/24/travel/footsteps-when-harry-met-sally-new-york.html)

Gergen, Kenneth J. 1991. *The Saturated Self.* New York: BasicBooks.

The Globe and Mail. 2015. "What Is the Dark Web and Who Uses It?" August 19. Retrieved June 14, 2016 (http://www.theglobeandmail.com/technology/tech-news/what-is-the-dark-web-and-who-uses-it/article26026082/).

Goffman, Erving. 1959. *The Presentation of Self in Everyday Life.* Garden City, NY: Anchor.

_____. 1961. *Encounters: Two Studies in the Sociology of Interaction—Fun in Games & Role Distance.* Indianapolis, IN: Bobbs-Merrill.

Goodman, Tim. 2013. "Manti Teʼo, 'Catfish,' Katie Couric, Oprah and the Sports World: Paging Dr. Phil!" *The Hollywood Reporter*, January 24. Retrieved June 18, 2015 (http://www. hollywoodreporter.com/bastard-machine/manti-teo-story-hooks-media-415094).

Grayling, A.C. 2013. *Friendship*. New Haven, CT: Yale University Press.

Greater Good Science Center. 2016a. "What Is Happiness?" Retrieved November 21, 2016 (http://greatergood.berkeley.edu/topic/happiness/definition#).

_____. 2016b. "Awe Narrative." Retrieved November 27, 2016 (http://ggia.berkeley.edu/ practice/awe_narrative).

Gregoire, Carolyn. 2013. "Happiness Index: Only 1 in 3 Americans Are Very Happy, According to Harris Poll." *Huffington Post*, June 1. Retrieved August 18, 2016 (http://www.huffington post.com/2013/06/01/happiness-index-only-1-in_n_3354524.html).

Grewen, Karen M., Susan S. Girdler, Janet Amico, and Kathleen C. Light. 2005. "Effects of Partner Support on Resting Oxytocin, Cortisol, Norephinephrine, and Blood Pressure Before and After Warm Partner Contact." *Psychosomatic Medicine*, 67(4): 531–538.

Griffin, James. 1986. *Well-being: Its Meaning, Measurement, and Moral Importance*. Oxford, England: Clarendon Press.

Gruber, H.A. 2000. "The Story of Greeks: Damon and Pythias." Retrieved July 2, 2016 (http:// www.mainlesson.com/display.php?author=guerber&book=greeks&story=damon).

Günter, Barrie, Caroline Oates, and Mark Blades. 2005. *Advertising to Children on TV: Content, Impact, and Regulation*. Mahwah, NJ: Lawrence Erlbaum.

Gurko, Miriam. 1974. *The Ladies of Seneca Falls*. New York: Schocken Books.

Haig, Ed. 2017. "Meet Aristotle, the Baby Monitor of the Future." *USA Today*. January 4: 4B.

Harlan, Jane, and Richard Pillard. 1976. *The Wild Boy of Aveyron*. Cambridge, MA: Harvard University Press.

The Harris Poll. 2016. "Latest Happiness Index Reveals American Happiness at All-Time Low." *The Harris Poll*, July 8. Retrieved August 18, 2016 (http://www.theharrispoll.com/ health-and-life/American-Happiness-at-All-Time-Low.html).

Healthline. 2012. "Did You Know 80% of Individuals Affected by Depression Do Not Receive Any Treatment? Learn More Depression Statistics & Facts." Retrieved August 21, 2016 (http://www.healthline.com/health/depression/statistics-infographic).

Helliwell, Cedric, and Haifang Huang. 2013. "Comparing the Happiness Effects of Real and On-line Friends." U.S. National Library of Medicine National Institute of Health, 8(9).

Henderson, Hannah. 2016. "Muhammad Ali was My Pen Pal for 30 Years." *BBC*, June 10. Retrieved June 10, 2016 (http://www.bbc.com/news/world-us-canada-36461015).

Hershfield, Hal E., Cassie Mogilner, and Uri Barnea. 2016. "People Who Choose Time Over Money Are Happier." *Social Psychological & Personality Science*. Retrieved November 26, 2016 (http://spp.sagepub.com/content/early/2016/05/18/1948550616649239.full).

Hitwise US. 2008. "Top 20 Websites—January, 2008." Retrieved circa January 2009 (www. hitwise.com/datacenter/rankings.php).

Holiday Insights. 2016. "Make a Friend Day." Retrieved July 26, 2016 (http://www.holiday insights.com/moreholidays/February/makeafriendday.htm).

Holmes, Mary. 2011. "Emotional Reflexivity in Contemporary Friendships: Understanding It Using Elias and Facebook Etiquette." *Sociological Research Online*, 16(1):11. Retrieved June 23, 2016 (http://www.socresonline.org.uk/16/1/11.html).

Homans, George. 1950. *The Human Group*. New York: Harcourt & Brace.

_____. 1961. *Social Behavior: Its Elementary Forms*. New York: Harcourt, Brace and World.

HubPages. 2015. "102 Fun Nicknames for Best Friends." Retrieved June 6, 2016 (http:// hubpages.com/relationships/nicknames-for-best-friends).

The Huffington Post. 2013. "How Stress Affects the Body." January 10. Retrieved August 21, 2016 (http://www.huffingtonpost.com/heartmath-llc/how-stress-affects-the-body_b_ 2422522.html).

Hughes, Clyde. 2015. "Selfie Deaths Beat Fatal Shark Attacks 12–8 So Far in 2015." *Newsmax*, September 23. Retrieved June 14, 2016 (http://www.newsmax.com/TheWire/selfie-deaths-fatal-shark/2015/09/23/id/692836/).

Humphreys, Joe. 2016. "What Aristotle Can Teach Us About Friendship." *Irish Times*, November 1. Retrieved November 3, 2016 (http://www.irishtimes.com/culture/what-aristotle-can-teach-us-about-friendship-1.2844486).

IMDb. 2016. "Avatar." Retrieved June 28, 2016 (http://www.imdb.com/title/tt0499549/).

Ingraham, Christopher. 2016. "Why Smart People are Better Off with Fewer Friends." *The Washington Post*, March 18. Retrieved June 24 (https://www.washingtonpost.com/news/wonk/wp/2016/03/18/why-smart…).

Inguaggiato, Brodie. 2014. "Yik Yak App May Perpetuate Cyberbullying." *The Stylus*, October 1: 10.

Jayson, Sharon. 2006. "Are Social Norms Steadily Unraveling?" *USA Today*, April 13: 4D.

Joel, Samantha. 2015. "Expressing Your Insecurities to Your Partner Can Actually Create More Insecurities." *Science of Relations*. Retrieved June 7, 2016 (http://www.scienceofrelationships.com/home/2015/2/23/expressing-your-insecurities-to-your-partner-can-actually-cr.html).

Juette, Melvin, and Ronald J. Berger. 2008. *Wheelchair Warrior: Gangs, Disability, and Basketball*. Philadelphia: Temple University Press.

Kahneman, Daniel, and Angus Deaton. 2010. "High Income Improves Evaluation of Life but Not Emotional Well-being." *Proceedings of the National Academy of Sciences*, 107(38): 16489–16493.

Kallen, Horace. 1956. *The Social Dynamics of George H. Mead*. Washington, D.C.: Public Affairs Press.

Karaian, Jason. 2015. "We Now Spend More than Eight Hours a Day Consuming Media." Quartzwww, June 1. Retrieved June 19 (http://qz.com/416416/we-now-spend-more-than-eight-hours-a-day-consuming-media/).

Kasser, Tim, and Kennon M. Sheldon. 2009. "Time Affluence as a Path Toward Personal Happiness and Ethical Business Practice: Empirical Evidence from Four Studies." *Journal of Business Ethics*, 84: 243–255.

Kelly, Maura. 2010. "The 3 Kinds of Friendship." *Marie Claire*, May 6. Retrieved December 14, 2016 (http://www.marieclaire.com/sex-love/a4028/friendships-aristotle-utility-ethics-lifestyles/).

Kelton Research and Support. 2008. "News & Information." Retrieved circa January 2009 (http://sev.prnewswire.com/computer-electronics).

Keyes, Alexa. 2014. "Top 15 Most Used Emojis on Twitter." *NBC News*, June 19. Retrieved June 14, 2016 (http://www.nbcnews.com/nightly-news/top-15-most-used-emojis-twitter-n135201).

Kopan, Tal. 2014. "Poll: Most Unhappy with Government." *Politico*, January 22. Retrieved August 22, 2016 (http://www.politico.com/story/2014/01/poll-government-satisfaction-102463).

Krotoski, Aleks. 2010. "Robin Dunbar: We Can Only Ever Have 150 Friends, At Most." *The Guardian*, March 13. Retrieved June 24, 2016 (https://www.theguardian.com/technology/2010/mar/14/my-bright-idea-robin-dunbar).

Krug, Gary. 2005. *Communication, Technology, and Cultural Change*. Thousand Oaks, CA: Sage.

Kumar, Amit, Matthew A. Killingsworth, and Thomas Gilovich. 2014. "Waiting for Merlot: Anticipatory Consumption of Experiential and Material Purchases." *Psychological Science*, 25(10): 1924–1931.

Leaf, Caroline. 2013. *Switch on Your Brain: The Key to Peak Happiness, Thinking, and Health*. Grand Rapids, MI: Baker Books.

Lee, BoNhia. 2007. "How 3 Girls from Korea Discovered Friendship and Their Heritage in CNY." *The Post-Standard*, March 30: A-1, A-4.

Leigh, Andrew. 2006. "Growth Matters." *Aurora Magazine*, Issue 3 (July). Retrieved circa August 2013 (http://people.anu.edu.au/andrew.leigh/pdf/GrowthMatters.pdf).

Leiner, Barry M., Vinton G. Cerf, David D. Clark, Robert E. Kahn, Leonard Kleinrock, Daniel C. Lynch, Jon Postel, Larry G. Roberts, and Stephen Wolff. 2014. "Brief History of the

Internet." *Internet Society*. Retrieved October 21, 2015 (http://www.internetsociety.org/internet/what-internet/history-internet/brief-history-internet).

Levine, Laura E., and Joyce Munsch. 2016. *Child Development from Infancy to Adolescence: An Active Learning Approach*. Thousand Oaks, CA: Sage.

Levit, Alexandra. 2011. "Work Friends vs. Real Friends." WetFeet.com, May 9. Retrieved June 6, 2016 (https://www.wetfeet.com/articles/work-friends-vs-real-friends).

Levy, Andrew. 2011. "Sorry Chaps, Women Only Get Dressed Up to Impress Each Other." *Daily Mail*, June 10. Retrieved April 25, 2016 (http://www.dailymail.co.uk/news/article-2002391/Sorry-chaps-women-dress-impress-other.html).

Lewis, Jane, and Anne West. 2009. "Friending: London-based Undergraduates' Experiences of Facebook." *New Media Society*, 11 (7): 1209–1229.

Li, Norman, and Satoshi Kanazawa. 2016. "Country Roads, Take Me Home…To My Friends: How Intelligence, Population Density, and Friendship Affect Modern Happiness." *British Journal of Psychology*. Retrieved June 24, 2016 (http://www.ncbi.nlm.nih.gov/pubmed/26847844).

Lien, Tracey. 2016. "A Breakout Hit for Augmented Reality." *Los Angeles Times*, July 12:C1.

Limbasiya, Nailesh. 2015. "The Views on Happiness: A Dialectic Approach." *International Journal of Computational Engineering & Management*, 18(5): 12–15.

Loy, John, and Alan Ingham. 1981. "Play, Games, and Sport in the Psychological Development of Children and Youth," pp. 189–216 in *Sport, Culture and Society*, edited by John Loy, Gerald Kenyon, and Barry McPherson. Philadelphia: Lea & Febiger.

Lyubomirsky, Sonja, Laura King, and Ed Diener. 2005. "The Benefits of Frequent Positive Affect: Does Happiness Lead to Success?" *Psychological Bulletin*, 131(6): 803–855.

Lyubomirsky, Sonja. 2008. *The How of Happiness: A Scientific Approach to Getting the Life You Want*. New York: Penguin.

Madigan, Tim, and Peter Stone. 2016. *Bertrand Russell, Public Intellectual*. Rochester, NY: Tiger Bark Press.

Madigan, Tim. 2007. "Aristotle's E-mail: Or, Friendship in the Cyber Age." *Philosophy Now*, 61, May/June: 13–15.

———. 2016. "Literary Philosophers: Irving Singer and George Santayana." *Overheard in Seville: The Bulletin of the George Santayana Society*, No. 34, Fall 2016: 17–22.

Maloney, Patricia. 2012. "Online Networks and Emotional Energy: How Pro-anorexic Websites Use Interaction Ritual Chains to (Re)form Identity." *Information, Communication & Society*, 16(1): 105–24.

Marche, Stephen. 2012 (May). "Is Facebook Making Us Lonely?" *The Atlantic*. Retrieved June 21, 2016 (http://www.theatlantic.com/magazine/archive/2012/05/is-facebook-making-us-lonely/308930/).

Marriott, Alexander. 2011. "The Curse of the Internet: Fake Historical Quotes." Retrieved November 21, 2016 (http://alexandermarriott.blogspot.com/2011/11/curse-of-internet-fake-historical.html).

Martindale, Don. 1988. *The Nature and Types of Sociological Theory*. Prospect Heights, IL: Waveland Press.

Mashable.com. 2016. "Augmented Reality." Retrieved June 27, 2016 (http://mashable.com/category/augmented-reality/).

Maslow, Abraham. 1954. *Motivation and Personality*. New York: Harper & Row.

Masten. Ann S., and Abigail H. Gewirtz. 2006. "Resilience in Development: The Importance of Early Childhood." *Encyclopedia on Early Childhood Development*. Retrieved circa September 2007 (www.child-encyclopedia.com/documents/Masten-GewritzANGxp.pdf).

Mayo Clinic. 2016. "Depression (Major Depressive Disorder)." Retrieved August 21, 2016 (http://www.mayoclinic.org/diseases-conditions/depression/basics/definition/con-20032977).

Mead, George Herbert. 1934. *Mind, Self & Society*, edited and with introduction by Charles W. Morris. Chicago: University of Chicago Press.

_____. 1964. *Selected Writings*, edited by Andrew Reck. Indianapolis, IN: Bobbs-Merrill.

Meath, Michael. 2016. "Beware of Facebook's Cultural Echo Chamber." *The Post-Standard*, June 2: A-14.

Medical-Dictionarywww. 2016. "Fatigue." Retrieved April 25, 2016 (http://medical-dictionary. thefreedictionary.com/Fatigue).

Medicine.Netwww. 2016. "Definition of Fatigue." Retrieved April 26, 2016 (http://www. medicinenet.com/script/main/art.asp?articlekey=9879).

Meltzer, Bernard, John Petras, and Larry Reynolds. 1975. *Symbolic Interactionism—Genesis, Varieties & Criticisms*. Boston: Routledge & Kegan Paul.

Merriam-Webster Dictionary. 2016a. "Bromance." Retrieved June 6, 2016 (http://www. merriam-webster.com/dictionary/bromance).

_____. 2016b. "Virtual." Retrieved June 23, 2016 (http://www.merriam-webster.com/dictionary/ virtual).

Meshi, Dar, Carmen Morawetz, and Hauke R. Heekeren. 2013 (Nov). "Facebook, Being Cool, and Your Brain: What Science Tells Us." *Frontiers in Human Neuroscience*, 1(4):1–17.

Milgram, Stanley. 1974. *Obedience to Authority*. New York: Harper Torchbooks.

Mill, John Stuart. 1863/1979. *Utilitarianism*. New York: Hackett Publishing Company.

Miller, David. 1973. *George Herbert Mead: Self, Language, and the World*. Austin: University of Texas Press.

Mohan, Geoffrey. 2013. "Why our Brains Like Facebook." *Los Angeles Times*, as it appeared in *The Post-Standard*, September 10: D-8.

Montaigne, Michel de. 1991. *On Friendship*. New York: Penguin Books.

Moreau, Elise. 2016. "The Top 25 Social Networking Sites People Are Using." Aboutwww, February 13. Retrieved June 20, 2016 (http://webtrends.about.com/od/socialnetworking reviews/tp/Social-Networking-Sites.htm).

Moriarty, Rick. 2009. "Facebook Co-founder's Preference: 'Defriend.'" *The Post-Standard*, November 18: A-3.

MTV. 2016. "Catfish: The TV Show." Retrieved June 18, 2016 (http://www.mtv.com/shows/ catfish-the-tv-show).

Murphy, Kate. 2016. "Do Your Friends Actually Like You?" *The New York Times*, August 7: A7.

Myers, Christi. 2013. "Report: Americans Most Unhappy People in the World." *ABC 13 Eye Witness News* (Houston), February 20. Retrieved August 21, 2016 (http://abc13.com/ archive/9000225/).

National Center for Education Statistics (NCES). 2014. *Indicators of School Crime and Safety: 2013*. "Key Findings." Retrieved June 20, 2015 (http://nces.ed.gov/programs/crime indicators/crimeindicators2013/key.asp).

National Conference of State Legislatures. 2015. "State Cyberstalking and Cyberharassment Laws." Retrieved June 20, 2015 (http://www.ncsl.org/research/telecommunications-and- information-technology/cyberstalking-and-cyberharassment-laws.aspx).

National Day Calendar (NDC). 2016. "Calendar at a Glance." Retrieved June 29, 2016 (http:// www.nationaldaycalendar.com/calendar-at-a-glance/).

National Down Syndrome Society (NDSS). 2012. "Positive Steps for Social Inclusion." Retrieved June 6, 2016 (http://www.ndss.org/Resources/Wellness/Recreation-Friendship/).

National Institute on Aging. 2009. "Research Shows that Happiness Spreads Through Social Groups. Retrieved June 5, 2016 (https://www.nia.nih.gov/newsroom/announcements/ 2009/05/research-shows-happiness-spreads-through-social-groups).

Nehamas, Alexander. 2016. *On Friendship*. New York: Basic Books.

Nelson, Dean. 2011. "Bhutan's 'Gross National Happiness Index.'" *The Telegraph*, March 2. Retrieved November 27, 2016 (http://www.telegraph.co.uk/news/worldnews/asia/ bhutan/8355028/Bhutans-Gross-National-Happiness-index.html).

Neuman, M. Gary. 2002. *Emotional Infidelity: How to Affair-Proof Your Marriage and 10 Other Secrets to a Great Relationship*. New York: Three Rivers Press.

Neus, Nora. 2015. "A Friendship Forged by Katrina." *CNN*, August 28. Retrieved June 6, 2016 (http://www.cnn.com/2015/08/28/us/mississippi-school-katrina/).

New World Encyclopedia. 2008. "Mass Media." Retrieved June 12, 2016 (http://www.new worldencyclopedia.org/entry/Mass_media).

_____. 2013. "Computer." Retrieved June 12, 2016 (http://www.newworldencyclopedia.org/ entry/Computer).

Newton, Michael. 2002. *Savage Girls and Wild Boys: A History of Feral Children*. London: Faber and Faber.

Nickles, Jesse. 2014. "Yik Yak: The Anonymous 'Shaming' App that Recalls Unpleasant Bullying Memories of JuicyCampus.com." *College Times*, March 15. Retrieved June 18, 2016 (https://collegetimes.co/yik-yak/).

Nixon, Howard II, and James H. Frey. 1996. *A Sociology of Sport*. Belmont, CA: Wadsworth.

Nussbaum, Martha. 1988. *The Fragility of Goodness*. New York: Cambridge University Press.

O'Connor, Lydia. 2014. "'Revenge Porn' Law Sees First Conviction in California." *Huffington Post*, December 2. Retrieved June 17, 2016 (http://www.huffingtonpost.com/2014/12/02/ revenge-porn-california-first-conviction_n_6258158.html).

Old Telephones. 2016. "The History." Retrieved June 12, 2016 (http://oldtelephones.com/the-history/).

Olds, Jacqueline, and Richard S. Schwartz. 2009. *The Lonely American*. Boston: Beacon Press.

O'Neill, Claire. 2012. "Are Your Facebook Friends Really Your Friends?" *NPR*, May 23. Retrieved June 23, 2016 (http://www.npr.org/sections/pictureshow/2012/04/23/151201002/ are-your-facebook-friends-really-your-friends).

Online Slang Dictionary. 2006. "Slang Words for Friend." Retrieved June 6, 2016 (http://onlineslangdictionary.com/thesaurus/words+meaning+friend,+friends.html).

Ophir, Eyal, Clifford Nass, and Anthony D. Wagner. 2009. "Cognitive Control in Media Multitaskers." *Proceedings of the National Academy of Sciences of the United States of America (PNAS)*, Sept, 106(37): 15583–15587. Retrieved June 19, 2016 (http://www.ncbi.nlm.nih. gov/pmc/articles/PMC2747164/).

O'Rourke, Fran. 2016. *Aristotelian Interpretations*. Kildare, Ireland: Irish Academic Press.

Ott, J.C. 2010. "Government and Happiness in 130 Nations: Good Governance Fosters Higher Level and More Equality of Happiness." *Social Indicators Research*, 102 (1): 3–32.

The Oxford English Dictionary. 2013. "The Oxford Dictionaries Word of the Year 2013 Is… Selfie." Retrieved January 12, 2014 (http://blog.oxforddictionaries.com/2013/11/word-of-the-year-2013-winner/).

Palmer, Roxanne. 2013. "Where Does 'Catfish' Come From? Online Hoax Movie Inspired by Fisherman's Lore." *International Business Times*, January 17. Retrieved June 18, 2015 (http://www.ibtimes.com/where-does-catfish-come-online-hoax-movie-inspired-fishermans-lore-1022374).

Pampel, Fred. 2000. *Sociological Lines and Ideas*. New York: Worth.

Parade. 2011. "Intelligence Report." April 3: 4.

Perry, Gina. 2013. *Behind the Shock Machine*. New York: The New Press.

Pfuetze, Paul. 1954. *Self, Society and Existence: Human Nature and Dialogue in the Thoughts of George Herbert Mead and Martin Buber*. New York: Harper Torch Books.

Piaget, Jean. [1936] 1952. *The Origins of Intelligence in Children*. New York: International Universities Press.

_____. 1954. *The Construction of Reality in the Child*. New York: Basic Books.

Piqueras, J.A., W. Kuhne, P. Vera-Villarroel, A. van Straten, and P. Cuijpers. 2011. "Happiness and Health Behaviors in Chilean College Students." *Journal of Religion and Health*, 52: 450–453.

Pleasant, Robert. 2016. "Pokemon GO: One Free App's Big Economic Impact." *Silicon Angle*, July 14. Retrieved July 26 (http://siliconangle.com/blog/2016/07/14/pokemon-go-one-free-apps-big-economic-impact/).

Pony Express National Museum. 2016. "The History of the Pony Express." Retrieved June 12, 2016 (http://ponyexpress.org/history/).

The Post-Standard. 2009. "What Word Sums up the Year 2009?" November, 17: A-1.

_____. 2010. "Anti-Facebook Pastor Was Once in Threesome." November, 21: A-4.

Powell, Hannah Lyons. 2014. "The Ultimate TV & Movie BFFs." *Glamour*, July 21. Retrieved June 9, 2016 (http://www.glamourmagazine.co.uk/celebrity/celebrity-galleries/2014/07/best-tv-and-movie-best-friendships-bffs/viewgallery/994856).

Price, A.W. 1989. *Love and Friendship in Plato and Aristotle*. New York: Oxford University Press.

Proctor, Carmel, P. Alex Linley, and John Maltby. 2010. "Very Happy Youths: Benefits of Very High Life Satisfaction Among Adolescents." *Social Indicators Research*, 98(3): 519–532.

Psychology Today. 2016. "Loneliness." Retrieved June 21, 2016 (https://www.psychologytoday.com/basics/loneliness).

Pyle, Richard. 2000. "Batch of New Words for Dictionary." *CBS News*, June 27. Retrieved circa July 14, 2008 (www.cbsnews.com/stories/2000/06/27/tech/main210016.shtml%20or%20www.merriam-webster.com/info/newworlds09.htm).

Quora. 2016. "What Is the Female Equivalent of 'Bros Before Hoes'"? Retrieved June 7, 2016 (https://www.quora.com/What-is-the-female-equivalent-of-bros-before-hoes).

ReachOutwww. 2016. "What Makes a Good Friend?" Retrieved June 5, 2016 (http://au.reachout.com/what-makes-a-good-friend).

Real, Michael R. 1996. *Exploring Media Culture: A Guide*. Thousand Oaks, CA: Sage.

Reynolds, Larry. 1993. *Interactionism: Exposition and Critique*, 3rd ed. Dix Hills, NY: General Hall.

Richter, Felix. 2015. "Americans Use Electronic Media 11+ Hours a Day." *Statista*. Retrieved December 14, 2015 (http://www.statista.com/chart/1971/electronic-media-use/).

Riparbelli, Laura. 2011. "12-Year-Old Sentenced for Cyberstalking Classmate." *ABC News*, July 14. Retrieved June 16 2016 (http://abcnews.go.com/Technology/12-year-sentenced-washington-cyberstalking-case/story?id=14072315).

Rist, John M. 1980. "Epicurus on Friendship." *Classical Philology*, 75(2): 121–129.

Ritzer, George. 2000. *Classical Social Theory*, 3rd ed. Boston: McGraw-Hill.

Roberts, Paul. 2014. *The Impulse Society: America in the Age of Instant Gratification*. New York: Bloomsbury.

Robinson, Laura. 2010. "Cyberself: The Self-ing Project Goes Online, Symbolic Interaction in the Digital Age." *New Media & Society*, 9(1): 93–110.

Russell, Bertrand. 1930. *The Conquest of Happiness*. London: Allen & Unwin.

Ruth, David. 2012. "Women Use Emoticons More Than Men in Text Messaging ;-)." *Current News* (Rice University News & Media). Retrieved June 14, 2016 (http://news.rice.edu/2012/10/10/women-use-emoticons-more-than-men-in-text-messaging-2/).

Rutledge, Pamela B. 2013. "Making Sense of Selfies." *Psychology Today*, July 6. Retrieved October 9, 2016 (https://www.psychologytoday.com/blog/positively-media/201307/making-sense-selfies).

Ryan, John, and William M. Wentworth. 1999. *Media and Society*. Boston: Allyn and Bacon.

Ryan, Patrick. 2016. "Billy Bob Thornton Suits Up for Battle in 'Goliath.'" *USA Today*, October 17: 6B.

Saad, Lydia. 2012. "U.S. Workers Least Happy with Their Work Stress and Pay." *Gallup*, November 12. Retrieved August 21, 2016 (http://www.gallup.com/poll/158723/workers-least-happy-work-stress-pay.aspx).

Saint-Exupéry, Antoine de. 1943/2000. *The Little Prince*. New York: Harcourt.

Sakaluk, M.A. 2012. "Breaking Up Bad: The Best and Worst Ways to Break Up." *Science of Relations*. Retrieved June 12, 2016 (http://www.scienceofrelationships.com/home/2012/10/1/breaking-up-bad-the-best-and-worst-ways-to-break-up.html).

Sanacore, Wendy. 2014. "Are Work Friends 'True' Friends?" Linkedinwww. Retrieved June 6, 2016 (https://www.linkedin.com/pulse/20140715200730-44541711-are-work-friends-true-friends).

Santrock. John W. 2007. *Children*, 10th ed. New York: McGraw-Hill.

Sarkisova, Gayana. 2012. "The 10 Commandments to Being Friends with Benefits." *Elite Daily*, November 8. Retrieved June 6, 2016 (http://elitedaily.com/dating/sex/10-commandments-friends-benefits/).

Saul, Heather. 2014. "Tiananmen Square: What Happened to Tank Man?" *The Independent*, June 4. Retrieved June 13, 2016 (http://www.independent.co.uk/news/world/asia/tiananmen-square-what-happened-to-tank-man-9483398.html).

Schaffer, H.R. 1984. *The Child's Entry into a Social World*. New York: Harcourt Brace Jovanovich.

Schaub, Diana J. 2003. *Aristotle and the Philosophy of Friendship*. New York: Cambridge University Press.

Scott, Paula Spencer. 2016. "Feeling Awe May Be the Secret to Health and Happiness." *Parade*, October 9: 6–8.

Seinfeld. 1992. "The Boyfriend." First air date, February 12. Retrieved July 3, 2016 (http://www.seinfeldscripts.com/TheBoyfriend2.htm).

Selfhout, Maarteen, Susan J.T. Branje, Tom F.M. ter Bogt, and Wim H.J. Meeus. 2009 (Feb). "The Role of Music Preferences in Early Adolescents' Friendship Formation and Stability." *Journal of Adolescence*, 32(1): 95–107.

Seligman, Martin E.P., and Ed Royzman. 2003 (July). "Authentic Happiness." University of Penn. Retrieved November 23, 2016 (https://www.authentichappiness.sas.upenn.edu/newsletters/authentichappiness/happiness).

Shaer, Matthew. 2009. "English Gets Millionth Word, Site Says." *Christian Science Monitor*, June 10. Retrieved circa November, 2009 (http://news.aol.com/article/one-millionth-word-web-20/5222727?cid+main).

Shaw, M., and D.W. Black. 2008. "Internet Addiction: Definition, Assessment, Epidemiology and Clinical Management." *CNS Drugs*, 22 (5): 353–65. Retrieved June 19, 2016 (http://www.ncbi.nlm.nih.gov/pubmed/18399706).

Shin, Paul H.B. 2014. "Tiananmen Square Tank Man: 25 Years Later, His Memory Lives On." *ABC News*, June 3. Retrieved June 13, 2016 (http://abcnews.go.com/International/tiananmen-square-tank-man-25-years-memory-lives/story?id=23965993).

Shontell, Alyson. 2010. "80% Hate Their Jobs—But Should You Choose a Passion or a Paycheck." *Business Insider*, October 4. Retrieved August 21, 2016 (http://www.businessinsider.com/what-do-you-do-when-you-hate-your-job-2010-10).

Simmel, Georg, and Everett C. Hughes. 1949. "The Sociology of Sociability." *American Journal of Sociology*, 55(3) (Nov.): 254–261.

Singer, Irving. 1984–1987. *The Nature of Love: The Modern World*, volumes 1–3. Cambridge, MA: MIT Press.

Singh, Maanvi. 2014. "You Can Buy Happiness, If It's an Experience." *NPR*, September 3. Retrieved November 24, 2016 (http://www.npr.org/sections/health-shots/2014/09/03/345540607/look-forward-to-the-trip-not-the-gadgets-to-be-truly-happy).

Smith, Craig. 2016. "By the Numbers: 80 Amazing Snapchat Statistics." *DMR Stats/Gadgets*. Retrieved June 21, 2016 (http://expandedramblings.com/index.php/snapchat-statistics/).

Sober Bastard. 2012. "Friends vs Drinking Buddies." Retrieved June 6, 2016 (http://soberbastard.com/friendsfamily/friends-vs-drinking-buddies/).

SpyBuddy. 2016. "SpyBuddy 2013." Retrieved June 16, 2016 (http://www.exploreanywhere.com/products/spybuddy/).

Statista. 2016a. "Number of Daily Active Snapchat Users from March 2014 to June 2016 (in millions)." Retrieved June 21, 2016 (http://www.statista.com/statistics/545967/snapchat-app-dau/).

_____. 2016b. "Distribution of Snapchat Users in the United States as of February 2016, by Age." Retrieved June 21, 2016 (http://www.statista.com/statistics/326452/snapchat-age-group-usa/).

_____. 2016c. "Number of World of Warcraft Subscribers from 1st Quarter to 3rd Quarter 2015 (in Millions." Retrieved June 28, 2016 (http://www.statista.com/statistics/276601/number-of-world-of-warcraft-subscribers-by-quarter/).

_____. 2016d. "Distribution of World of Warcraft Players in 2013, By Age Group." Retrieved June 28, 2016 (http://www.statista.com/statistics/327283/wow-players-age/).

Stebner, Beth. 2013. "Over 70% of U.S. Workers Unhappy About Their Job: Poll." *Daily News*,

June 24. Retrieved August 21, 2016 (http://www.nydailynews.com/news/national/70-u-s-workers-hate-job-poll-article-1.1381297).

Steinberg, Laurence, Marc H. Bornstein, Deborah Lowe Vandell, and Karen S. Rook. 2011. *Lifespan Development: Infancy Through Adulthood*. Belmont, CA: Cengage.

Steiner-Adair, Catherine. 2015. "Are You Addicted to the Internet?" *CNN*, July 17. Retrieved June 19, 2016 (http://www.cnn.com/2015/07/17/opinions/steiner-adair-internet-addiction/).

Stinson, Barney, with Matt Kuhn. 2008. *The Bro Code*. New York: Simon & Schuster.

Stockton, Nick. 2014. "What's Up with That: Why Do All My Friends Like the Same Music?" Wiredwww, September 16. Retrieved June 6, 2016 (http://www.wired.com/2014/09/whats-friends-like-music/).

Stokel-Walker, Chris. 2013. "Second Life's Strange Second Life." TheVerge.com, September 24. Retrieved June 28, 2016 (http://www.theverge.com/2013/9/24/4698382/second-lifes-strange-second-life).

StopBullying.gov. 2015. "What Is Cyberbullying?" Retrieved June 19, 2015 (http://www.stopbullying.gov/cyberbullying/what-is-it/).

Stout, Hilary. 2010. "Antisocial Networking?" *New York Times*, as it appeared in *The Post-Standard*, June 3: C-2.

Thai, Michael, Matthew J. Hornsey, and Fiona Kate Barlow. 2016. "Friends with Moral Credentials: Minority Friendships Reduce Attributions of Racism for Majority Group Members Who Make Conceivably Racist Statements." *Social Psychosocial & Personality Science*, February. Retrieved June 6, 2016 (http://spp.sagepub.com/content/early/2016/01/27/1948550615624140.abstract).

Thayer, H.S. 1968. *Meaning and Action: A Critical History of Pragmatism*. New York: Bobbs-Merrill.

Thelwall, Mike. 2010. "Emotion Homophily in Social Network Site Messages." *First Monday*, 15(4–5). Retrieved June 23, 2016 (http://journals.uic.edu/ojs/index.php/fm/article/view/2897/2483).

Think Exist. 2016. "Benjamin Franklin Quotes." Retrieved November 21, 2016 (http://thinkexist.com/quotation/our_new_constitution_is_now_established-and_has/154933.html).

Time and Date. 2016. "International Day of Friendship." Retrieved June 29, 2016 (http://www.timeanddate.com/holidays/un/friendship-day).

Tinder. 2016. "By the Numbers: 41 Impressive Tinder Statistics." Retrieved June 21, 2016 (http://expandedramblings.com/index.php/tinder-statistics/).

Today. 2016. "Death of the Mall." Original airdate, June 19, on NBC.

True Activist. 2014. "Scientists Link Selfies to Narcissism, Addiction & Mental Illness." Retrieved October 9, 2016 (http://www.trueactivist.com/scientists-link-selfies-to-narcissism-addiction-mental-illness/).

Tugade, Michele M., and Barbara L. Fredrickson. 2004. "Resilient Individuals Use Positive Emotions to Bounce Back from Negative Emotional Experiences." *Journal of Personality and Social Psychology*, 86(2): 320–333.

Turner, Jonathan H. 2006. *Sociology*. Upper Saddle River, NJ: Pearson/Prentice Hall.

Twenge, Jean M. 2006. *Generation Me*. New York: Free Press.

Twenge, Jean, and W. Keith Campbell. 2009. *The Narcissism Epidemic: Living in the Age of Entitlement*. New York: Simon & Schuster.

Twitter. 2016. "Twitter Statistics." Retrieved June 21, 2016 (http://www.statisticbrain.com/twitter-statistics/).

UNESCO. 2016. "Anniversaries 2016—2400th Anniversary of the Birth of Aristotle." Retrieved October 20, 2016 (http://en.unesco.org/celebrations/anniversaries/2016/all?page=1).

United States Postal Service (USPS). 2012. "The United States Postal Service: An American History 1775–2006." Retrieved June 11, 2016 (https://about.usps.com/publications/pub100.pdf).

_____. 2016. "About: A Decade of Facts and Figures." Retrieved June 11, 2016 (https://about.usps.com/who-we-are/postal-facts/decade-of-facts-and-figures.htm).

Urban Dictionary. 2010. "Bromance." Retrieved June 6, 2016 (http://www.urbandictionary.com/define.php?term=Bromance).

_____. 2013a. "Bro Code." Retrieved June 7, 2016 (http://www.urbandictionary.com/define.php?term=Bro%20Code).

_____. 2013b. "Broette." Retrieved June 7, 2016 (http://www.urbandictionary.com/define.php?term=broette).

_____. 2015. "Catfishing." Retrieved June 18, 2015 (http://www.urbandictionary.com/define.php?term=Catfishing).

_____. 2016a. "Best Friend." Retrieved June 6, 2016 (http://www.urbandictionary.com/define.php?term=Best%20Friend).

_____. 2016b. "Ex-Friend." Retrieved June 6, 2016 (http://www.urbandictionary.com/define.php?term=ex-friend).

Vanier, Jean. 2012. *Happiness: A Guide to the Good Life*. New York: Arcade Publishing.

Veblen, Thorstein. 1899. *The Theory of the Leisure Class*. New York: Macmillan.

Vedantam, Shankar. 2010. "Happiness and Selfishness: A Paradox: Are Happier People Unselfish?" *Psychology Today*, March 27. Retrieved November 21, 2016 (https://www.psychologytoday.com/blog/the-hidden-brain/201003/happiness-and-selfishness-paradox).

Vernon, Mark. 2010. *The Meaning of Friendship*. New York: Palgrave MacMillan.

Virtual Reality Society. 2016a. "Applications of Virtual Reality." Retrieved June 27, 2016 (http://www.vrs.org.uk/virtual-reality-applications/).

_____. 2016b. "Second Life." Retrieved June 28, 2016 (http://www.vrs.org.uk/virtual-reality-games/second-life.html).

Wallace, Kelly. 2015. "Teens Spend a 'Mind-Boggling' 9 Hours a Day Using Media, Report Says." *CNN*, November 3. Retrieved June 19, 2016 (http://www.cnn.com/2015/11/03/health/teens-tweens-media-screen-use-report/index.html).

Warrell, Margie. 2014. "Unhappy at Work? Either Change What You Do or Change How You Do It." *Forbes*, July 16. Retrieved August 21, 2016 (http://www.forbes.com/sites/margiewarrell/2014/07/16/unhappy-at-work-either-change-what-you-do-or-change-how-you-do-it/#40750649485e).

Watts, Duncan J. 2003. *Six Degrees: The Science of a Connected Age*. New York: W.W. Norton & Company.

Weinberger, Matt. 2015. "This Company was 13 Years Early to Virtual Reality—And It's Getting Ready to Try Again. *Business Insider*, March 29. Retrieved June 28, 2016 (http://www.businessinsider.com/second-life-is-still-around-and-getting-ready-to-conquer-virtual-reality-2015-3).

What National Day Is It. 2016. "When is National Selfie Day?" Retrieved June 29, 2016 (http://whatnationaldayisit.com/day/Selfie/).

When Harry Met Sally: Quotes. 2016. Retrieved October 10 (http://m.imdb.com/title/tt0098635/quotes).

White, Tyler. 2015. "Belgian Student Travels 5,000 Miles to Austin to Meet Facebook Friend Suggestion." MySanAntoniowww, January 7. Retrieved June 23, 2016 (http://www.mysanantonio.com/news/us-world/article/Belgian-student-travels-to-Austin-to-meet-5999335.php).

Whitehouse, Tom. 1998. "From the Wild: Feral Boy Prefers Living with Dogs." *Daily Breeze*, July 7: A7.

Whitty, Monica Therese. 2003. "Cyber-Flirting: Playing at Love on the Internet." *Theory Psychology*, 13(3) (June): 339–357.

Wihbey, John. 2011. "Cognitive Control in Media Multitaskers." *Journalist Resource*, August 1. Retrieved June 19, 2016 (http://journalistsresource.org/studies/society/internet/cognitive-control-in-media-multitaskers).

Williams, Dmitri, Nicolas Ducheneaut, Li Xiong, Nick Yee, and Eric Nickell. 2006. "From Tree House to Barracks: The Social Life of Guilds in World of Warcraft." *Games and Culture*, 1(4):338–361.

Williams, Rhiannon. 2014. "Facebook Isn't Dying. It's Just Changing." *The Telegraph*, November 26. Retrieved June 21, 2016. (http://www.telegraph.co.uk/technology/facebook/11252782/Facebook-isnt-dying.-Its-just-changing.html).

Wilson, Chris. 2014. "The Selfiest Cities in the World: TIME's Definitive Ranking." *TIME*, March 10. Retrieved June 14, 2016 (http://time.com/selfies-cities-world-rankings/).

Woollaston, Victoria. 2015. "Queen's Don't Stop Me Now Is the Top Feel-good Song of the Past 50 Years…and a Scientific Formula Has Proved It." *Daily Mail*, September 17. Retrieved December 15, 2016 (http://www.dailymail.co.uk/sciencetech/article-3238679/Queen-s-Don-t-Stop-feel-good-song-past-50-years-scientific-formula-proved-it.html).

World Database of Happiness. 2011. "Continuous Register of Scientific Research on Subjective Appreciation of Life." Retrieved circa March 2013 (http://worlddatabaseofhappiness.eur.nl/).

World Health Organization (WHO). 2016a. "Health Impact Assessment (HIA): The Determinants of Health." Retrieved June 5, 2016 (http://www.who.int/hia/evidence/doh/en/).

_____. 2016b. "Depression." Retrieved August 21, 2016 (http://www.who.int/mediacentre/factsheets/fs369/en/).

World of Warcraft. 2016. "What Is World of Warcraft?" Retrieved June 28, 2016 (http://us.battle.net/wow/en/game/guide/).

Wortham, Jenna. 2016. "B.F.F. Tattoos." *New York Times Magazine*, May 29: 20–21.

YouTube. 2009. "Virtual Dinosaur Revival Hits Japan." Retrieved June 27, 2016 (https://www.youtube.com/watch?v=i2RqDTYYoFc).

Zelenski, John Michael, Steven A. Murphy, and David A. Jenkins. 2008 (Dec). "The Happy-Productive Worker Thesis Revisited." *Journal of Happiness Studies*, 9(4): 521–537.

Zigterman, Ben. 2013. "How We Stopped Communicating Like Animals: 15 Ways Phones Have Evolved." *BGR*, December 13. Retrieved June 12, 2016 (http://bgr.com/2013/12/13/telephone-timeline-a-brief-history-of-the-phone/).

Zuckerberg, Mark. 2015. "Facebook Post Made by Mark Zuckerberg." February 4. Retrieved June 29, 2016 (https://www.facebook.com/zuck/posts/10101889611150901).

Index